Gout, Hyperuricemia, and Other Crystal-Associated Arthropathies

Gout, Hyperuricemia, and Other Crystal-Associated Arthropathies

edited by

Charley J. Smyth

V. Michael Holers

University of Colorado Health Sciences Center
Denver, Colorado

MARCEL DEKKER, INC. NEW YORK • BASEL • HONG KONG

ISBN: 0-8247-0210-7

This book is printed on acid-free paper.

Headquarters
Marcel Dekker, Inc.
270 Madison Avenue, New York, NY 10016
tel: 212-696-9000; fax: 212-685-4540

Eastern Hemisphere Distribution
Marcel Dekker AG
Hutgasse 4, Postfach 812, CH-4001 Basel, Switzerland
tel: 44-61-261-8482; fax: 44-61-261-8896

World Wide Web
http://www.dekker.com

The publisher offers discounts on this book when ordered in bulk quantities. For more information, write to Special Sales/Professional Marketing at the headquarters address above.

Current printing (last digit):
10 9 8 7 6 5 4 3 2 1

PRINTED IN THE UNITED STATES OF AMERICA

VMH and CJS dedicate this book to our wives, Jill and Laura, who have provided invaluable support and taught us so much. We also wish to recognize our families, patients, the many supportive members of the Rocky Mountain Chapter of the Arthritis Foundation, and the collegial faculty and staff of the Rheumatology Division of the University of Colorado Health Sciences Center for all of their contributions to this project.

In Memoriam: Charley J. Smyth

Dr. Charley J. Smyth died unexpectedly on December 20, 1997 during the final editing and initial production phase of this book. It was Dr. Smyth's dream during the last several years of his life to see this book published, and it will serve as a tribute to his determination as well as to his long and distinguished career. It is important to realize that Dr. Smyth saw this book not only as a didactic presentation of the crystal-associated arthropathies but also as a blueprint for others to follow that had resulted in the conquering of a severe affliction. He was convinced that investigators interested in studying the more than 100 other forms of arthritis could learn much by following the broad-based strategies applied to the conquest of gout.

Dr. Smyth was born into a medical career, with a father who was a practicing physician and a mother who ran the office, as well as several additional ancestors in the profession. He received his undergraduate education at the University of Michigan, where he was a star runner on the track team who lost only occasionally, but once to a youngster named Jesse Owens of Ohio State University (but reportedly not by much). He attended Jefferson Medical College, his father's alma mater, and then returned to Ann Arbor for his Internal Medicine training. Dr. Smyth was the first fellow in the then new Rackham Arthritis Unit. Following training under Dr. Freyberg and an additional year in the unit, he moved to Detroit during the second World War, where he was the medical director at Wayne County General Hospital.

Dr. Smyth moved in 1949 to the Department of Medicine at the University of Colorado School of Medicine in Denver to direct graduate and postgraduate medical education efforts. After five years in this role, he founded the Division of Rheumatology and served as its director for 20 years. As such, he traveled throughout Colorado and trained many of the currently practicing rheumatologists in this state. In 1974 he became Medical Director of the Alpert Arthritis Treatment Center at the affiliated Rose Medical Center. From 1974 to 1991 he had a part-time medical practice. In 1991 he "retired" to a life consisting of continuing his extraordinarily hard work for two of his lifelong passions—the University of Colorado Health Sciences Center and the Arthritis Foundation—in addition to making sure that trout in the streams of Colorado did not sleep comfortably.

Anyone who ever had the opportunity to meet Dr. Smyth was undoubtedly struck by his charismatic personality and boundless enthusiasm (with the rough edges smoothed by his lovely and warm wife, Laura). His life was also characterized by his love for his large immediate and extended family, his tireless dedication to the causes he chose to promote, and his intense interest in the opinions and lives of others around him. He was a born leader, recognizing the unique skills inherent in each person and seeking to help one use them effectively.

Dr. Smyth was a pioneer in the field of arthritis research and patient care. His interests were wide, ranging from the physiology of gout to better defining how rheumatologists and orthopedists could collaboratively care for patients. He also had the foresight to realize that effective organizations were necessary in order for all patients with rheumatic diseases to receive optimal care. He was one of the founders of the National Arthritis Foundation in 1948, and was also a founding member of both the Michigan and Rocky Mountain Chapters. Dr. Smyth had been a member of the American Rheumatism Association (now the American College of Rheumatology) since 1940 and served as its President in 1959–1960. He also played a central role in the mid-1970s in promoting the creation of an independent National Institutes of Health entity dedicated to arthritis research. His efforts, along with those many other supporters, were rewarded by the creation of the National Institute of Arthritis and Musculoskeletal and Skin Diseases (NIAMS), which today plays a central role in funding studies of rheumatic diseases. Dr. Smyth also served many other organizations, such as the American College of Physicians, and was a major contributor to medical education at all levels. Finally, he was very moved by the establishment by his friends, supporters, and patients of an endowed chair in rheumatology research at the University of Colorado School of Medicine, which I have had the privilege to hold.

Befitting his career, Dr. Smyth was given many awards, which he greatly appreciated. However, like many overly modest men of his era, he was likely to lose the physical award piece amid the clutter of his office and basement. His honors included a Commendation for Exceptional Service from President Gerald Ford in 1976 for his work promoting the creation of NIAMS. He was a Master of the American College of Physicians and the American College of Rheumatology. In 1995 he received the Sewall Award for exceptional contributions to the University of Colorado Health Sciences Center. In 1981 Dr. Smyth received the Harding Award for Distinguished Service from the Arthritis Foundation, which is its highest honor. Shortly before his death, he was recognized at the National Arthritis Foundation meeting as the organization was entering its 50th year. He was greatly pleased at this occasion to see how large and vital the organization had become.

In the end, it was clear to all who knew him that a day with Dr. Smyth was a day one would not soon forget. He always believed and taught everyone around him that one's life was dictated by the attitude with which it was embraced. Imbued with this approach, his life was fulfilling and productive until his very last hour. Because of this, his family, friends, patients, colleagues, and community have benefited immeasurably. He is and will be greatly missed by all of us.

V. Michael Holers

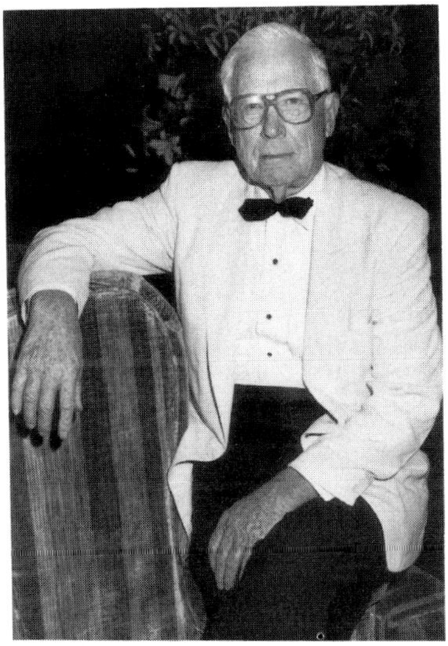

Preface

The concept for *Gout, Hyperuricemia, and Other Crystal-Associated Arthropathies* originated from discussions between the editors about the history of gout and how this illness fits into the contemporary clinical and scientific environment. Gout is one of the few arthritidies whose pathophysiology is relatively well understood and for which curative therapy is available. One of us (CJS) had been diagnosed with gout and was a noted author and expert who had written extensively on the clinical aspects of the topic. The other editor (VMH) had worked in the basic science of acute inflammation and was very well aware of the major role that crystal-induced disease still plays in this field.

Several decades have passed since the last publication of a book that comprehensively reviewed crystal-associated diseases. Our goal in editing this book was to provide a multifaceted resource for clinicians interested in contemporary concepts of diagnosis and treatment of gout and other crystal-associated diseases. However, we also wanted to provide a text of substantial usefulness for scientists interested in inflammation research, for students of all types interested in acquiring an elegant pathophysiological understanding of these illnesses, and for genetic epidemiologists interested in the many groundbreaking studies of these complex illnesses.

Each chapter in the text is written by a well-recognized expert in that particular area. In addition, two of the three sections are introduced by noted contributors Dr. Daniel J. McCarty and Dr. H. Ralph Schumacher, Jr., who have both published extensively in their respective areas of expertise. These introductions have provided additional points for the reader to consider. We have also attempted to minimize redundancy but have allowed each chapter to stand as an independent contribution.

The first part describes general features of the crystal-associated arthropathies. The second part is introduced by Dr. McCarty, and focuses on gout. The chapters describe the history, diagnosis, treatment options, epidemiology, pathophysiology, associated conditions, and radiographical changes. The third part, introduced by Dr. Schumacher, discusses other crystal-associated diseases, including those that have been more recently described. These include calcium pyrophosphate deposition disease and basic calcium phosphate crystal deposition diseases as well as other less frequently encountered conditions.

Although gout has been a longstanding affliction, each new patient with podagra reminds us that it is an illness still affecting mankind. However, as has been demonstrated countless times in clinical settings, with appropriate therapy gout, as well as many other crystal-associated diseases, can be effectively controlled. We hope that the information in this book is of value to many individuals.

We would like to express our appreciation to all the contributing authors, who have demonstrated so much enthusiasm and interest in this project. In addition, we thank Michele Sinoway, Marilyn Ludzki, and especially Lia Pelosi of Marcel Dekker, Inc., for their invaluable help with this project. We also wish to thank Ellen Stumer for her outstanding secretarial assistance.

Charley J. Smyth
V. Michael Holers

Contents

Contributors

JOHN H. BLAND, M.D., M.A.C.R. Professor, Department of Medicine, Rheumatology and Clinical Immunology Unit, University of Vermont College of Medicine, Burlington, Vermont

BRUCE N. CRONSTEIN, M.D. Professor, Department of Medicine, New York University School of Medicine, New York, New York

JAN DEQUEKER, M.D., PH.D., F.R.C.P. Professor, Department of Rheumatology, University Hospitals, University Ziekenhuizen Leuven, Lubbeek, Belgium

HERBERT S. DIAMOND, M.D. Chairman, Department of Medicine, The Western Pennsylvania Hospital, and Clinical Professor of Medicine, University of Pittsburgh School of Medicine, Pittsburgh, Pennsylvania

BRYAN T. EMMERSON, M.D., PH.D., F.R.A.C.P. Professor and Research Consultant, Department of Medicine, University of Queensland at the Princess Alexandra Hospital, Brisbane, Queensland, Australia

GERALD F. FALASCA, M.D. Associate Professor, Division of Rheumatology, Department of Medicine, Cooper Hospital/University Medical Center, Robert Wood Johnson Medical School at Camden, University of Medicine and Dentistry at New Jersey, Camden, New Jersey

ADEL G. FAM, M.D., F.R.C.P.(C), F.A.C.P. Professor and Head, Division of Rheumatology, Department of Medicine, Sunnybrook Health Science Centre, University of Toronto, Toronto, Ontario, Canada

ROBERT A. GATTER, M.D.* Chief, Department of Rheumatology, Abington Memorial Hospital, and Associate Clinical Professor, University of Pennsylvania, Philadelphia, Pennsylvania

*Retired.

LOUIS A. HEALEY, M.D. Clinical Professor Emeritus, Department of Medicine, University of Washington, Seattle, Washington

A. TAREQ KHAWAJA, M.D. Chief Resident, Department of Medicine, The Western Pennsylvania Hospital, and Clinical Instructor, Department of Medicine, University of Pittsburgh School of Medicine, Pittsburgh, Pennsylvania

JAMES R. KLINENBERG, M.D. F.A.C.P. Senior Vice President and Director, Division of Rheumatology, Cedars Sinai Medical Center, and Professor and Assistant Dean, University of California at Los Angeles School of Medicine, Los Angeles, California

STEPHEN E. MALAWISTA, M.D. Professor, Department of Internal Medicine, Yale University School of Medicine, New Haven, Connecticut

WILLIAM MARTEL, M.D. Professor Emeritus, Department of Radiology, University of Michigan Hospital, Ann Arbor, Michigan

IKUKO MASUDA, M.D., PH.D. Assistant Professor, Division of Rheumatology, Department of Medicine, Medical College of Wisconsin, Milwaukee, Wisconsin

GERALDINE M. MCCARTHY, M.D., F.R.C.P.I.* Associate Professor, Division of Rheumatology, Department of Medicine, Medical College of Wisconsin, Milwaukee, Wisconsin

DANIEL J. MCCARTY, M.D. Ross Professor of Medicine Emeritus, Division of Rheumatology, Department of Medicine, Medical College of Wisconsin, Milwaukee, Wisconsin

WILLIAM M. MIKKELSEN, M.D. Professor Emeritus, Department of Internal Medicine and Rheumatology, The University of Michigan Medical School, Ann Arbor, Michigan

CHRISTIAN MOENS, M.D. Rheumatologist, Brussels, Belgium

PHILIPPE J. MOENS, M.D. Department of Rheumatology and Readaptation, St. Elisabeth Clinic, Brussels, Belgium

YAIR MOLAD, M.D. Lecturer, Sackler School of Medicine, Tel Aviv University, Tel Aviv, Israel

J. DESMOND O'DUFFY, M.B. Consultant, Division of Rheumatology, Mayo Clinic, Rochester, Minnesota

DUNCAN S. OWEN, JR., M.D. Professor, Department of Internal Medicine, Virginia Commonwealth University, Richmond, Virginia

*Current affiliation: Department of Clinical Pharmacology, Royal College of Surgeons in Ireland, Dublin, Ireland.

ANTONIO J. REGINATO, M.D. Professor of Medicine and Chief, Division of Rheumatology, Department of Medicine, Cooper Hospital/University Medical Center, Robert Wood Johnson Medical School at Camden, University of Medicine and Dentistry at New Jersey, Camden, New Jersey

DONALD RESNICK, M.D. Professor, Department of Radiology, University of California—San Diego and Veterans Affairs Medical Center, San Diego, California

A. LEÓN RIVELIS, M.D.[†] Rheumatologist, Department of Rheumatology, Hospital for Special Surgery, New York, New York, and Instituto de Reumatología, Buenos Aires, Argentina

ANA CARINA RIVELIS, M.D. Rheumatologist, Department of Rheumatology, Hospital Ramos Mejía, Buenos Aires, Argentina

LAWRENCE M. RYAN, M.D. Will and Cava Ross Professor of Medicine and Chief, Division of Rheumatology, Department of Medicine, Medical College of Wisconsin, Milwaukee, Wisconsin

H. RALPH SCHUMACHER, JR., M.D. Professor, Division of Rheumatology, University of Pennsylvania School of Medicine, Philadelphia, Pennsylvania

J. EDWIN SEEGMILLER, M.D. Professor Emeritus, Stein Institute for Research on Aging, Department of Medicine, University of California—San Diego, La Jolla, California

HARRY SPIERA, M.D. Clinical Professor, Department of Medicine/Rheumatology, Mount Sinai School of Medicine, New York, New York

LYNNE S. STEINBACH, M.D. Professor, Department of Radiology, University of California—San Francisco, San Francisco, California

ROBERT TERKELTAUB, M.D. Chief, Rheumatology Section, and Associate Professor in Residence, Department of Medicine, Veterans Affairs Medical Center, University of California—San Diego, San Diego, California

DANIEL S. URI, M.D. Presbyterian Orthopedic Hospital, Charlotte, North Carolina

PASCALE VOLDERS, M.D. Department of Rheumatology, University Hospitals, University Ziekenhuizen Leuven, Lubbeek, Belgium

JEFFREY H. WIMSATT, D.V.M., PH.D. Assistant Professor, Department of Clinical Sciences, College of Veterinary Medicine and Biomedical Sciences, Colorado State University, Fort Collins, Colorado

TSAI-FAN YÜ, M.D. Emeritus Professor, Department of Medicine, Mount Sinai School of Medicine, New York, New York

---

[†]Retired.

1

Pathogenesis of Inflammatory Manifestations Caused by Crystals

ROBERT TERKELTAUB
Veterans Affairs Medical Center, University of California—San Diego, San Diego, California

Crystals deposited in joints can cause a variety of articular problems, including acute inflammatory arthritis, chronic inflammatory joint disease with synovial proliferation, and degenerative arthropathy primarily affecting cartilage. This chapter concentrates on the current understanding of the mechanisms by which crystals can cause inflammation, and in particular the acute neutrophil-mediated synovitis characteristic of acute gout and pseudogout. A major focus of this review is on recent advances in the cellular and molecular biology of crystal-cell interaction, which is central to clinical sequelae and cartilage degradation in all forms of crystal-induced arthritis.

I. GOUT AND PSEUDOGOUT AS PARADIGMS OF ACUTE CRYSTAL-INDUCED INFLAMMATION

The acute, intense, but self-limiting character of paroxysms of gouty joint inflammation has been recognized since antiquity. Pseudogout as well as acute articular and periarticular inflammation caused by basic calcium phosphate (BCP) crystals can behave similarly, reflecting the fact that CPPD and BCP crystals share many of the fundamental mechanisms of cell activation utilized by urate crystals.

It is believed that acute crystal-induced synovitis is triggered by factors that include the availability (or de novo liberation or formation) of free crystals. Other precipitating factors include the generation of a sufficient body of proinflammatory mediators in response to free crystals or to other events such as local trauma or intercurrent systemic stress (e.g., the postoperative state) (1).

Free crystals can induce the release of proinflammatory mediators by catalyzing the release of active proteolytic cleavage fragments from complement and coagulation proteins and by directly and indirectly stimulating resident synovial fluid mononuclear cells, synovial lining cells, mast cells, and chondrocytes (Figure 1). In this regard, striking joint pain and articular and periarticular swelling and erythema—characteristic of acute gout and pseudogout—are likely mediated in part by vasoactive prostaglandins, kinins (which also potentiate prostaglandin synthesis via release of membrane arachidonate), complement-derived peptides (including C3a and C5a), and histamine (Figure 1). Pain signals also likely prompt the release from nociceptive afferent sensory nerves of substance P, which has several proinflammatory actions. Nitric oxide production can be triggered by certain inflammatory mediators [including interleukin-1 (IL-1)], and has the potential to play a vasoactive and proinflammatory role in crystal-induced arthritis.

Free crystals can induce the transcription and release from phagocytes and synovial lining cells of cytokines (1–3) including IL-1β, transforming growth factor alpha (TNFα) IL-6, and IL-8, which may spill into the circulation and promote systemic manifestations such as fever, leukocytosis, and the hepatic acute phase protein response.

IL-1 and TNFα, by activating the endothelial cells of postcapillary venules and promoting neutrophil adhesion, are believed to provide crucial signals for neutrophil influx in acute crystal-induced arthritis. Specifically, the injection of free urate crystals into the joint space rapidly upregulates the expression by the synovial microvascular endothelium of E-selectin, a major adhesion ligand for neutrophils. Furthermore, Dorian Haskard and associates have proven a role for TNFα in this process in vivo (4).

Crystal-associated IL-1 and TNFα production may be a product of direct and indirect effects of crystal-cell interaction. For example, John Bomalaski and coworkers demonstrated that inflammatory crystals and IL-1 are both capable of inducing phospholipase A2-activating protein (PLAP) (5) in leukocytes, and PLAP can in turn induce IL-1 and TNFα expression in monocytes.

Neutrophils, which are virtually absent in the normal joint, are required for the development of the full-blown gouty attack (1). Specifically, Paulding Phelps and Daniel McCarty first established that experimental urate crystal-induced arthritis is markedly diminished in neutrophil-depleted animals. Histopathological studies of acute gout have revealed that neutrophils accumulate in both the joint fluid and the synovial membrane, where they aggregate in the microvasculature. Neutrophils that enter the joint in acute gout and pseudogout can be activated by exposure to numerous soluble inflammatory mediators and by direct encounters with crystals, which are phagocytosed by neutrophils (Table 1). Urate crystals have a particularly potent ability to lyse cell membranes, thereby con-

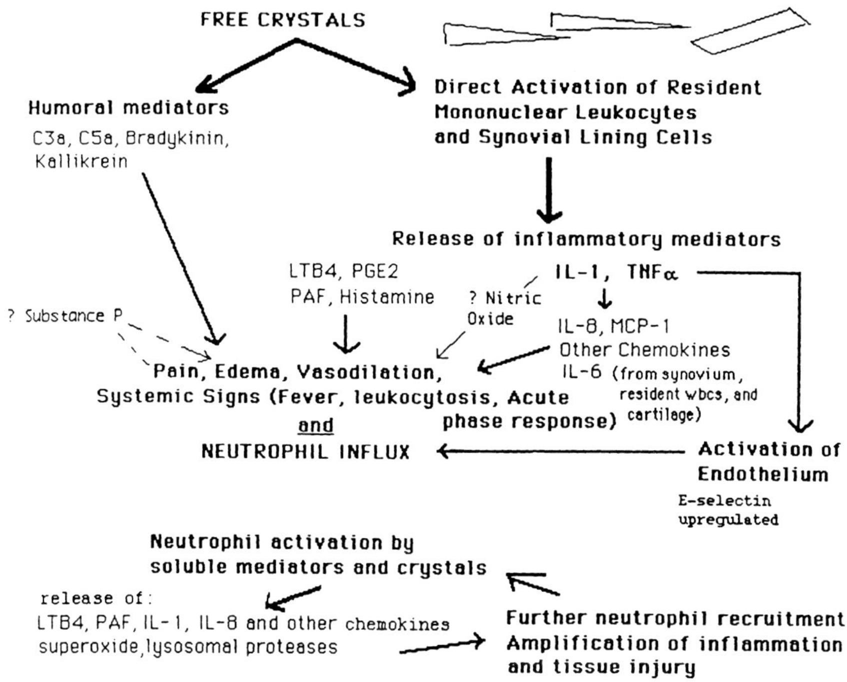

FIGURE 1 Model for pathogenesis of acute crystal-induced inflammatory arthritis (discussed in text).

tributing to lysosomal protease release by cytolysis in phagocytes that have ingested the crystals. This process, characterized in elegant detail by Gerald Weissmann and coworkers (21), has been termed the "suicide sad."

Leukocytes that encounter crystals release more chemotactic factors for neutrophils, thus amplifying crystal-induced arthritis. The neutrophil chemotaxins released by phagocytes exposed to crystals include leukotriene B4 (LTB4), as first elucidated by Weissmann and coworkers (21), and low molecular weight inducible secreted polypeptides, first discovered and characterized by Paulding Phelps, Dan McCarty, Isaias Spilberg, and others more than two decades ago. These polypeptides, were initially termed crystal-induced chemotactic factors (CCF) (1).

Spilberg and others recognized that CCF activity is newly transcribed by phagocytes that meet urate crystals, and that this response is largely dependent on phagocytosis. However, it is now appreciated that CCF almost certainly represents an early description of members of the chemotactic cytokine (chemokine) family (2, 6–9), which are also transcriptionally regulated. Specifically, my laboratory observed that the chemokine IL-8 is the major neutrophil

TABLE I Some of the Known Inflammatory Mediators Induced by Monosodium Urate and CPPD Crystals[a]

Coagulation proteins: including bradykinin, kallikrein
Complement peptides: including C3a, C5a
Eicosanoids: including prostaglandin E2 (PGE2) and leukotriene B4 (LTB4)
Oxygen radicals derived from NADPH oxidase: e.g., $O_2\cdot$ (and H_2O_2 and OH· radical from $O_2\cdot$)
Phosphoplipase A2 (PLA2) and phospholipase A2-activating protein (PLAP)
Platelet activating factor (PAF)
Released leukocyte lysosomal proteases and platelet granule proteins
Cytokines: including IL-1, TNFα, IL-6, IL-8, GROα

[a]Most of these mediators are detected in the synovial fluid in patients with acute pseudogout and gout, but crystal-related temporal and quantitative differences in the generation of these mediators are observed.

chemotaxin released from urate and CPPD crystal-stimulated monocyte-macrophages (2). IL-8 is similarly expressed and released from neutrophils activated by crystals (8), and IL-8 is abundant in the joint fluid in both acute gout and pseudogout (2).

II. IL-8, CHEMOKINES, AND OTHER NEUTROPHIL CHEMOTAXINS IN CRYSTAL-INDUCED ARTHRITIS

IL-8 not only provides a chemotactic gradient for neutrophil movement into the joint space, but also promotes neutrophil adhesion to the endothelium by activating neutrophil integrins and enhances neutrophil inflammatory functions that contribute to matrix degradation, including lysosomal protease release and the production of oxygen radicals through the NADPH oxidase (6). Because IL-8 is relatively resistant to proteolytic inactivation, it has the potential to be more long-lived than neutrophil chemotactic mediators derived from complement peptides (including C5a) or from phospholipids [including LTB4 and platelet activating factor (PAF)], a notion supported by the observation that immunoadsorption of IL-8 from an acute pseudogout synovial fluid removed most neutrophil chemotactic activity (1).

Infusion of IL-8 into the joint space induces marked neutrophil ingress associated with release of neutrophil elastase and accelerated cartilage degradation in rabbits (9). IL-8 also can chemoattract T lymphocytes and is a particularly potent angiogenic factor, thereby giving it the potential to contribute to the chronic proliferative synovitis that can develop in crystal deposition diseases. IL-8 also can suppress collagen synthesis in fibroblasts, consistent with a larger role in tissue repair. Adel Fam and coworkers have demonstrated that recurrent episodes of experimental pseudogout can accelerate lapine osteoarthritis. Thus, it is likely that crystal-induced IL-8 expression is a factor in the negative prognostic implications of secondary chondrocalcinosis in osteoarthritis.

A. The Chemokine Subfamilies

Chemokines are divided into subfamilies; the major ones are designated as C-C and C-X-C, according to whether the first two of four conserved cysteines are separated by an amino acid (6). The human C-X-C chemokines, which include IL-8, are predominantly recognized for effects on neutrophils. Only two human high-affinity IL-8 receptors (designated CXCR-1 and CXCR-2) exist (6). However, a subgroup of chemokines share an IL-8 ELR sequence motif that allows binding to the promiscuous CXCR-2. These include ENA-78, which is abundant and functionally active in RA synovial fluid, NAP-2, which is derived from platelet β-thromboglobulin, and GRO α, β, γ. It is highly likely that several of these neutrophil chemotactic chemokines related to IL-8 play a role in crystal-induced inflammation. For example, urate and CPPD crystals are known to induce GROα expression by neutrophils, though GROα is produced much less abundantly than IL-8 under these circumstances (8).

The C-C chemokines, which include MCP-1 and MIP-1 α,β, act predominantly on monocytes, T lymphocytes, and eosinophils but not on neutrophils. However, because MCP-1 and certain other C-C chemokines can be induced by IL-1 and TNFα, it is likely that some chemokines in this subfamily play a role in crystal-induced inflammation.

Importantly, resident cells in the joint other than mononuclear leukocytes (i.e., synovial lining cells and chondrocytes) also can express IL-8 (and other chemokines) in vitro and in the course of inflammatory arthritides, including rheumatoid arthritis. Furthermore, concordant expression of a broad array of chemokines, including IL-8, GRO genes, and MCP-1, is now recognized to arise following stimulation by IL-1 and certain other cytokines and by several growth factors, including platelet derived growth factor (PDGF) and transforming growth factor β (TGFβ). In this regard, concomitant expression of IL-8 and GROα, β, γ is described in the synovium in vitro and in vivo in rheumatoid arthritis (7), possibly because these chemokines share the ability to be induced in response to both IL-1β and TNFα.

Significantly, nonchemokine mediators released in direct response to free crystals, including C5a, LTB4, and PAF, might be sufficient to initiate or perpetuate a chemotactic gradient for neutrophils to enter the joint. Furthermore, C5a and LTB4 can induce IL-8 expression in neutrophils that have entered the joint, and IL-8 can in turn induce LTB4 and PAF production by activated neutrophils. In addition, crystal-induced PLAP can turn on LTB4 production by neutrophils.

Thus, given the synergistic and redundant inflammatory pathways activated by crystals, further studies will be needed to determine if a single chemokine, or subgroup of chemokines, is critical for crystal-induced synovitis. Our latest studies suggest that IL-8 receptor-binding C-X-C chemokines, as a group, appear essential for neutrophil influx.

III. MECHANISM OF CRYSTAL-INDUCED INFLAMMATORY MEDIATOR PRODUCTION BY CELLS

Crystals have the ability to nonspecifically bind and crosslink membrane and plasma proteins and perturb lipid bilayers. In this regard, Bryon Jaques and Mark Ginsberg first demonstrated that the binding by naked urate crystals of platelet membrane glycoproteins, and particularly of integrins, contributes substantially to cell activation.

Recent studies have further elucidated the fundamental mechanism by which crystals induce expression of inflammatory cytokines and metalloproteinases in phagocytes, chondrocytes, and synovial lining cells. My laboratory, and that of Paul Naccache, demonstrated that urate and CPPD crystals also trigger signal transduction pathways physiologically employed by specific ligand-receptor interactions in phagocytes. These include the membrane heterotrimeric G protein Giα2, phospholipases A2 (5), D, and C [the latter with attendant phosphatidylinositol (PI) 4,5 bisphosphate hydrolysis and activation of protein kinase C (PKC) and cytosolic Ca^{++} mobilization] (1,10–12) (Figure 2).

Significantly, we observed that urate crystal-induced phospholipase C-catalyzed PI 4,5 bisphosphate hydrolysis and cytosolic calcium mobilization do not require membrane G protein activation in neutrophils, unlike the case for activation by chemotactic peptides. Furthermore, we observed that uncoated urate crystals, unlike chemotactic peptides, do not induce rapid activation of PI-3 kinase in neutrophils, again pointing to a signal transduction pathway partially unique from that used by chemotactic peptides (11).

Naccache and coworkers discovered that urate and crystals induce stimulus-specific patterns of tyrosine kinase signaling in neutrophils, including common activation of the *src* family nonreceptor tyrosine kinase *lyn* (13–15). Some evidence suggests that tyrosine kinase signaling may be critical to certain leukocyte responses to CPPD crystals, including activation of the NADPH oxidase and degranulation. Furthermore, the microtubule antagonist colchicine, at micromolar concentrations achievable in cells during the primary treatment of acute pseudogout and gout with high doses of the drug, selectively suppresses CPPD and urate crystal-induced tyrosine kinase activation in leukocytes and inhibits crystal-induced IL-1 expression in neutrophils (14,16).

Ligand-induced dimerization is an important step in activation of receptor

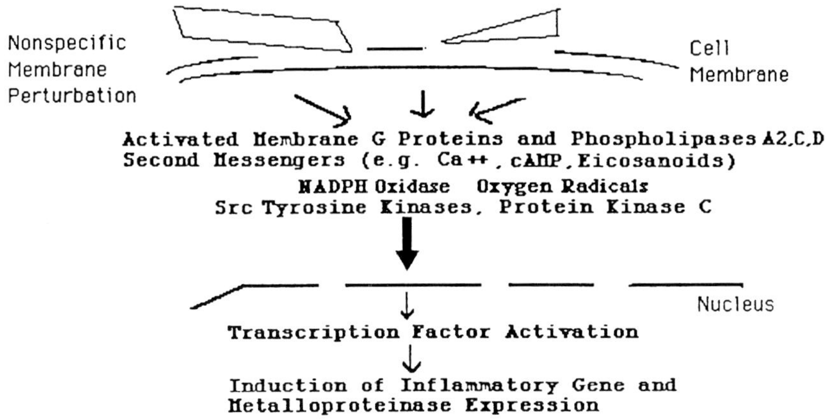

FIGURE 2 Model for crystal-induced inflammatory gene expression (discussed in text).

tyrosine kinases. Thus, collectively, the observations cited above suggest that the ability of naked urate crystals to crosslink and cluster membrane proteins and to activate the cytoskeleton may be critical mechanisms for crystal-induced cell activation. In this regard, membrane protein crosslinking could be enhanced by opsonization of the crystals with IgG. However, it is not likely that a single membrane receptor is critical for urate crystals to activate phagocytes.

Significantly, Malawista and coworkers have determined that the capacity of CPPD crystals to directly induce IL-1β and TNFα in macrophages is weak and inconsistent compared to that of urate crystals (3). Furthermore, under conditions where CPPD crystals are potent inducers of IL-8 in neutrophils, GROα is induced more weakly and expression of the C-C chemokine MIP-1α is inhibited (8). Thus, CPPD crystal-induced IL-8 expression, which helps to promote the clinical phenotype of neutrophil-mediated joint inflammation in microcrystalline arthritis, also reinforces the partial selectivity of cellular signal transduction mechanism triggered by crystals.

A. Crystal-Induced Activation of Transcription Factors

The pathway from crystal-induced membrane stimulation to inflammatory genes expression includes, by necessity, the activation of transcription factors. In this regard, the seminal work of Herman Cheung and coworkers has suggested that CPPD and hydroxyapatite crystals have the potential to enhance activation of AP-1 in fibroblasts and chondrocytes, partially through induction of fos and jun expression, and that CPPD and hydroxyapatite-induced AP-1 activation mediates crystal-induced metalloproteinase expression (17,18).

The work of Cheung and associates suggests that AP-1 activation also might play an additive role with intracellular calcium from crystal dissolution, and with PKC activation, in the mitogenic activity of basic calcium phosphate and CPPD crystals for fibroblasts. In this regard, signaling through crystal-induced activation of plasma membrane heterotrimeric G proteins (such as crystal-activated Giα2 in phagocytes) could be a factor in promoting AP-1 activation through stimulation of the mitogen activated protein kinase (MAPK) pathway.

IL-8 expression, generally silent in resting cells, is transcriptionally regulated in a manner that generally depends on activation of latent cytosolic transcription factors of the NFκB/rel family. Thus, NFκB is likely to be one of the transcription factors other than AP-1 involved in crystal-induced inflammatory gene expression.

IV. INITIATION OF ACUTE CRYSTAL-INDUCED SYNOVITIS AND FACTORS DETERMINING INTENSITY OF INFLAMMATION

Though crystals consistently induce inflammatory mediators in vitro, the degree of inflammation provoked experimentally by crystals in vivo is more variable. Furthermore, it is common to observe free and phagocytosed urate crystals in asymptomatic or subclinically inflamed joints and subcutaneous tophi. Thus, the precise trigger for acute gout and pseudogout remains unidentified. The triggering of crystal-induced inflammation is not an "all or nothing" state related to the new appearance of free crystals.

Acute gout and pseudogout are frequently precipitated by local trauma or intercurrent medical illness, or in the postoperative state. Furthermore, subclinical synovial inflammation clearly exists in gout, evidenced by Pascual's observations of mildly elevated leukocyte and absolute neutrophil counts that decrease in response to prophylactic colchicine in the synovial fluids of asymptomatic knees (19). These observations collectively suggest that local or systemic inflammatory cytokine release, by "priming" articular inflammatory cells to heightened responsiveness to local stimuli, can ignite a smoldering subclinical inflammatory response to crystals in otherwise asymptomatic joints. Such effects also likely explain the occurrence of polyarticular gout and pseudogout attacks beyond a single region of the body.

A. Surface Properties and Crystal-Bound Proteins

Variation in the surface properties and morphology of crystals likely influences the course of acute microcrystalline arthritis. In this regard, Paul Dieppe and other investigators have shown that monoclinic (plate-like) CPPD crystals are more inflammatory in vivo and in vitro than triclinic (rod-like) CPPD crystals. Furthermore, monoclinic CPPD crystals appear to be significantly enriched relative to triclinic crystals in the joint fluid in acute pseudogout (20).

Urate, CPPD, and basic calcium phosphate crystals differentially bind substantial amounts of certain proteins from plasma including the opsonins IgG, C3b, C1q, and fibronectin. Furthermore, precoating of crystals with whole plasma or serum can markedly alter their ability to activate neutrophils (1).

Significantly, plasma low-density lipoprotein (LDL) binds avidly to monosodium urate crystals; we demonstrated that this molecule markedly attenuates urate crystal-induced phagocyte activation and largely accounts for the inhibitory activity of whole serum on this activity. The high molecular weight, hydrophobic apolipoprotein B moiety of LDL appears to be responsible by hindering physical crystal-cell interaction. Ralph Schumacher and coworkers have demonstrated a decrease in crystal-bound IgG and a progressive, marked increase in crystal-bound LDL during the evolution of acute gout and experimental urate crystal-induced inflammation in vivo. Recently, we observed that oxidation of LDL lipids, which has been documented in inflammatory joint fluids, actually renders LDL capable of inducing monocyte-macrophages to express several inflammatory cytokines, including IL-8.

Hydroxyapatite and CPPD crystals bind protein less avidly than urate crystals. However, we demonstrated that adsorption of the plasma protein α2-HS glycoprotein to hydroxyapatite crystals markedly inhibits the ability of the crystals to activate neutrophils.

V. MECHANISMS THAT LIMIT ACUTE CRYSTAL-INDUCED ARTHRITIS

Fundamental anti-inflammatory mechanisms are reflected in the spontaneous self-limitation characteristic of acute gout, initially described by Hippocrates. Factors other than crystal sequestration or oxidative crystal dissolution must play a role in terminating gouty attacks, because free urate crystals are usually present in synovial fluid for many weeks after subsidence of an acute gouty paroxysm. Changes in the balance between pro- and anti-inflammatory effects that could regulate acute crystal-induced arthritis may include expression of peptidases that can inactivate IL-1, substance P, C5a, and certain other mediators. Tachyphylaxis and cross-desensitization of leukocytes to chemotactic mediators may be particularly significant because IL-8 and certain other chemokines are relatively resistant to proteolytic inactivation.

My laboratory has noted that urate crystals induce TGFβ production by synovial lining cells (R. Terkeltaub, unpublished observations). TGFβ, which can be abundant in acute gout synovial fluids, can exert several proinflammatory activities (including induction of IL-8 expression by chondrocytes). However, TGFβ also can inhibit IL-1 and IL-1 receptor expression, and TGFβ induces IL-1 receptor antagonist expression. In this regard, the IL-1 receptor antagonist also can be present in synovial fluids in acute crystal-induced arthritis. Interestingly, Liote and coworkers have observed that exogenous TGFβ can block the development of experimental urate crystal-induced inflammation in vivo. Thus, de novo production and release of TGFβ may act predominantly to limit crystal-induced synovitis.

Because the continuing ingress of neutrophils is likely essential for perpetuation of acute gouty inflammation, the relatively short functional lifespan of neutrophils (which is limited to a maximum of a few days) must play an important role in limiting gouty inflammation. In this regard, the neutrophil life span in inflammatory loci is limited in large part by apoptotic programmed cell death, an integral process in the resolution of several forms of tissue inflammation. Though neutrophil apoptosis can be delayed by many mediators, including C5a, TGFβ, IL-1, and IL-8, under certain conditions, IL-6, TNFα, and some other mediators accelerate neutrophil apoptosis.

VI. FUNDAMENTAL BASIS FOR THE SUCCESS OF PHARMACOLOGIC TREATMENT OF ACUTE CRYSTAL-INDUCED ARTHRITIS

Current understanding of the pathogenesis of acute crystal-induced inflammation and the natural mechanisms that limit this process is consistent with the observations that agents that suppress neutrophil adhesion and activation are particularly effective in treating and preventing acute gout and pseudogout. The disproportionately strong effectiveness in both the prophylaxis and treatment of acute gout and pseudogout of colchicine, a relatively weak general anti-inflammatory drug is noteworthy.

The efficacy of colchicine as a treatment for established acute crystal-induced arthritis is diminished when the clinical inflammation has become prolonged, probably because of a heightened contribution of the synovium relative to that of neutrophils. The effects of synovial mitogenesis promoted by the ingestion of CPPD crystals by the synovial membrane (with subsequent intracellular crystal dissolution and liberation of calcium) may similarly promote a relative refractoriness to therapy in some cases of CPPD crystal-induced inflammatory arthritis.

Recent work by Bruce Cronstein and associates has provided fresh insight into the basis for the prophylactic effects of low doses of colchicine for gout and pseudogout (21) (Table 2). Specifically, at nanomolar concentrations

TABLE 2 Proposed Mechanisms for Efficacy of Colchicine in Acute Crystal-Induced Arthritis

Inhibits neutrophil inflammatory function
Inhibits upregulated neutrophil-endothelial adhesion (particularly potent effect)
Increases cAMP
Inhibits crystal-induced tyrosine kinase activation
Selectively inhibits mediator release (e.g., decreases IL-1 and chemotactic cytokine release, but not IL-1 receptor antagonist release)
Inhibits crystal-induced PLA2 activity, and PLAP and LTB4 release
Inhibits migration
Inhibits phagocytosis
Other inhibitory effects:
Inhibits expression of TNFα receptors in macrophages and endothelium (not in neutrophils)
Supresses histamine release from mast cells

of the drug, achievable with low-dose daily oral colchicine regimens, colchicine inhibits E-selectin–mediated endothelial adhesiveness for neutrophils. Colchicine, and other agents that disrupt microtubules, critically alter the surface topography, but not the quantity of E-selectin molecules on the surface of the endothelial cells (21).

Recent studies have further documented the broad array of effects of colchicine on neutrophil function and adhesion to the endothelium at micromolar therapeutic concentrations achievable with high-dose primary treatment regimens for acute gout and pseudogout. In this regard, the in vitro effects of colchicine are consistent with the particularly rapid therapeutic efficacy of high-dose colchicine. Specifically, colchicine diminishes the expression by neutrophils (but not lymphocytes) of L-selectin, which mediates neutrophil sticking to the endothelium, and colchicine also inhibits endothelial ICAM-1 expression. In addition, colchicine increases the rolling velocity of neutrophils on the endothelium in the microvasculature in vivo.

High doses of colchicine also suppress random motility, chemotaxis, PLA2 activation, and the stimulated elaboration of PLAP and of certain chemotactic factors (CCF, LTB4) by neutrophils in response to certain agonists, including several soluble chemotactic factors. Colchicine also appears to inhibit IL-1 production (but not IL-1 receptor antagonist release) by activated neutrophils. However, the drug may have different effects on IL-1 production by other cells. Colchicine inhibits phagocytosis of certain particulates, but these effects are relatively weak and colchicine does not inhibit superoxide generation by neutrophils.

Colchicine also can inhibit mast cell histamine release, and the drug can directly downregulate TNFα receptors in macrophages and endothelial cells. Significantly, neutrophil TNFα receptors are unaffected under identical conditions.

Thus, colchicine has many potentially pivotal effects on neutrophils and endothelial cells that underlie its remarkable effectiveness in both controlling and preventing acute gout and pseudogout. The basis for many of these effects lies in the ability of colchicine to inhibit the assembly of microtubules, cytoskeletal polymers of tubulin dimers that can alter the distribution of membrane glycoproteins. The stabilization of labile microtubules normally needed for leukocyte motility helps block chemotaxis, phagocytosis, and adhesiveness. Reibman and coworkers have demonstrated that intact microtubule function clearly contributes to optimum expression of neutrophil 5- and 15-lipoxygenase activity, and, furthermore, that colchicine markedly suppresses these activities in neutrophils (21). As mentioned above, colchicine (at micromolar levels) inhibits MSU and CPPD crystal-induced tyrosine kinase activation in neutrophils, but not tyrosine kinase activation induced by chemotactic factors such as FMLP and C5a. These observations suggest inhibition of crystal-induced and microtubule-mediated membrane protein clustering by colchicine. The ability of colchicine to bind to certain leukocyte membrane proteins that may be tubulin-like attachment points for microtubules may play a role in these effects.

The basic mechanisms by which colchicine can suppress acute inflammation are not limited to effects on microtubules. In this regard, elevation of cAMP can globally depress neutrophil function and colchicine directly elevates cyclic AMP levels and potentiates prostaglandin E-induced and beta-adrenergic-induced rises in neutrophil cyclic AMP, probably by stimulating the GTPase activity of tubulin. Colchicine may alter diacylglycerol generation and thus modulate certain stimulus-response coupling mechanisms. Furthermore, certain colchicine analogs that do not effectively bind to tubulin, and which are not metabolized to colchicine in humans, appear to have anti-inflammatory effects in animal model systems and possibly in patients with acute gout.

Nonsteroidal anti-inflammatory drugs (NSAIDs) and high doses of local or systemic glucocorticoids or adrenocorticotrophic hormone (ACTH) also are quite effective in treating crystal-induced inflammation, and their potential for toxicity is often lower than that of high-dose colchicine. The ability of NSAIDs and glucocorticoids to attenuate acute gouty inflammation is now believed to partially reflect the capacity of many of these agents to inhibit neutrophil adhesion to the endothelium, to suppress neutrophil activation, to decrease nitric oxide generation, and to hinder inflammatory cytokine gene expression.

New modalities under investigation as potential therapeutic agents for crystal-induced inflammation include phosphocitrate, an inhibitor of calcium phosphate crystallization that is constitutively present in mitochondria and the urine. Herman Cheung and coworkers have shown that phosphocitrate has the capacity to diminish the formation of CPPD and basic calcium phosphate crystals and to make these crystal surfaces less activating for cell membranes, with resultant inhibition of crystal-induced fibroblast mitogenesis and metalloproteinase expression (18).

Further studies specifying the structural and molecular means by which crystals activate cells should identify novel targets for inhibition of the inflammatory and degenerative consequences of articular crystal deposition diseases.

REFERENCES

1. R. Terkeltaub. Pathogenesis and treatment of crystal-induced inflammation, In: Arthritis and Allied Conditions, 13th Edition (W. J. Koopman, ed.), Williams and Wilkins, Baltimore, MD, 1996, p. 2085.
2. R. Terkeltaub, C. Zachariae, D. Santoro, J. Martin, P. Peveri, and K. Matsushima. Monocyte-derived Neutrophil Chemotactic Factor/IL-8 is a potential mediator of crystal-induced inflammation, *Arthritis Rheum 34*:894 (1991).
3. F.S. di Giovine, S.E. Malawista, E. Thornton, and G.W. Duff. Urate crystals stimulate production of TNFα from human blood monocytes and synovial cells, *J Clin Invest 87*:1375 (1991).
4. P.T. Chapman, F. Jamar, A.A. Harrison, J.B. Schofield, A.M. Peters, R.M. Binns, and D.O. Haskard. Characterization of E-selection expression, leucocyte traffic and clinical sequelae in urate crystal-induced inflammation: an insight into gout, *Br J Rheumatol 35*:323 (1996).
5. J.S. Bomalaski, D.G. Baker, L.M. Brophy, and M.A. Clark. Monosodium urate crystals stimulate phospholipase A2 enzyme activities and the synthesis of a phospholipase A2-activating protein, *J Immunol 145*:3391 (1990).
6. R.C. Hoch, I.U. Schraufstatter, and C.G. Cochrane. In vivo, in vitro, and molecular aspects of interleukin-8 and the interleukin-8 receptors, *J Lab Clin Med 128*:134 (1996).
7. M. Hogan, B. Sherry, C. Ritchlin, M. Fabre, R. Winchester, A. Cerami, and R. Bucala. Differential expression of the small inducible cytokines GRO alpha and GRO beta by synovial fibroblasts in chronic arthritis: possible role in growth regulation, *Cytokine 6*:61 (1994).
8. M. Hachicha, P.H. Naccache, S.R. McColl. Inflammatory microcrystals differentially regulate the secretion of macrophage inflammatory protein 1 and interleukin 8 by human neutrophils: a possible mechanism of neutrophil recruitment to sites of inflammation in synovitis, *J Exp Med 182*:2019 (1995).
9. A. Matsukawa, T. Yoshimura, T. Maeda, S. Ohkawara, K. Takagi, and M. Yoshinaga. Neutrophil accumulation and activation by homologous IL-8 in rabbits: IL-8 induces destruction of cartilage and production of IL-1 and IL-1 receptor antagonist in vivo, *J Immunol 154*:5418 (1995).
10. R. Terkeltaub, L.A. Sklar, and H. Mueller. Neutrophil activation by inflammatory microcrystals of monosodium urate monohydrate utilizes pertussis toxin-insensitive and sensitive pathways, *J Immunol 144*:2719 (1990).
11. E. Onello, A. Traynor-Kaplan, L. Sklar, and R. Terkeltaub. Mechanism of neutrophil

activation by an unopsonized inflammatory particulate: Monosodium urate crystals induce pertussis toxin-insensitive hydrolysis of phosphatidylinositol 4,5-bisphosphate, *J Immunol 146*:4289 (1991).

12. P.H. Naccache, S. Bourgoin, and E. Plante. Crystal-induced neutrophil activation, role of phospholipase D, *Arthritis Rheum 36*:117 (1993).
13. M. Gaudry, C. Roberge, R. Medicis, A. Lussier, P. Poubelle, and P. Naccache. Crystal-induced neutrophil activation III. Inflammatory microcrystals induce a distinct pattern of tyrosine phosphorylation in human neutrophils, *J Clin Invest 91*:1649 (1993).
14. C. Roberge, M. Gaudry, R. Medicis, A. Lussier, P. Poubelle, and P. Naccache. Crystal-induced neutrophil activation. IV. Specific inhibition of tyrosine phosphorylation by colchicine, *J Clin Invest 92*:1722 (1993).
15. M. Gaudry, C. Gilbert, F. Barabe, P.E. Poubelle, and P.H. Naccache. Activation of Lyn is a common element of the stimulation of human neutrophils by soluble and particulate agonists, *Blood 86*:3567 (1995).
16. C.J. Roberge, M. Gaudry, C. Gilbert, S.E. Malawista, R. de Medicis, A. Lussler, P.E. Poubelle, and P.H. Naccache. Paradoxical effects of colchicine on the activation of human neutrophils by chemotactic factors and inflammatory microcrystal, *J Leukocyte Biol 59*:864 (1996).
17. P.G. Mitchell, J.A. Struve, G.M. McCarthy, and H.S. Cheung. Basic calcium phosphate crystals stimulate cell proliferation and collagenase message accumulation in cultured adult articular chondrocytes, *Arthritis Rheum 35*:343 (1992).
18. H.S. Cheung, J.D. Sallis, and J.A. Struve. Specific inhibition of basic calcium phosphate and calcium pyrophosphate crystal-induction of metalloproteinase synthesis by phosphocitrate, *Biochim Biophysica Acta 1315*:105 (1996).
19. E. Pascual and J.A. Castellano. Treatment with colchicine decreases white cell counts in synovial fluid of asymptomatic knees that contain monosodium urate crystals, *J Rheumatology 19*:600 (1992).
20. A. Swan, B. Heywood, B. Chapman, H. Seward, and P. Dieppe. Evidence for a causal relationship between the structure, size, and load of calcium pyrophosphate dihydrate crystals, and attacks of pseudogout, *Ann Rheum Dis 54*:825 (1995).
21. B.N. Cronstein, Y. Molad, J. Reibman, E. Balakhane, R.I. Levin, and G. Weissmann. Colchicine alters the quantitative and qualitative display of selectins on endothelial cells and neutrophils, *J Clin Invest 96*:994 (1995).

2
Crystal Identification and Joint Fluid Analysis

ROBERT A. GATTER*
Abington Memorial Hospital and University of Pennsylvania, Philadelphia, Pennsylvania

DUNCAN S. OWEN, JR.
Virginia Commonwealth University, Richmond, Virginia

I. CRYSTAL IDENTIFICATION

A. Urate Crystals and Acute Gout

Hollander's and McCarty's work (1) was the catalyst for other investigators to focus on joint fluid to diagnose and confirm specific diseases. Awareness that crystals in joint fluid could cause arthritis in man occurred in 1961. McCarty and Hollander described urate crystals in the joint fluid and/or tophi in 15 of 18 patients with known gout (1).

Two Swiss investigators, Freudweiler and His, working with gouty tophi in 1899 and 1900, respectively, showed that urate crystals caused gouty inflammation in man and animal (2,3). Their work was not recognized at that time. Urate aggregates were held to be secondary to local necrotic processes. Crystals were seen in 1959 by Bauer but were considered to be infrequent and of little assistance in diagnosis (4). Hollander reported crystals in 8 of 17 joint fluids from gouty patients in 1960 using ordinary light microscopy (5).

Dr. McCarty stated that on the first day of his rheumatology fellowship in 1959 at the University of Pennsylvania, his mentor, Dr. Joseph Hollander, showed him crystals in a drop of joint fluid from an inflamed joint under ordinary light mi-

*Retired.

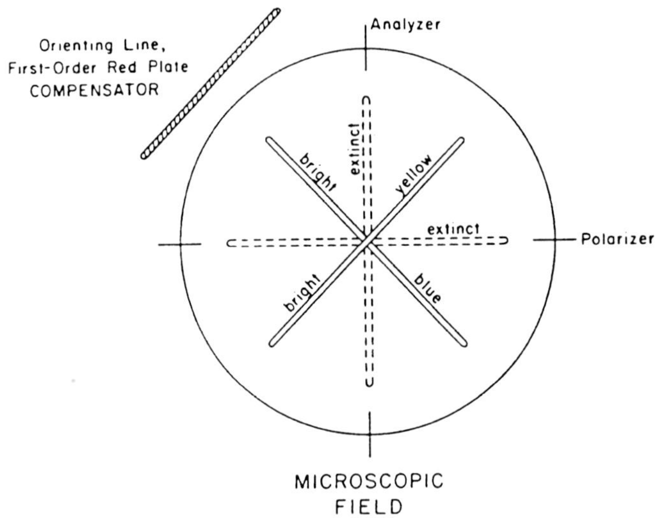

FIGURE 1 Microscopic field with monosodium urate monohydrate crystal rotating 360° under compensated polarized light. Maximum brilliance occurs parallel and perperdicular to the compensator; extinction occurs in the plane of the polarizer and analyzer. (From Ref. 61.)

croscopy (6). Hollander assumed that these crystals were sodium urate. McCarty then undertook the further study of these crystals. He characterized tophaceous material microscopically, using polarized light with a first-order red retardation plate (compensator). The crystals were needle shaped, having strong negative elongation with extinction on the axes (Figure 1, Table 1). They disappeared when stimulated by uricase. Phagocytosis of these crystals occurred in gouty synovia (7). McCarty applied the same methods of identification to the reported 18 patients. The joint fluid crystals behaved identically to the tophaceous crystals in the control material.

B. Calcium Pyrophosphate Crystals and Pseudogout

Subsequently, two hyperuricemic men were seen with acute arthritis of the knees. Joint fluid was examined from these patients. Crystals were found but they exhibited different properties from urates. These crystals showed weak positive elongation or were nearly colorless (isotropic). Extinction was gradual ("oblique") about the axes (Figure 2). Crystal morphology was mixed: needle shaped (acicular) and rhomboid. These crystals were not digested by uricase. Phase light combined with compensated polarized light microscopy (CPLM) helped reveal the thin and small isotropic crystals. Crystals were added to buffy coat and prompt phagocytosis resulted. This observation suggested a mechanism for the observed intracellular positioning of these crystals. The acute attacks were called "pseudogout" (8). McCarty, his fellows, and his associates at the University of Pennsylvania studied these nonurate crystals. They treated

TABLE 1 Joint Fluid Crystal Characteristics

Crystal	Elongation	Brightness (intensity)	Morphology	Extinction	Size (estimation)
MSUM	Negative	Strong	Needle, rod, spherule	On axis sharply	Submicroscopic—40 μm
CPPD	Positive	Weak	Rod and rhomboid	Gradual	Submicroscopic—40 μm
HA[a] individual			Rod		Submicroscopic— 1.9–15.6 μm
crystal clusters			Shiny coins		
$CaHPO_4 2H_2O$	Positive	Strong	Rod		
Calcium oxalate	Position	Variable	Tetrahedron, rod		1.0–2.0 μm
Cholesterol	Negative or positive	Weak or strong	Plates (notched corners)		5–40 μm
			Few rods		
Lipid liquid	Maltese cross positive	Variable	Round extracellular or intracellular		0.5–30 μm
Lithium heparin	Positive	Weak	Polymorphic		2–5 μm
Talc or starch	Maltese cross positive	Strong	Ovoid		
Corticosteroid	Variable	Usually strong	Polymorphic		1–40 μm
Nail polish	Positive	Strong	Rod		5–10 μm

[a]HA = BCP, 'apatite."
Source: Ref. 63.

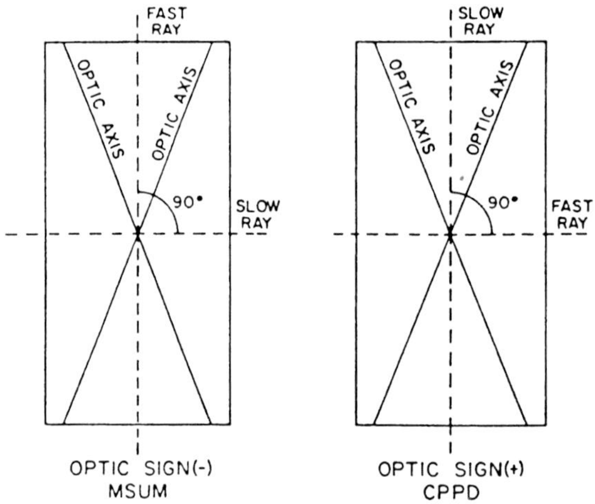

FIGURE 2 Optical sign determination in biaxial crystals. The sign is positive (+) when the slow ray is the acute bisectrix of the optical axes and negative (–) when the fast ray is the acute bisectrix. (From Ref. 40.)

them with hyaluronidase, pelleted the crystals by centrifugation and ruptured the pellet by freeze thawing. The liquid was removed by ether and the protein was digested by trypsin. The solid material remaining was studied by infrared spectrophotometry. It revealed absorption bands characteristic of pyrophosphate (9). X-ray diffraction showed interplanar spacings identical to those of synthetic calcium pyrophosphate dihydrate (CPPD) as published by the National Fertilizer Center in Alabama (10). Pathologic sodium urate crystals were determined to be monosodium urate monohydrate (MSUM) by x-ray diffraction.

C. Crystal-Induced Inflammation

This was a time of intense activity. Many new and important questions needed answers, but only a few people were working on the solutions. In 1961, Dr. McCarty, then Chief of Rheumatology at Hahnemann Medical College and Hospitals, and Dr. Faires, his rheumatology fellow, injected their own knees with sodium urate crystals to prove that these crystals caused acute gout (11). Experiments in both man and animals documented that urate, calcium oxalate, CPPD, and corticosteroid crystals caused inflammation and acute inflammatory arthritis (12).

D. Other Pathological Crystals in Man

The search for pathological crystals was then widened. The orthophosphate, calcium hydrogen phosphate dihydrate (a dimorph of brushite), and the basic calcium phosphates (BCPs), hydroxy-apatite and carbonate-apatite, were initially found in the menisci of cadavers (13,14). Other tissues also revealed hydroxy-apatite and carbonate-apatite plus another tricalcium phosphate (Whitlockite) (15). "Apatite" was first associated with human disease in acute inflammation of soft tissues. The clumped crystals could be seen as "shiny coins" under phase microscopy (16). Subsequently, apatite deposition disease was described (17). Apatite arthropathy was documented (18,19,20,21,22). "Milwaukee shoulder" arthropathy with BCP associated rotator cuff destruction was described (23). BCP has been reported in association with CPPD and MSUM crystals in the same joint (24).

Dicalcium phosphate dihydrate was found in human joint fluid (25). Octacalcium phosphate and calcite were found in the olecranon bursa of a long-term dialysis patient (26). Calcium oxalate related arthritis was found in end-stage renal disease (27,28,29). Urate crystals were found in spherulite form (30).

BCPs remain the most common crystals associated with subcutaneous calcification, tendinitis, bursitis, and severe osteoarthritis.

Cholesterol crystals were noted in chronic effusions of bursi and joints. They are large, plate-like, and appear notched (31) (Table 1). They are not thought to initiate inflammation.

E. Other Joint Fluid Crystals and Findings

Other important findings include lipid liquid crystals (32,33), cryoprotein crystals (34), Charcot-Leyden crystals (35,36), amyloid fragments (37,38), ochronotic shards (39), hemoglobin and hematoidin crystals (40), collagen fibrils (41), prosthetic fragments (42,43), silicone (44), and aluminum (45).

F. Joint Fluid Artifacts

Important artifacts have been described such as: oxalate anticoagulant associated, calcium oxalate crystals (47,48), lithium heparin crystals (49), storage artifacts (49–51), starch from surgical gloves, nail polish, lens paper, dust, fiber, and cover slip glass (52).

The investigators mentioned above utilized technologies from other fields and adapted them to joint fluid research. In addition to the CPLM, x-ray diffraction, and infrared spectrophotometry, electron microscopy in several forms (including scanning, rapid transmission, electron probe analysis, x-ray energy dispersion analysis), Fourier transformed infrared spectrophotometry, and (14CN) diphosphonate binding assay have also played a part. Newer technology such as atomic force spectroscopy (53) and extraction methods (54) may add further information.

II. SYNOVIANALYSIS

A. A Systematic Approach

Paracelsus named joint fluid "synovia" (like "egg white") (55). In 1960, Coggeshall suggested that the analysis of joint fluid was as important a test for joint diseases as urinalysis was for urinary tract disease (56). In 1961, Hollander coined the term "synovianalysis" to reflect this analogy (57).

Prior to 1953, joint fluid was examined mainly in cases of suspected infection. Tests performed usually were Gram stain, culture, and glucose. Although interested in the nature of joint fluid since 1940 (58), it was in 1953 that Ropes and Bauer's extensive study divided pathological joint fluid into two "groups": noninflammatory (Group I), and inflammatory (Group II) (59). In spite of this book, little attention was focused on joint fluid in the 1950s. Because of the diagnostic implications, in 1960 Coggeshall separated purulent fluid (Group III) from the original Group II fluid category (57); and in 1964, Gatter and McCarty separated "hemorrhagic" fluids from Group I and Group II (60). Therefore, "routine" synovianalysis expanded to include gross analysis for volume, viscosity, color, and clarity; and microscopic analysis for white blood cell (WBC) count, differential WBC, and crystal analysis by "wet preparation" under CPLM. Gram stain and culture are added if needed. Tables 2A and B show these groups and how the they relate to disease entities.

Only a few milliliters of joint fluid are needed to perform all of these tests and a single small drop is sufficient for a WBC estimate, WBC differential count, crystal analysis, and Gram stain. Other tests performed, such as mucin clot, rheumatoid factor, antinuclear antibodies, complement, and globulins, are no longer recommended (61). Aspiration of a dry inactive joint can provide the crystal diagnosis of gout (62) or pseudogout (63) by flushing the needle tip contents onto a slide for examination under CPLM.

B. From Research to Clinical Test

The initial research on MSUM and CPPD correlating CPLM with x-ray diffraction findings clearly showed the specificity of the CPLM findings. Now that gout and pseudogout could be diagnosed by finding the characteristic crystals under CPLM without further sophisticated study, keen interest developed in synovianalysis among clinicians. The advent of a test that was pathognomonic, rapid, and simple and that could be performed routinely in the office was a true breakthrough in diagnostic rheumatology. The clinical use of CPLM was described in the literature (64,65,66), but the expense was a drawback to its use. Inexpensive adaptations for ordinary light microscopes were developed and helped to bridge the gap until less-expensive reliable clinical microscopes were available (67,68).

C. Gross Findings

Rice bodies, first noted in 1895 by Riege (69), were associated with rheumatoid arthritis (70,71). Gross changes in synovia were noted with particles from failed prosthesis (42), and from the presence of lipids (72,73), amyloid (38), and ochronotic shards ("ground pepper" sign) (74).

TABLE 2A Joint Fluid Characteristics

	Normal	Group I (noninflammatory)	Group II (inflammatory)	Group III (septic)
Volume (knee, in ml)	<3.5	>3.5	>3.5	>3.5
Viscosity	Very high	High[a]	Low	Variable
Color	Clear	Straw	Straw to opalescent	Variable with organisms
Clarity	Transparent	Transparent	Translucent, opaque at times	Opaque
Mucin clot	Firm	Firm	Friable	Friable
WBC/mm^3	200	200–2,000[b]	2,000–100,000	>50,000[c] usually >100,000
PMN (%)	<25	<25	>50 often	>75[c]
Culture	Negative	Negative	Negative	Usually positive

[a]Rapid accumulation of fluid will lower viscosity.
[b]2000 is an approximation.
[c]May be lower with partially treated or low-virulence organisms.
Source: Ref. 63.

D. Cellular Findings

Investigations into cellular elements of synovia also were renewed. Cytoplasmic inclusion bodies ("RA cells") (75,76), Reiter's cells (77), lupus erythematosus (LE) cells (78), sickle cells (79), tumor cells (80), "stimulated" monocytes in rheumatoid arthritis (81), the predominance of lymphocytes in early rheumatoid arthritis (82), lymphoblasts associated with rheumatoid arthritis (83), acute monocytic arthritis (84) and eosinophilic synovitis (85) were some of the new findings. Many other interesting studies have been reported subsequently; however, no findings except LE cells, tumor cells, and sickle cells have been diagnostically significant.

E. Other Studies

Numerous chemical, biochemical, and immunological studies have been reported. None have proven to be clinically helpful to date, but they have added to our basic knowledge of synovia.

Common histological stains have been used successfully, some with modification, for joint fluid study. Congo red and amyloid, alizarin red S for calcium, prussian blue for iron, sudan black III for lipid, Wright stain for cellular morphology, and Gram stain for bacteria have been employed.

TABLE 2B Differential Diagnosis by Joint Fluid Groups[a]

Group I (noninflammatory)	Group II (inflammatory)	Group III (septic)	Group IV (hemorrhagic)
Osteoarthritis	Rheumatoid disease	Bacterial infections	Trauma with or without fracture
Traumatic arthritis	Crystal-induced synovitis		Charcot's arthropathy
Avascular necrosis	Gout		Hemorrhagic diathesis
Internal derangement	Pseudogout		Anticoagulant therapy
Osteochondritis dissecans	Hydroxyapatite		von Willebrand's
Osteochondromatosis	Corticosteroid injection		Hemophilia
Charcot's arthropathy	Psoriatic arthritis		Scurvy
Subsiding inflammation	Reactive arthritis		Thrombocytopenia
Villonodular synovitis	Reiter's syndrome		Hemangioma
Hypertrophic pulmonary osteoarthropathy	Regional enteritis		Tumor
Systemic lupus erythematosus[b]	Ulcerative colitis		Pigmented villonodular synovitis
Rheumatic fever[b]	Postileal bypass		Synovioma
Scleroderma[b]	Yersinia		
Amyloidosis[b]	Campylobacter		
Myxedema	Whipple's disease		
Acromegaly	Connective tissue disease		
Hemochromatosis	Systemic lupus		
Gaucher's disease	Polyarteritis		
Ochronosis	Scleroderma		

Paget's disease of bone	Polymyositis	
Sickle cell disease	Vasculitis (nonspecific)	
Milwaukee shoulder	Polymyalgia rheumatica	
	Polychondritis	
	Sarcoidosis	
		Behçet's syndrome
	Ankylosing spondylitis	
	Juvenile rheumatoid arthritis	
	Rheumatic fever	
	Agammaglobulinemia	
	Infectious arthritis (low-virulence)	
	Viral	
	Fungal	
	Bacterial	
	Mycobacterial	
	Mycoplasmal	
	Hypersensitivity	
	Serum sickness	
	Erythema multiforme	
	Lyme disease	
	Leukemia	

[a]Partial listing.
[b]May be Group I or II.
Source Ref. 63.

III. QUALITY CONTROL AND CONTINUING EDUCATION

Variation in results was addressed as synovianalysis became a frequent and common procedure. Viscosity seemed to be less reliable than initially had been supposed (86). Quality control studies were performed, but considerable variation was found among laboratories (87–92).

Educational efforts include joint fluid specific self-learning series (93), courses (94), books (95–97), and guidelines (62). Many articles and textbook chapters have been published as well. Hopefully, these endeavors will continue to improve the accuracy, efficiency, reproducibility, and cost-effectiveness of synovianalysis.

IV. SUMMARY

The second half of the 20th century has been a time of great interest, activity, and progress in the study of joint fluid. Synovianalysis, a simple, rapid and diagnostic test, was brought to a field where previously few diagnostic tests had existed. Mechanisms of crystal-induced joint inflammation were elucidated and previously unknown crystal-induced disorders were discovered and defined.

REFERENCES

1. D.J. McCarty and J.L. Hollander. Identification of urate crystals in gouty synovial fluid, *Ann Int Med 54*:452 (1961).
2. M. Freudweiler. Studies on the nature of gouty tophi, *Dtsch Arch Klin Med 63*:266 (1899).
3. W. His. Fate and effects of the uric acid sodium in the abdominal and joint cavities of the robbit, *Dtsch Arch Klin Med 67*:81 (1900).
4. W. Bauer and E. Calkins. *Diseases of Metabolism* (G.G. Duncan, ed.), W.B. Saunders, Philadelphia, PA, 1959, p. 659.
5. J.L. Hollander. *Arthritis and Allied Conditions* (J.L. Hollander, ed.), Lea and Febiger, Philadelphia, PA, 1960, p. 77.
6. D.J. McCarty. *Personal Communication*, 1962.
7. D.J. McCarty. Phagocytosis of urate crystals in gouty synovial fluid, *Arthritis Rheum. 4*:425–425 (1961).
8. D.J. McCarty, Jr., N.N. Kohn, and J.S. Faires. The significance of calcium phosphate crystals in the synovial fluid of arthritic patients: The "pseudogout syndrome" I: Clinical Aspects, *Ann Int Med 56*:711 (1962).
9. N.N. Kohn, R.E. Hughes, D.J. McCarty, Jr., and J.S. Fares. The significance of calcium phosphate crystals in the synovial fluid of arthritic patients: The "pseudogout syndrome" II: Identification of crystals, *Ann Int Med 56*:738 (1962).
10. E.H. Brown, J.R. Lehr, J.P. Smith, et al. Crystalline intermediates in the hydrologic degradation of calcium polymetaphosphate, *J Phys Chem 61*:1669 (1957).
11. J.S. Faires and D.J. McCarty. Acute arthritis in man and dog produced by intrasynovial injection of sodium urate crystals, *Clin Res 9*:329 (1961).
12. J.S. Faires and D.J. McCarty. Acute synovitis in normal joints and dogs produced by

the injection of microcrystalline sodium urate, calcium oxalate and corticosteroid esters, *Arthritis Rheum 5*:295–296 (1962).
13. D.J. McCarty and R.A. Gatter. Identification of calcium hydrogen phosphate dihydrate crystals in human fibro-cartilage, *Nature 201*:391 (1964).
14. D.J. McCarty, J.M. Hogan, and R.A. Gatter. Studies in pathological calcifications in human cartilages. I: Prevalence and types of crystal deposits in the menisci of two hundred fifteen cadavers, *J Bone Joint Surg 48A*:309–325 (1966).
15. R.A. Gatter and J.D. McCarty. Pathological tissue calcification in man, *Arch Pathol 84*:346–353, 1967.
16. D.J. McCarty and R.A. Gatter. Recurrent acute inflammation associated with focal apatite crystal deposition, *Arthritis Rheum 9*:804 (1966).
17. P.A. Dieppe, E.C. Huskisson, P. Crocker, et al. Apatite deposition disease-a new anthropathy, *Lancet 1*:266 (1976).
18. H.R. Schumacher, R. Tse, A.J. Reginato. Hydroxyapatite-like crystals in synovial fluid cell vacuoles, a suspected new cause for crystal-induced arthritis, *Arthritis Rheum 7*:821 (1976).
19. P.B. Halverson. Arthropathies associated with basic calcium phosphate crystals, *Scanning Microsc 6*:791 (1992).
20. A.G. Fam and J. Stein. Hydroxyapatite pseudopodagra in young women, *J Rheumatol 19*:662 (1992).
21. A.J. Reginato and H.R. Schumacher. Apatite crystals in joint fluid, clinical relevance and the search for a simple and accurate diagnostic test, *Rheumatol Rev 3*:9 (1994).
22. J.C. Marcos, A.S. Arturi, C. Bambini, et al. Familial hydroxyapatite chondrocalcinosis: Clinical course and lack of genetic linkage with the type II procollagen gene, *J Clin Rheumatol 1*:171 (1995).
23. P.B. Halverson, H.S. Cheung, D.J. McCarty, J Garancis, and N. Mandel. "Milwaukee Shoulder"—Association of microspheroids containing hydroxyapatite crystals, active collagenase, and neutral protease with rotator cuff detects, *Arthritis Rheum 24*:474 (1981).
24. P.B. Halverson and L.E. Ryan. Triple crystal disease: monosodium urate monohydrate, calcium pyrophosphate dihydrate, and basic calcium phosphate in a single joint, *Ann Rheum Dis 47*:864 (1988).
25. P.D. Utsinger. Dicalcium phosphate deposition disease: A suspected new crystal-induced arthritis, XIV International Congress of Rheumatology, San Francisco, California, 1977.
26. R. Irby, W. Edwards, and R.A. Gatter. Articular complications of homotransplantation and chronic hemodialysis, *J Rheum 2*:340 (1975).
27. G.S. Hoffman, H.R. Schumacher, H. Paul, et al. Calcium oxalate microcrystalline associated arthritis in end stage renal diseases, *Ann Int Med 97*:36 (1982).
28. A.J. Reginato, J.L. Ferreiro Seone, C. Barbaza Alvarez, et al. Arthropathy and cutaneous calcinosis in hemodialysis oxalosis, *Arthritis Rheum 29*:1387 (1986).
29. H.R. Schumacher, A.J. Reginato, S. Pullman. Synovial fluid oxalate deposition complicating rheumatoid arthritis with amyloidosis and renal failure: demonstration of intracellular oxalate crystals, *J Rheumatol 14*:361–366 (1987).
30. J.J. Fiechtner and P.A. Simkin. Urate spherulites in gouty synovia, *JAMA 245*:1533 (1981).
31. J. Zuckner, J. Uddin, G. Gantner, et al. Cholesterol crystals in synovial fluid, *Ann Int Med 60*:436 (1964).

32. P.A. Schlesinger, M.T. Stillman, and L. Peterson. Polyarthritis with birefringent lipid with synovial fluid macrophages: case study report and ultrastructural study, *Arthritis Rheum 25*:1365 (1982).
33. H.J. Reginato, H.R. Schumacher, D. Allan, and J.L. Rabinowitz. Acute monoarthritis associated with lipid liquid crystals, *Arthritis Rheum 25*:S35 (1982).
34. D.R. Langlands, R.J. Dawkins, L.R. Metz, et al. Arthritis associated with crystallizing cryoprecipitable IgG paraprotein, *Amer J Med 68*:461–465 (1980).
35. H.A. Menard, et al. Charcot-Leyden crystals in synovial fluid, *Arthritis Rheum 24*:1591 (1981).
36. M. Dougados, L. Benhamov, and B. Amar. Charcot-Leyden crystals in synovial fluid, *Arthritis Rheum 26*:1 (1983).
37. D.A. Gordon, W. Pruzanski, and M.A. Ogryzlo. Synovial fluid examination for the diagnosis of amyloidosis, *Ann Rheum Dis 32*:248 (1973).
38. S. Lakhanpal, et al. Synovial fluid examination for the diagnosis of amyloidosis, *Ann Rheum Dis 32*:248 (1973).
39. H.R. Schumacher and D.E. Holdsworth. Ochronotic arthropathy. I. Clinicopathologic studies, Semin. *Arthritis Rheum 6*:207 (1977).
40. G.A. Tate, et al. Four patients with synovial fluid crystals derived from hemoglobin degradation products, *Arthritis Rheum 31*:S24 (1988).
41. R.C. Kitridou, et al. Identification of collagen in synovial fluid, *Arthritis Rheum 12*:580 (1969).
42. R.C. Kitridou, H.R. Schumacher, J.L. Sbarbaro, and J.L. Hollander. Recurrent hemarthrosis after prosthetic knee arthroplasty: Identification of metal particles in the synovial fluid, *Arthritis Rheum 12*:520 (1969).
43. A. Crugnola, A. Schiller, and E. Radin. Polymeric debris in synovium after total hip replacement: histological identification, *J Bone Joint Surg [Am]59*:860 (1977).
44. D.E. Rosenthal, A.E. Rosenberg, A.L. Schiller, R.J. Smith. Destructive arthritis due to silicone: A foreign body reaction, *Radiology 149*:69 (1983).
45. P. Netter, J.L. Delongeas, and G. Faure. Inflammatory effect of aluminum phosphate, *Ann Rheum Dis 42 (S)*:114 (1983).
46. R.A. Gatter and D.J. McCarty. Synovianalysis, a rapid clinical diagnostic procedure, *Rheumatism 20*:2–6 (1964).
47. H.R. Schumacher. Intracellular crystals in synovial fluid anticoagulated with oxalate, *N Engl J Med 274*:1372 (1966).
48. K. Tanphaichitr, I. Spilberg, and B. Hahn. Lithium heparin crystals simulating calcium pyrophosphate dihydrate crystals in synovial fluid, *Arthritis Rheum 19*:966 (1976).
49. G. Kerolous, G. Clayburne, and H.R. Schumacher. Is it necessary to examine synovial fluid promptly after arthrocentesis? *Arthritis Rheum 32*:271–278 (1989).
50. H.R. Schumacher and A.J. Reginato. *Atlas of Synovial Fluid Analysis Analysis and Crystal Identification*, Lea and Febiger, Philadelphia, PA, 1991, 9. 232–238.
51. N.W. McGill, A. Swan, P.A. Diepper. Survival of calcium pyrophosphate crystals in stored synovial fluids, *Ann Rheum Dis 50*:939–941 (1991).
52. R.A. Gatter. *A Practical Handbook of Joint Fluid Analysis*, Lea and Febiger, Philadelphia, PA, 1984, pp. 43–44.
53. J.M. Blair, L. Tarneswar, L.B. Sorenson, M. Arnsdorf. Identification of hydroxyapatite and other microcrystals by application of atomic force spectroscopy, *Arthritis Rheum 35*:R27 (1992).

54. A.J. Swan, B.R. Haywood, P.A. Dieppe. Extraction of calcium containing crystal from synovial fluids and articular cartilage, *J Rheumatol 19*:1763–1773, 1992.
55. E.J. Field, R.J. Harrison. *Anatomical Terms: Their origin and derivation*, 2nd edition, Cambridge-Heffer, 1957.
56. H.C. Coggeshall. *Arthritis and Allied Conditions*, 6th edition, (J.L. Hollander, ed.), Lea and Febiger, Philadelphia, PA, 1960.
57. J.L. Hollander, R.A. Jessar, D.J. McCarty. Synovianalysis: An aid in arthritis diagnosis, *Bull Rheum Dis 12*:263 (1961).
58. M.W. Ropes, E.C. Rossmeisl, and W. Bauer. The origin and nature of normal synovial fluid, *J Clin Invest 19*:795 (1940).
59. M.W. Ropes and W. Bauer. *Synovial Fluid Changes in Joint Disease*, Harvard University Press, Cambridge, MA, 1953.
60. R.A. Gatter and D.J. McCarty. Synovianalysis, a rapid clinical diagnostic procedure, *Rheumatism 20*:2–6 (1964).
61. R.A. Gatter, R.P. Andrews, D.A. Cooley, J.J. Fiechtner, D.A. Minna, P. Phelps, and C. Wasner. American College of Rheumatology guidelines for performing office synovial fluid examinations, *J Clin Rheum 1*:194–195 (1995).
62. A. Weinberg, H.R. Schumacher, and C.A. Agudelo. Urate crystals in asymptomatic metatarsal phalangeal joints, *Ann Intern Med 91*:56 (1979).
63. B.B. Dorwart. Pseudogout crystals in asymptomatic toe joints, American Rheumatism Association Southeastern meeting, Charleston, South Carolina, 1980.
64. P. Phelps, A.D. Steele, D.J. McCarty. Compensated polarized light microscopy: Identification of crystals in synovial fluids from gout and pseudogout, *JAMA 203*:508–512 (1968).
65. R.A. Gatter. The compensated polarized light microscope in clinical rheumatology, *Arthritis Rheum 17*:253 (1974).
66. R.A. Gatter. Use of the compensated polarized microscope, *Clin Rheum Dis 3*:91 (1977).
67. D.S. Owen. A cheap and useful compensated polarizing microscope, *New England J of Med 285*:1152 (1971).
68. T.J. Fagan and M.D. Lidsky. Compensated polarized light microscopy using cellophane adhesive tape, *Arthritis Rheum 17*:256–262 (1974).
69. H. Riege. Die reiskorperchen in tuberculos erkrankten synovalsacken, *Deutsch Z Chir 42*:1 (1895).
70. H.S. Cheung, et al. Synovial origins of rice bodies in joint fluid, *Arthritis Rheum 23*:72–76 (1980).
71. J. Galvez, J. Sola, G. Ortuno, et al. Microscopic rice bodies in rheumatoid synovial fluid sediments nearly specific for RA, *J Rheumatol 19*:1851–1858 (1992).
72. C. Lawrence and B. Seife. Bone marrow in joint fluid: A clue to fracture, *Ann Intern Med 74*:740 (1971).
73. W.E. Ryan, R.D. Ellefson, and L.L. Ward. Lipid synovial effusion. Unique occurrence in systemic lupud erythematosus, *Arthritis Rheum 16*:759 (1973).
74. T. Hunter, W. Pruzanski, and M.A. Ogryzlo, the ground pepper sign of synovial fluid; A now diagnostic feature of ochronosis, *J Rheumatol 1*:45 (1974).
75. R.A. Gatter and D.J. McCarty. Presented as a supplement to Pseudogout Syndrome V: A Clinical Analysis of 30 Cases, American Rheumatism Association Annual Scientific Session, Atlantic City, 1963.
76. J.L. Hollander and D.J. McCarty. Studies on the pathogenesis of rheumatoid joint

fluid inflammation. I. The "RA cell" and a working hypothesis, *Ann Intern Med 62*:271 (1965).
77. T.J. Pekin, T.I. Malinin, and M.J. Zvaifler. Unusual synovial fluid in Reiter's syndrome, *Ann Intern Med 66*:677, 1967.
78. G.C. Hunder and R.V. Pierce. In vivo LE cell formation in synovial fluid, *Arthritis Rheum 13*:448 (1970).
79. H.R. Schumacher. Arthropathy of sickle cell diseases, *Ann Intern Med 78*:203 (1973).
80. A.G. Fam, A. Kolin, and A.J. Lewis. Metastatic carcinomatous arthritis and carcinoma of the lung. A report of two cases diagnosed by synovial fluid cytology, *J Rheumatol 7*:98 (1980).
81. K. Takasugi and J.W. Hollingsworth. Morphologic studies of mononuclear cells of human synovial fluid, *Arthritis Rheum 10*:495 (1967).
82. R.A. Gatter and J.D. Richmond. The predominance of synovial fluid lymphocytes in early rheumatoid arthritis, *J Rheumatol 2*:340–345 (1975).
83. R.B. Trayroff, E. Pascual, and H.R. Schumacher. Mononuclear cells in human synovial fluid. Identification of lymphoblasts in rheumatoid arthritis, *Arthritis Rheum 19*:743 (1976).
84. A.E. Brawer and E.S. Catheart. Acute monocytic arthritis, *Arthritis Rheum 22*:294 (1979).
85. J.P. Brown, M. Rola-Pleszoynski, and H. Menard. Eosinophilic synovitis: clinical observations on a newly recognized subset of patients with dermatographism, *Arthritis Rheum 29*:1147–1161 (1986).
86. P. Hasselbacher. Measuring synovial fluid viscosity with a white blood cell diluting pipette, *Arthritis Rheum 19*:1358 (1976).
87. J.M. Eisenberg, H.R. Schumacher, P.K. Davidson, and L. Kauffman. Usefulness of synovial fluid analysis in the evaluation of joint effusions: Use of threshold analysis and the likelihood ratios to assess a diagnostic test, *Arch Intern Med 144*:715 (1984).
88. H.R. Schumacher, M.S. Sieck, S. Rothfuss, et al. Reproducibility of synovial fluid analysis. A study among four laboratories, *Arthritis Rheum 29*:770–774 (1986).
89. P. Hasselbacher. Variation in synovial fluid analysis by hospital laboratories, *Arthritis Rheum 30*:637–342 (1987).
90. H.R. Schumacher, M. Sieck, and G. Clayburne. Quality control in synovial fluid analysis. Development of a testing mechanism, *Arthritis Rheum 30*:S101 (1988).
91. C. Gordan, A. Swan, P. Dieppe. Detection of crystals in synovial fluids by light microscopy: sensitivity and reliability, *Ann Rheum Dis 48*:737–742 (1989).
92. R. Von Essen, et al. Quality control of the laboratory diagnosis of gout by synovial fluid microscopy, *Scand J Rheumatol 19*:232–234 (1990).
93. D.S. Owen, Jr., B.F. Germain, and H.R. Schumacher. *Synovial Fluid Analysis, Self-Learning Series*, American College of Physicians, Philadelphia, PA, July, 1978.
94. H.R. Schumacher, Jr., M.D. Workshop on practical synovial fluid analysis, University of Pennsylvania, Philadelphia.
95. P. Dieppe and P. Calvert. *Crystals and Joint Diseases*, Chapman and Hall, London and New York, 1983.
96. R.A. Gatter, H.R. Schumacher. *A Practical Handbook of Joint Fluid Analysis*. 2nd Ed., Lea and Febiger, Philadelphia, Pennsylvania, 1991.
97. H.R. Schumacher and A.J. Reginato. *Atlas of Synovial Fluid Analysis and Crystal Identification*, Lea and Febiger, Philadelphia, 1991.

3
The Pathogenesis of Bone Changes Due to Crystals

Jan Dequeker and Pascale Volders
University Hospitals, University Ziekenhuizen Leuven, Lubbeek, Belgium

I. BONE CHANGES IN GOUT

In crystal arthropathies, in particular chronic gouty arthritis, clinicians have noted that the reactions of the bone subchondral and at the joint margins are hypertrophic with exuberant osteophytosis and sclerosis (1). These osteosclerotic changes are more marked in gout than in osteoarthritis and are in contrast to the bone loss and decalcification observed in rheumatoid arthritis and related diseases. Juxta-articular osteoporosis, which is a common early finding in rheumatoid arthritis, is typically absent or mild in gouty arthritis, unless disuse osteoporosis supervenes. The joint space in gout is very characteristically well maintained in contrast to the early joint-space narrowing of rheumatoid arthritis. Repeated gouty attacks of the midfoot joints lead to typical radiological signs of moderate joint-space narrowing and formation of multiple osteophytes along the dorsum of the foot, which gives a spike appearance resembling the back of the hedgehog, hence the French term *pied hérissé*. Despite the striking radiological abnormalities, sufferers from gout maintain very good function outside the acute attacks.

The pathogenesis of osteolytic lesions in gout is linked to the chronic biologic effects of crystals on synovial cells, fibroblasts, macrophages, and chrondrocytes. Each crystal type is opsonized with various proteins: some are prophlogistic, others are antiphlogistic. The crystals can undergo endocytosis by macrophages or monocytes in the synovial fluid or by fixed synovial cells, and can activate phospholipase A2, which generates arachidonic acid substrate for the cyclooxygenase and lipoxygenase pathways. They stimulate an increase of mRNA for collagenase, stromelysin, and gelatinase [matrixmetalloproteinases (MMP)] (2). The increased enzyme release continues as long as the crystal is in the cell and, if there is an increased protease release over a long period, it contributes to the destruction of joint tissues. If there is an increased synthesis of MMP, induced by monosodium urate (MSU) crystals, it is carving out the space in bone, cartilage, and other hard tissues to make room for the deposition of tophaceous masses.

The inflammation-induced localized bone resorption is also due to activation and recruitment of osteoclasts by locally produced inflammatory mediators and cytokines. Several interleukins (IL-1, -3, -4, -6, and -11), TNF (α, β), γ-interferon, and TGF-β have effects on bone resorption and bone formation (3). Ohashi et al. (4) found that gelatinase B was strongly positive in osteoclasts. Conway and coworkers (5) showed that MMP inhibitors (e.g., butanediamide) are osteo- and chrondroprotective and that they induce a significant reduction in osteoclasts. In chronic gout, lesions in the soft tissues adjacent to bone can also induce areas of pressure erosions. These defects are typically in a periarticular position.

In conclusion, we can say that the rate of bone resorption in inflammation-induced bone loss may not be due to a single factor, but to the concerted action of several local or systemic factors.

Although during the gouty arthritis there are generally crystal/cell attacks, a variety of inflammatory mediators may be released as PGE-2, LTB-4, IL-1–IL-6, oxygen radicals, and collagenases, which might have also an effect, mostly negative, on bone. The bone compartment in gout reacts in an opposite direction as compared to other inflammatory rheumatic diseases, resulting in sclerosis and osteophytes. What makes the difference between gout and, for example, rheumatoid arthritis in the host reaction? Duration of inflammation, age, gender, hormonal environment, genetics?

II. GOUT COMORBIDITY: OBESITY, DIABETES MELLITUS TYPE II, DIFFUSE IDIOPATHIC SKELETAL HYPEROSTOSIS, GENERALIZED OSTEOARTHRITIS

The link to the solution may be comorbidity. There is a strong relationship between gout and obesity, and a less strong correlation between gout and diabetes mellitus type II (Figure 1). Bone diseases with hypertrophic reactions such as hyperostosis vertebralis (Forestier's disease, more commonly called diffuse idiopathic skeletal hyperostosis (DISH)] and generalized osteoarthritis are also associated with obesity (6) and diabetes mellitus type II. Generalized DISH is characterized by the following radiographic criteria: calcification/ossification along the anterolateral aspects of at least four contiguous vertebral bodies,

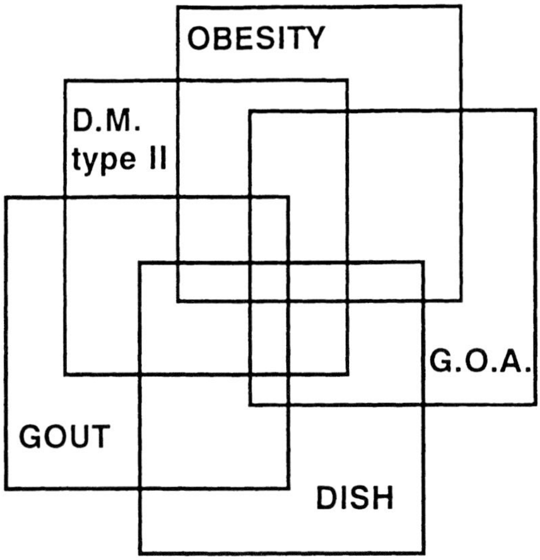

FIGURE 1 Venn diagram illustrating comorbity and overlapping bone features between gout and diabetes mellitus type II (DM), obesity, diffuse idiopathic skeletal hyperostosis (DISH), and generalized osteoarthritis (GOA).

preservation of intervertebral disc height, and absence of apophyseal joint bony ankylosis and sacroiliac joint erosions, sclerosis, or osseous fusion (7).

Generalized osteoarthritis (GOA) is characterized by hand osteoarthritis (Heberden and Bouchard nodes) and at least two other locations of osteoarthritis (knee, hip, spine) (8). Hyperuricemia and/or gout is found more often than expected in diabetes mellitus type II, in DISH (9,10), and in GOA; inversely, the incidence of diabetes mellitus or glucose intolerance is found more often than expected in gout (11) and in DISH (10,12), and obesity is also associated with abnormalities of insulin metabolism. The relationship between gout, diabetes mellitus, DISH, and GOA may provide seminal clues as to the pathophysiological factors involved in hypertrophic (OA-like) changes observed in the above conditions.

III. GROWTH FACTORS: GROWTH HORMONE, INSULIN-LIKE GROWTH FACTORS, AND TRANSFORMING GROWTH FACTOR β

A. Growth Factors in Aging and Hypertrophic Bone Disease

Because of the resemblance of bone-joint changes in acromegaly with osteoarthritis, abnormal growth hormone (GH) levels have been studied first. We found some alterations in fasting GH levels and after insulin-induced hypoglycemia in generalized osteoarthritis compared to osteoporosis cases. Osteoarthritis cases had a significantly higher fasting GH level and response (13).

In DISH, one study (14) found high levels of GH, which could not be confirmed by Littlejohn and coworkers (15). Physiological GH secretion follows a circadian rhythm in addition to internal or external stimulating factors, which complicate the study unless 24-hour patterns are analyzed.

If the disease association of DISH, GOA, obesity, diabetes mellitus, and gout is not spurious, a common factor may be an abnormality in insulin metabolism. Insulin is structurally closely related to the somatomedins and may have growth factor–like activity. The two best identified insulin-like growth factors are IGF-I and IGF-II. Aging is associated with a decrease in growth hormone secretion (16) and lowered serum levels of insulin-like growth factor-I (IGF-I) (17,18), endocrine factors considered to be anabolic for the bone tissue (19). Circulating IGF-I represents a reliable index of GH status and is mainly of hepatic origin (20). In addition, GH stimulates, at its target sites, local synthesis and release of IGF-I, which acts in an autocrine or paracrine way at the tissue-level (21), implying that serum IGF-I levels do not completely account for IGF-I tissue effects. We have shown, using multiple response analysis, a positive relationship between serum IGF-I as an integrated measure of GH secretion and bone density at the hip in healthy community-dwelling older women (22). Changes in the IGF-I regulatory system over time could be an important pathophysiologic component of age-related diseases such as osteoarthritis, DISH, and osteoporosis. In femoral neck fracture cases, we found a significant deficit of the serum stimulating component of the IGF system (23). Serum levels of IGF-I are elevated in patients with acromegaly, a disease associated with the development of secondary osteoarthritis (24). New bone formation has also been related to increased serum levels of IGF-I in patients with diffuse idiopathic skeletal hyperostosis (25). In one study, both the size and the growth of osteophytes were directly correlated with serum levels of IGF-I in subjects with osteoarthritis of the knee (26). Other studies, however, have yielded conflicting results (27–29).

Hochberg et al. (28) examined the relationship between serum levels of IGF-I and the presence and severity of radiographic changes of knee osteoarthritis in subjects participating in the Baltimore Longitudinal Study of Aging. Mean serum IGF-I levels were significantly lower in subjects with knee osteoarthritis; however, after adjustment for age-related changes in IGF-I levels, these differences were no longer significant.

We examined serum levels of IGF-I in osteoarthritis and osteoporosis cases and did not find significant differences, even after stimulation with growth hormone releasing factor (30).

Another important member of the family of anabolic growth factors is transforming growth factor β (TGFβ) induced by many cell types including the osteoblast. This has an autocrine and paracrine function, and can be studied by serum levels or by tissue levels. The latter levels are important because the growth factors as IGFs and TGFβ can be released from the matrix because they are acid-resistant and become activated to stimulate the repairing cell population (coupling factor in bone disease?) (Figure 2).

We found a significantly high level of IGF-I and -II and TGFβ (27) and of osteocalcin, a specific bone protein involved in calcification of the matrix, in the matrix from the iliac crest in necropsy cases with hand osteoarthritis compared to age-matched controls (28). Recently, we found significant variations in trabecular bone composition including IGF-II with anatomical site and age, suggesting potential implications for bone quality assessment (29).

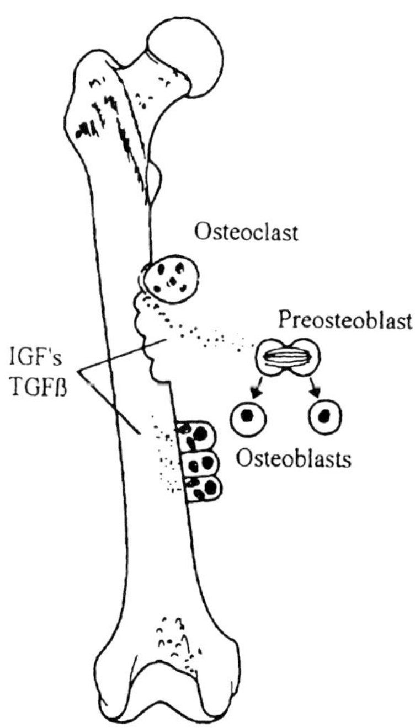

FIGURE 2 Schematic diagram of the metabolic circle (IGFs and TGFβ) of mitogenic growth factors (IGFs and TGFβ). These proteins are released by the osteoclasts in the process of bone resorption and stimulate preosteoblasts to divide and form new osteoblasts, which incorporate new growth factor in the matrix.

B. Osteophytes

In studies with experimentally induced osteoarthritis in animals and studies of human osteoarthritis chondrocytes in cell culture, there is ample evidence that OA chondrocytes display deranged reactivity to IGF and TGFβ (34–37). In human osteophyte formation, locally produced IGFs are important regulators of bone formation (38). Throughout the developing osteophyte there was a strong association between osteogenesis and the expression of mRNA transcripts for IGF-I, IGF-II, and the IGF-receptor. In the murine knee model, it was found that TGFβ1 stimulates articular chondrocyte proteoglycan synthesis and induces osteophyte formation (39).

Elucidation of the action and interaction of these growth factors and cytokines may be expected to clarify the etiopathogenesis of (secondary) osteoarthritis and possibly offer novel models for its treatment.

IV. BONE DENSITY AND BONE QUALITY

The role of bone in particular subchondral bone in the pathogenesis of primary and/or secondary osteoarthritis is controversial. Osteoarthritis is usually considered to be a primary disorder of chondrocyte function with secondary change in bones. However, a defect in the subchondral bone, resulting in the loss of its shock-absorbing capacity, could transfer the stress of loading directly to the articular cartilage with secondary change in the cartilage.

The secondary occurrence of marked hypertrophic OA changes in chronic gout could also be based on a bone predisposition facilitating the occurrence of hyperostotic reaction. To determine whether bone changes may precede injury to the cartilage and metabolic and systemic influences can also alter the subchondral bone, rendering it less able to withstand normal mechanical stresses, bone at different sites in the body has been studied extensively by the authors (40). Epidemiological and case-control studies have revealed that osteoarthritis cases have more bone at all sites than expected and that bone in cases with generalized osteoarthritis shows both quantitative and qualitative differences, including increased contents of growth factors and hypermineralization (41). The observation that not only apparent bone density, but also pure bone density, cortical as well as trabecular, is increased as measured by gradient density centrifugation (32) or with backscattered electronic microscopy (42,43) in GOA is of particular biomechanical importance. These findings suggest that a more generalized bone alteration may be on the basis of the pathogenesis of osteoarthritis and related generalized hyperostotic changes as seen in chronic gout, DISH, diabetes mellitus, and obesity.

Mechanical properties of iliac crest trabecular bones have been tested in OA and controls. A significant difference in stiffness elastic modulus as measured by compression tests was found, the osteoarthritic trabecular bone being significantly stiffer than the nonosteoarthritic trabecular bone. A significant correlation was found between elastic modulus, apparent density, percentage pure to crude bone volume, and cortical thickness and trabecular width, the latter two evaluated by quantitative histomorphometry. Compressive strength was higher in osteoarthritic bone, but not significantly. A significant correlation between trabecular bone volume and trabecular width and maximum compressive strength was established (44).

V. CONCLUSIONS

The multiplicity of significant alterations found in patients with hypertrophic bone alterations as primary osteoarthritis and in osteoarthritic bone far away from the articular lesion indicates that osteoarthritis is part of a more generalized bone disease.

These quantitative and qualitative differences in bone may produce disease by increasing subchondral bone stiffness and by making subchondral bone less deformable to impact loads. This stiff bone transmits more force to overlying cartilage, making it more vulnerable. In contrast to Radin's hypothesis (45,46), we hypothesize that subchondral bone stiffness is part of a more general bone alteration instead of healing of local microfractures.

In line with our observations of a generalized change in bone osteoarthritis, Doherty et al. (47) demonstrated that the predisposition to "primary" osteoarthritis influences the development and severity of "secondary" osteoarthritis. Patients who had undergone unilateral meniscetomy 19 years or more before and who had x-ray changes in the hands consistent with generalized osteoarthritis showed more frequently a more severe knee osteoarthritis, judged clinically and radiologically in both unoperated knees. In relation to the above observed alterations in GOA, we hypothesize that the bone alterations observed in gout, diabetes mellitus type II, obesity, and DISH are part of a constitutional genetic determined predisposition to develop in certain environmental conditions hypertropic bone and osteophytes mediated by anabolic growth factors IGF-I and -II and TGFβ.

REFERENCES

1. J. Dequeker. An Atlas of Radiology of Rheumatic Disorders, Wolf Medical Publication, London, 1982, 163–169.
2. A.J. Fam. Calcium pyrophosphate crystal deposition disease and other crystal deposition diseases. *Curr Opin Rheumatol 4*:574–582 (1992).

3. U.H. Lerner. Regulation of bone metabolism by the kallikrein-kinin system, the coagulation cascade, and the acute-phase reactants. *Oral Surg Oral Med Oral Pathol 78*:481–493 (1994).
4. K. Ohashi, R. Kawai, and M. Hara. Increased matrix metalloproteinases as possible cause of osteoarticular tissue destruction in long-term haemodialysis and beta2-microglobulin amyloidosis. *Virchows Arch 428*:37–46 (1996).
5. J.G. Conway, J.A. Wakefield, and R.H. Brown. Inhibition of cartilage and bone destruction in adjuvant arthritis in the rat by a matrix metalloproteinase inhibitor. *J Exp Med 182*:449–457 (1995).
6. J. Dequeker, P. Goris, and R. Uytterhoeven. Osteoporosis and osteoarthritis (osteoarthrosis): Anthropometric distinctions. *JAMA 249*:1448–1451 (1983).
7. D. Resnick and G. Niwayama. Radiographic and pathologic features of spinal involvement in diffuse idiopathic skeletal hyperostosis (DISH). *Radiology 146*:1 (1976).
8. J.H. Kellgren and J.S. Lawrence. Radiological assessment of osteoarthrosis. *Ann Rheum Dis 16*:494–502 (1957).
9. G.O. Littlejohn and S. Hall. Diffuse idiopathic skeletal hyperostosis and new bone formation in male gouty subjects. A radiologic study. *Rheumatol Int 2*:83–86 (1982).
10. G. Vezyroglou, A. Mitropoulos, N. Kyriazis, and C. Antoniadis. A metabolic syndrome in diffuse idiopathic skeletal hyperostosis. A controlled study. *J Rheumatol 23*:672–676 (1996).
11. J.B. Hezman and U. Goldcourt. Uric acid and diabetes observations in a population study. *Lancet 2*:240–241 (1982).
12. G.O. Littlejohn and H.H. Smyth. Marked hyperinsulinemia after glucose, challenge in patients with diffuse idiopathic skeletal hyperostosis. *J Rheumatol 8*:965–968 (1981).
13. J. Dequeker, A. Burssens, and R. Bouillon. Dynamics of growth hormone secretion in patients with osteoporosis and in patients with osteoarthritis. *Hormone Res 16*:353–356 (1982).
14. P.D. Utsinger, D. Resnick, and R. Shapiro. Diffuse skeletal abnormalities in Forestier's disease. *Arch of Int Med 136*:763–768 (1976).
15. G.O. Littlejohn, A.C. Herrington, and H.A. Smithe. Studies into various growth factors in diffuse idiopathic skeletal hyperostosis (DISH) (Forestier's disease). Abstract Bulletin #987, 15th International Congress of Rheumatology, Paris 1981.
16. A. Vermeulen. Nyctohemeral growth hormone profiles in young and aged men: correlation with somatomedin-C levels. *J Clin Endocrinol Metab 64*:884–888 (1987).
17. D. Rudman, M.H. Kutner, C.M. Roger, et al. Impaired growth hormone secretion in the adult population: relation to age and adiposity. *J Clin Invest 67*:1361–1369 (1981).
18. D. Clemmons and J. Van Wyck. Factors controlling blood concentration of somatomedin. *J Clin Endocrinol Metab 13*:113–143 (1984).
19. R. Bouillon. Growth hormone and bone. *Horm Res 6*:49–55 (1991).
20. K. Hall, J. Brandt, G. Enberg, and L. Gryklund. Immunoreactive somatomedin A in human serum. *J Clin Endocrinol Metab 48*:271–278 (1979).

21. E. Corpas, S. Harman, and M. Blackman. Human growth hormone and human aging. *Endocrinol Rev 14*:20–39 (1993).
22. S. Boonen, E. Lesaffre, J. Dequeker, J. Aerssens, J. Nijs, W. Pelemans, and R. Bouillon. Relationship between baseline insulin-like growth factor-I (IGF-I) and femoral bone density in women aged over 70 years: Potential implications for the prevention of age-related bone loss. *JAGS 44*:1301–1306 (1996).
23. S. Boonen, S. Mohan, J. Dequeker, J. Aerssens, G. Verbeke, P. Broos, R. Bouillon, and D.J. Baylink. Down-regulation of the serum stimulatory components of the insulin-like growth factor (IGF) system (IGF-I, IGF-II, IGF binding protein (BP)-3 and IGFBP-5) in age-related (type II) femoral neck osteoporosis. *J Clin Endocrinol Metab* 1997, submitted.
24. R. Bluestone, E.G.L. Bywaters, M. Hartog, P.J.L. Holt, and S. Hyde. Acro-megalic arthropathy. *Ann Rheum Dis 30*:243–258 (1972).
25. G.O. Littlejohn, S. Hall, C.A. Brand, and A. Davidson. New bone formation in acromegaly: Pathogenetic implications for diffuse idiopathic skeletal hyperostosis. *Clin Exp Rheumatol 4*:99–104 (1986).
26. J.S.A.G. Schouten, F.A. Van den Ouweland, H.A. Valkenburg, and S.W. Lamberts. Insulin-like growth factor-1: A prognostic factor of knee osteoarthritis. *Br J Rheumatol 32*:274–280 (1993).
27. C.W. Denko, B. Boja, and R.X. Moskowitz. Growth promoting peptides in osteoarthritis: Insulin, insulin-like growth factor-1, growth hormone. *J Rheumatol 17*:1217–1221 (1990).
28. M.C. Hochberg, M. Lethbridge-Cejku, W.W. Scott, R. Reichle, C.C. Plato, and J.D. Tobin. Serum levels of insulin-like growth factor 1 in subjects with osteoarthritis of the knee. *Arthritis Rheum 37*:1177–1180 (1994).
29. T.E. McAlindon, D. Teale, and P.A. Dieppe. Insulin-like growth factor 1: Effect of age accounts for apparent correlation with sclerosis and osteophytosis in osteoarthritis of the knee (abstract). *Br J Rheumatol 31*:213 (1992).
30. J. Dequeker, J. Lenaerts, and R. Bouillon. Alteration growth hormone/IGF axis in osteoarthritis. *Clin Rheumatol 13*:163 (1994).
31. J. Dequeker, S. Mohan, R.D. Finkelman, J. Aerssens, and D.J. Baylink. Generalized osteoarthritis associated with increased insulin-like growth factor types I and II and transforming growth factor β in cortical bone from the iliac crest. *Arthritis Rheum 36*:1702–1708 (1993).
32. G. Raymaekers, J. Aerssens, R. Van den Eynde, J. Peeters, P. Geusens, P. Devos, and J. Dequeker. Alterations of the mineralization profile and osteocalcin concentrations in osteoarthritic cortical iliac crest bone. *Calcif Tissue Int 51*:269–275 (1992).
33. J. Aerssens, S. Boonen, G. Lowet, and J. Dequeker. Interspecies differences in bone composition, density, and quality: Potential implications for in vivo bone research. *Endocrinology* 1997, submitted.
34. W. Van den Berg. Chondrocyte-cytokine interactions in OA. Osteoarthritis and Cartilage 5 (Suppl. A-abstract 24), 1997, 31.
35. S. Doré, T. Abribat, N. Rousseau, P. Brazeau, G. Tardif, J.A. DiBattista, J.M. Cloutier, J.P. Pelletier, and J. Martel-Pelletier. Increased insulin-like growth factor 1

production by human osteoarthritic chondrocytes is not dependent on growth hormone action. *Arthritis Rheum 3*:413–419 (1995).

36. G. Tardif, P. Reboul, J.P. Pelletier, C. Geng, J.M. Cloutier, and J. Martel-Pelletier. Normal expression of type 1 insulin-like growth factor receptor by human osteoarthritic chondrocytes with increased expression and synthesis of insulin-like growth factor binding proteins. *Arthritis Rheum 39*:968–978 (1996).
37. F.P.J.G. Lafeber, H.L.A.M. Van Roy, P.M. Van der Kraan, W.B. Van den Berg, and J.W.J. Bijlsma. Transforming growth factor-β predominantly stimulates phenotypically changed chondrocytes in osteoarthritic human cartilage. *J Rheumatol 24*:536–542 (1997).
38. J. Middleton, N. Arnott, S. Walsh, and J. Bersford. Osteoblasts and osteoclasts in adult human osteophyte tissue express the mRNAs for insulin-like growth factors I and II and the type 1 IGF receptor. *Bone 16(3)*:287–293 (1995).
39. H.M. Van Beuningen, P.M. Van der Kraan, and W.B. Van den Berg. TGFβ1 stimulates articular chondrocyte proteoglycan synthesis and induces osteophyte formation in the murine knee. *Lab Invest 71*:279–90 (1994).
40. J. Dequeker, L. Mokassa, J. Aerssens, and S. Boonen. Bone density and local growth factors in generalized osteoarthritis. *Microscopy Res Tech 37*:358–371 (1997).
41. J. Dequeker, S. Boonen, J. Aerssens, R. Westhovens. Inverse relationship osteoarthritis–osteoporosis: What is the evidence? What are the consequences? *Br J Rheumatol 35*:813–820 (1996).
42. A. Boyde, S.A. Jones, J. Aerssens, J. Dequeker. Mineral density quantitation of the human cortical iliac crest by backscattered electron image analysis: Variations with age, sex and degree of osteoarthritis. *Bone 16(6)*:619–327 (1995).
43. X.G. Cheng, A. Boyde, S. Jones, J. Aerssens, and J. Dequeker. Osteoarthritis increases bone matrix mineralisation. A backscattered electron microscope (BSE) study. *Osteoarthritis and Cartilage 5 Suppl* (abstract #100), 1997, 50.
44. G. Gevers, J. Dequeker, M. Martens, and R. Van Audekercke. Biomechanical characteristics of iliac crest bone in elderly women, according to osteoarthritis gade at the hand joints. *J Rheumatol 16*:660–663 (1989).
45. E.L. Radin and I.L. Paul. Does cartilage compliance reduce skeletal impact loads? *Arthritis Rheum 13*:139–144 (1970).
46. E. Radin and R. Rose. Role of subchondral bone in the initiation and progression of cartilage damage. *Clin Orth Rel Res 213*:34–40 (1986).
47. M. Doherty, I. Watt, and P. Dieppe. Influence of primary generalized osteoarthritis on development of secondary osteoarthritis. *Lancet II*:8–11 (1983).

4
Crystal-Related Tissue Damage

GERALDINE M. MCCARTHY
Medical College of Wisconsin, Milwaukee, Wisconsin

Concurrence of calcium-containing crystals such as basic calcium phosphate (BCP) (hydroxyapatite, octacalcium phosphate, tricalcium phosphate) and calcium pyrophosphate dihydrate (CPPD) deposition and degenerative joint disease is well established. The basis of cartilage damage by crystals has been the subject of numerous investigations. Although ample data support their role in cartilage degeneration, controversies persist concerning the relationship between calcium-containing crystals and cartilage degeneration (1).

I. CLINICAL ASSOCIATIONS

A distinctive type of destructive arthropathy described by our group in 1981 [Milwaukee Shoulder Syndrome (MSS)] (2), by Neer et al. in 1983 (cuff tear arthropathy) (3), and by Dieppe et al. in 1984 apatite associated destructive arthritis is prototypic of other arthritides associated with calcium-containing crystal deposition (4). The gross anatomical features of MSS are often bilateral and include disappearance of the superior part of the fibrous rotator cuff and intra-articular portion of the tendon of the long head of biceps; glenohumeral degenerative changes with loss of articular cartilage, marginal osteophytes, and bony remodeling of both the humeral head and the glenoid fascia; upward subluxation of the humeral head with eburnation of the superior aspect as it forms a pseudoarthrosis with the coracoacromial vault and medial clavicle; and synovial hypertrophy with frequent formation of pedunculated loose bodies and separation of the acromion into two parts along the plane of the original epiphysis. Frequently, large, noninflammatory joint effusions are associated.

The etiologic role of BCP crystals in MSS was first observed in our laboratory. Synovial fluid studies of patients with MSS showed microaggregates of BCP crystals and particulate collagens with few leukocytes (5). Synovial biopsies from patients with MSS showed increased numbers of villi, focal synovial lining hyperplasia, and chondromatosis associated with intra- and extracellular BCP crystal deposits (6). It was therefore postulated that BCP crystals play an important pathogenic role in MSS since BCP crystals are identified from all affected joints.

Several other patterns of arthritis have been associated with BCP crystals including primary osteoarthritis, an erosive polyarthritis, and an acute inflammatory arthritis. Articular BCP crystal deposition also occurs as a consequence of several other conditions and may be termed secondary BCP arthropathies or periarthropathies. (Table 1) (7).

BCP crystals are common in osteoarthritic knee effusions, often associated with synovial proliferation and severe degenerative arthritis. Several studies have suggested that the incidence of BCP crystals in synovial fluid from patients with knee osteoarthritis (OA) is between 30% and 60% (8,9). Indeed, it has been suggested that many osteoarthritis joint fluids contain CPPD or BCP crystals that are too small or too few in number to be identified by conventional techniques (10). The presence of BCP crystals correlates strongly with radiographic evi-

TABLE 1 Basic Calcium Crystal-Associated Joint Disease

Calcific periarthritis
Unifocal
Multifocal
Familial
Calcific tendonitis and bursitis
Intra-articular BCP arthropathies
Acute (gout-like) attacks
Milwaukee shoulder/knee syndrome
(Idiopathic destructive arthritis; cuff tear arthropathy)
Erosive polyarticular disease
Mixed crystal deposition disease (BCP and CPPD)
Secondary BCP crystal arthropathies/periarthropathies
Chronic renal failure
Calcinosis
Sequal to neurological injury
Following local corticosteroid injection
Miscellaneous
Tumoral calcinosis
Hyperphosphatemic
Nonhyperphosphatemic

dence of cartilaginous degeneration (11) and is associated with larger joint effusions when compared with joint fluid from OA knees without crystals (12).

A polyarticular erosive form of arthritis associated with BCP crystals has also been described. Pain and swelling were most prominent in the wrists, metacarpophalangeal joints, and proximal interphalangeal joints. Massive articular calcification was observed radiographically and joint damage was progressive (13). Periarticular BCP arthropathies include calcific periarthritis, tendonitis, and bursitis (7). For the most part, these appear to be related to isolated local dystrophic calcifications, the etiology of which remains obscure, and, in general, these calcifications appear to be asymptomatic. In some individuals, however, dramatic inflammatory episodes may occur with severe pain, swelling, and erythema resembling gout.

CPPD crystal deposition has been associated with the acute inflammatory arthritis of pseudogout. It is also associated with chronic pyrophosphate arthropathy, which is clinically distinguished from primary OA by its pattern of affected joints, greater severity, and prominent inflammatory component (Figure 1).

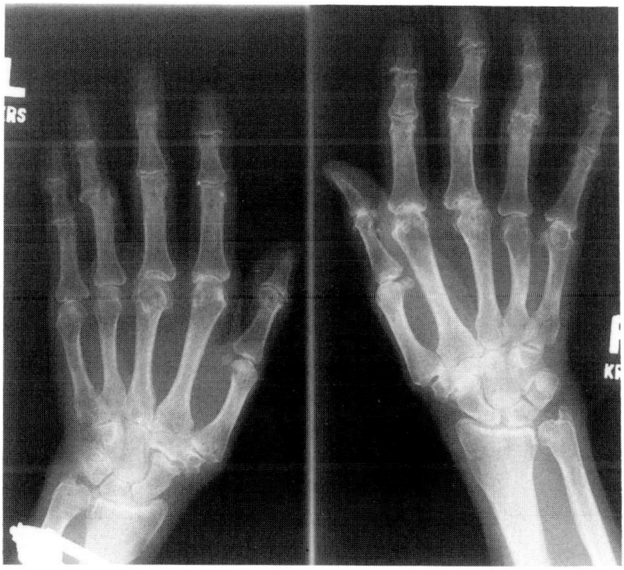

FIGURE 1 Radiographs of both hands of a patient with osteoarthritis complicated by CPPD deposition disease. Erosions are noted, especially at the 4th proximal interphalangeal and 3rd metacarpophalangeal joints bilaterally, associated with widespread subchondral cysts. Cystic degeneration is also noted in the wrists. Hook-like osteophytes are seen arising from the radial aspect of some metacarpal heads, in particular the right 5th metacarpal.

Inflammatory features may be sufficiently severe to cause confusion with rheumatoid disease (14). A study of factors affecting radiographic progression of knee osteoarthritis showed that CPPD crystal deposition predicted poor clinical and radiographic outcome (15).

BCP crystals are frequently observed together with CPPD and under these circumstances have been referred to as mixed crystal deposition disease. In pathological joint effusions, the mixture is as common as the presence of either crystal alone (16).

II. CALCIUM-CONTAINING CRYSTAL LOCATION AND IDENTIFICATION

Basic calcium phosphate crystals consist of partially carbonate substituted hydroxyapatite, octacalcium phosphate, and, rarely, tricalcium phosphate (17). Pathological calcifications in a wide variety of human tissues are composed of BCP crystals. They have long been known to deposit in periarticular locations in conditions such as calcific periarthritis and tendonitis. More recently, BCP crystals have also been found in intra-articular locations including synovial fluid, synovium, and hyaline cartilage (18). They are ultramicroscopic in size and therefore can be seen as individual particles only by transmission electron microscopy (TEM). These crystals have a remarkable tendency to clump as spheroidal microaggregates, which vary from about 1 to 50 μm in diameter. These clumps may be seen by light microscopy or by scanning electron microscope (SEM), where they look like snowballs. They are invariably associated with particulate collagens in synovial fluid (19).

Deposition of BCP cuboid crystals, identified as magnesium whitlockite, has been reported in OA and elderly normal femoral head articular cartilage and also in normal femoral head articular cartilage from a range of joint sites across a broad patient age spectrum (20). An active role of these crystals in the propagation of cartilage degeneration has been suggested but remains to be confirmed (21).

Calcium pyrophosphate dihydrate ($Ca_2P_2O_7 \cdot 2H_2O$) crystals are relatively specific for articular tissue although periarticular deposits of CPPD have been reported in tendons, dura mater, ligamenta flava and the olecranon bursa, as well as in isolated tophi (14).

BCP crystals obtained from joint fluid have been carefully identified by SEM and TEM, X-ray energy dispersive analysis, direct chemical analysis for calcium and phosphate, X-ray diffraction by the powder method, and Fourier transform infrared spectroscopy (19). Alizarin red S staining of synovial fluid pellets has been suggested as a screening technique for BCP crystals (22). This method is sensitive to 0.005 μg of hydroxyapatite (HA) standard per milliliter, but it is not specific for calcium phosphates and may provide many false positive results. A semiquantitative technique using the binding of (^{14}C) ethane-1-hydroxyl-1, 1-diphosphonate (EHDP) to BCP crystals has proved useful as a screening test and is sensitive to about 2 μg of HA standard (23). Diphosphonates are analogs of inorganic pyrophosphate (PP_i) that adsorb to the surface of calcium phosphate crystals but not to MSU, CPPD, cartilage fragments, particulate collagens, or to any other known particulate in joint fluid. Such adsorption is not inhibited to any significant extent by PP_i at the levels found in synovial fluid. Synovial fluid pellets that bound EHDP were examined routinely by SEM. Microspheroidal aggregates approximately 1 to 19 μm in diameter were generally found and were further characterized by X-ray energy dispersive analysis. The molar calcium/phosphorus was virtually identical to that of an HA standard (5).

Using TEM, magnesium whitlockite crystals have been frequently observed scattered among intramatrical lipidic debris, particularly pericellularly, in areas of cell necrosis and among close-packed tangential fibers between the articular surface and initial superficial zone chondrocytes of articular cartilage (21).

CPPD crystals can be identified by polarized light microscopy when they appear as anisotropic (nonrefractile) or positively birefringent rhomboidal crystals. Most patients whose joint fluid contains CPPD crystals will have radiographic evidence of calcified fibrocartilage and/or of hyaline articular cartilage, although some will appear radiographically normal (14).

III. CURRENT CONCEPTS OF THE PATHOPHYSIOLOGY OF CALCIUM-CONTAINING CRYSTAL DEPOSITION DISEASES

Concurrence of articular calcium-containing crystal deposition and degenerative joint disease is well established and ample data support their role in cartilage degeneration. Clinically, the joint degeneration of calcium-containing crystal deposition differs from the joint degeneration of primary OA (14). If crystals were simply an epiphenomenon of cartilage degeneration, we would expect to see CPPD or BCP crystals in the joints most commonly affected by primary OA. Instead, crystal deposition disease frequently involves shoulders, wrists, and elbows, sites rarely affected by primary OA. Not only is the distribution of joint involvement distinct, but the severity of joint degeneration is magnified in the presence of calcium-containing crystals. Some investigators speculate that articular crystals cause cartilage degeneration directly, whereas others hypothesize that clinically undetectable cartilage metabolic or structural aberrations are primary and these aberrations cause defects in matrix or chondrocyte metabolism that favor both crystal formation and degeneration. Thus, degeneration and crystal formation would be viewed as parallel events of common derivation (24). An intermediate view is that a primary metabolic abnormality leads to degeneration but that secondary crystal deposits accelerate deterioration—the "amplification loop" hypothesis (25).

The basis of cartilage damage by calcium-containing crystals remains somewhat speculative. Theoretically, crystals in cartilage may directly injure chondrocytes. However, in pathological specimens crystals are rarely seen in immediate contact with chondrocytes and even less frequently found engulfed by chondrocytes (26). It is more likely that cartilage damage results when synovial lining cells ingest crystals and then release matrix-degrading enzymes or secrete cytokines that stimulate chondrocytes to release matrix-degrading enzymes. This concept is further supported by data from a study of the role of CPPD crystal-induced synovitis in the development of accelerated OA in CPPD deposition disease (27). A lapine model of OA, induced by partial lateral meniscectomy and section of the fibular collateral and sesamoid ligaments, was used in the study. In meniscectomized right knees, following repeated (weekly) injections of CPPD crystals (either 1 or 10 mg), there was more severe OA at 8 weeks compared with noninjected contralateral meniscectomized left knees. The intensity of associated synovial inflammation correlated with intra-articular CPPD administration and dosage. Although the doses administered were considerably higher than concentrations found in vivo, the data support a worsening effect of chronic CPPD crystal-induced synovitis on experimental OA and suggest a role for CPPD crystal-induced inflammation in the progression of OA lesions in clinical CPPD crystal deposition disease.

IV. IN VITRO STUDIES

Potential mechanisms by which calcium-containing crystals may promote articular damage have been studied in our laboratories and will be presented below. These include their mitogenic properties and their ability to induce metalloproteases and to stimulate prostaglandin synthesis.

A. Mitogenic Effect of BCP Crystals

Synovial lining proliferation of varying degrees is common in crystal-associated arthritis and the crystals themselves are at least partly responsible for proliferation (6). Increased cell numbers in the synovial lining enhance the capacity for secretion of cytokines, which may promote chondrolysis and cause secretion of proteolytic enzymes.

BCP crystals in concentrations found in pathologic human joint fluids stimulated mitogenesis in quiescent cultured human skin fibroblasts, canine synovial fibroblasts, and mouse 3T3 cells in a concentration-dependent manner (28,29). Growth stimulation also occurred with CPPD, calcium urate, calcium sulfate, calcium carbonate, and calcium diphosphonate crystals (28,30). Both onset and peak (^{3}H)-thymidine incorporation induced by these crystals was delayed 2–3 hours compared to cells stimulated with serum. This lag time may in part represent time required for phagocytosis and intracellular dissolution of crystals. Addition of control particles of similar size such as diamond dust or latex beads did not stimulate mitogenesis. Monosodium urate monohydrate (MSU) crystals were weakly mitogenic and much less so than calcium urate, suggesting that the calcium content of crystals is important for mitogenesis. Synthetic BCP was as mitogenic as BCP obtained from a patient with calcinosis, indicating that the crystal and not a contaminant was responsible (28). The mitogenic effect of the calcium-containing crystals was not the result of increased ambient medium calcium concentration from crystal dissolution, since conditioned medium from cells that had been exposed to and dissolved BCP crystals did not stimulate (^{3}H)-thymidine incorporation by fibroblasts (30).

The mechanism of BCP crystal-induced mitogenesis has been explored. First, it was hypothesized that the abnormal proliferation of synovial cells may be at least in part due to endocytosis and intracellular dissolution of crystals producing an increased cytoplasmic calcium concentration that activates a calcium-dependent pathway leading to mitogenesis. This concept was supported by the following evidence. Direct cell-crystal contact is required for crystal-induced mitogenesis since cultures exposed to crystals were growth-stimulated, but in cultures inverted to prevent cell-crystal contact, no growth stimulation occured (31). To study the requirement for crystal phagocytosis following cell-crystal interaction, cells were exposed to ^{45}Ca-labeled BCP and (^{3}H)-thymidine. Cells containing ^{45}Ca-labeled BCP were separated by gradient centrifugation and found to have incorporated significantly more (^{3}H)-thymidine than those without BCP [32]. In cultured macrophages, inhibition of crystal endocytosis with cytochalasin B inhibited crystal dissolution, further supporting the requirement of phagocytosis (33). Calcium-containing crystals are acid soluble. Following phagocytosis, intracellular crystal dissolution likely occurs in the acid medium of the phagolysosomes. Chloroquine, ammonium chloride, and bafilomycin A_1, all lysosomotrophic agents that raise lysosomal pH, significantly inhibit intracellular crystal dissolution and (^{3}H)-thymidine uptake in a dose-dependent manner in fibroblasts exposed to BCP crystals (34). Current evidence suggests, therefore, that phagocytosis followed by intracellular crystal dissolution is necessary for BCP crystal-induced mitogenesis.

Second, it was noted that BCP crystals also stimulate mitogenesis by a process similar to platelet-derived growth factor (PDGF). PDGF is a peptide growth factor that renders quiescent fibroblasts and many other anchorage-dependent cell lines "competent" to respond to "progression" growth factors such as insulin-like growth factor-1 (IGF-1), which are required for progression through the cell cycle. BCP crystals could substitute for PDGF as a competence growth factor and, like PDGF, act synergistically with IGF-1 or plasma. Furthermore, blocking antibodies against IGF-1 diminished the mitogenic response of 3T3 cells to BCP (35). Some differences have been observed between the biochemical and cellular mechanisms of action of PDGF and BCP crystals. Mitchell et al. (36) demonstrated that BCP crystal induced mitogenesis in Balb/c-3T3 fibroblasts involves a rapid membrane-associated event which requires the presence of the serine/threonine protein kinase C (PKC), one of the major mediators of signals generated upon external stimulation of cells by hormones, neurotransmitters and growth factors. Downregulation of PKC activity in Balb/c-3T3 cells inhibited BCP crystal-mediated induction of the proto-oncogenes c-*fos* and c-*myc* but had no effect on that stimulated by PDGF (36).

It was therefore recognized that the increased intracellular calcium concentration that occurs as phagocytosed crystals dissolve is only one signal for mitogenesis. When growth factors such as PDGF bind to their membrane receptors, phospholipase C (a phosphodiesterase) is stimulated to hydrolyze phosphatidylinositol 4,5-bisphosphate (PIP_2) to the intracellular messengers, inosital triphosphate (IP_3), and diacylglycerol (DAG) (37). IP_3 releases calcium from the endoplasmic reticulum, modulating the activities of calcium-dependent and calcium/calmodulin-dependent enzymes such as protein kinases and proteases (38).

DAG, the other hydrolysis product of PIP_2, is a potent activator of PKC (39). Rothenberg and Cheung reported elevated phospholipase C degradation of inosital phospholipid in rabbit synovial cells in response to BCP crystal stimulation (40). BCP crystals significantly increased inosital-1-phosphate in (^{3}H)-inosital-labeled cells within 1 minute, and levels were maximum at 1 hour. Increased amounts of inositol mono-, bis-, and trisphosphates were all measured after crystal ingestion supporting the concept that BCP crystals enhance phospholipase C activity in synovial fibroblasts.

Since BCP crystals increased phospholipase C activity, resultant increased DAG accumulation and finally increased PKC activity was expected. Accordingly, the role of PKC in BCP-induced mitogenesis was examined. The effects of BCP crystals and PDGF on DNA synthesis were compared in Balb/c-3T3 fibroblasts. In some cultures, PKC was depleted by incubation of the cells with a high concentration of tumor-promoting phorbol diester (TPA), an analog of DAG. Chronic TPA stimulation down-regulates PKC, in contrast to acute treatment which activates PKC. Stimulation of DNA synthesis by BCP was inhibited after downregulation of PKC, implying an important role for PKC in BCP-induced mitogenesis. As noted above, no effect on PDGF-stimulated DNA synthesis was observed under the same conditions (36).

A class of genes known as proto-oncogenes play an important role in controlling cell proliferation. *Fos* and *myc* proteins, both products of the proto-oncogenes c-*fos* and c-*myc*, are localized to the cell nucleus and bind to specific DNA sequences (41,42). Stimulation of 3T3 fibroblasts with either BCP crystals or PDGF results in the expression of c-*fos* within minutes, reaching maximal expression approximately 30 minutes after stimulation. Induction of c-*myc* transcription by BCP or PDGF occurs within 1 hour and is maximal at about 3 hours after stimulation. Such stimulated cells maintain elevated transcription of c-*myc* for at least 5 hours [43]. The expression of c-*fos* and c-*myc* is increased in response to BCP crystal stimulation in a manner similar to the increase produced by PDGF. However, in PKC downregulated cells, both TPA and BCP crystal stimulation of c-*fos* and c-*myc* are markedly inhibited, whereas in contrast, the induction of these transcripts by PDGF is unaffected.

Members of the mitogen activated protein kinases (MAPK) family are key regulators of a variety of intracellular signal transduction cascades. One subclass of this family, the p42/p44 MAPKs, is believed to regulate cell proliferation by a mechanism that includes the activation of proto-oncogenes c-*fos* and c-*jun*. BCP and CPPD crystals both activate a protein kinase signal transduction pathway involving p42 and p44 MAPKs, suggesting that this pathway may contribute to calcium-containing crystal-induced mitogenesis (44).

Finally, the transcription factor nuclear factor κB (NF-κB) appears to contribute to BCP crystal-induced mitogenesis. NF-κB, first described as a regulator of the immunoglobulin kappa (Igκ) light-chain gene, is an inducible transcription factor critical to many signal transduction pathways because it regulates the expression of a wide variety of important genes. Induction of NF-κB ordinarily involves release from cytoplasmic inhibitory proteins, collectively referred to as IκB. NF-κB induction is followed by translocation of the active transcription factor complex into the nucleus. One mechanism of NF-κB induction involves the modification of IκB by direct PKC-catalyzed phosphorylation which causes it to lose its NF-κB inhibitory activity. Since BCP crystals activate PKC, concurrent induction of NF-κB is expected. BCP crystals induce NF-κB in Balb-c/3T3 fibroblasts and human foreskin fibroblasts (HFF). When HFF were treated with BCP crystals in the presence of the PKC inhibitor staurosporine, the induction of NF-κB was inhibited in a concentration-dependent fashion (45).

The mechanism of BCP crystal-induced mitogenesis in fibroblasts has therefore been shown to involve at least two distinct, but necessary, processes. The first is a fast, membrane-associated event resulting in PKC and MAPK activation, NF-κB induction, and proto-oncogene induction. The second event is a slower intracellular dissolution of the crystals that raises intracellular calcium

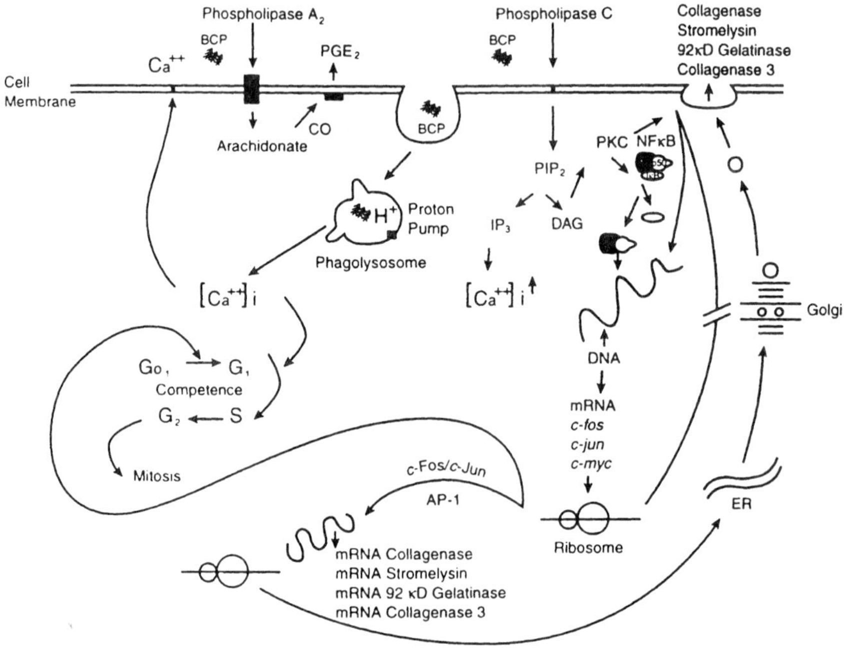

FIGURE 2 Some biological effects of calcium-containing crystals. BCP = basic calcium phosphate; CO = cyclo-oxygenase; ER = endoplasmic reticulum; PKC = protein kinase C; DAG = diacylglycerol; PIP_2 = phosphatidylinositol 4,5-bisphosphate; IP_3 = inositol 1,4,5-triphosphate; NF-κB = nuclear factor κB.

leading to the activation of a number of calcium-dependent processes stimulating mitogenesis. Figure 2 depicts our current concept of the biologic effects of calcium-containing crystals.

B. Matrix Metalloprotease Induction by BCP Crystals

Potential mediators of tissue damage from calcium-containing crystals are the matrix metalloproteases (MMP) collagenase-1 (MMP -1), stromelysin (transin, MMP 3), 92 kD gelatinase (gelatinase B/MMP 9) and collagenase-3 (MMP 13). The MMP family share a number of chief characteristics. The enzymes cleave one or more components of the extracellular matrix. Activity is inhibited by tissue inhibitor of metalloproteinases (TIMP). The proteinases are secreted in zymogen form, which can be activated by proteinases or by organomercurials. The catalytic mechanism depends on zinc at the active site. The cDNA sequences of the MMP family all show homology to that of collagenase (46).

Collagenase is a critical regulator of extracellular matrix remodeling because of its unique ability to degrade the native collagen fibril (46). Stromelysin degrades type 4 collagen and many other components of extracellular matrix including proteoglycan and laminin (47). 92 kD gelatinase accelerates the breakdown of matrix components such as gelatin, collagens type IV, V, and XI, and elastin [48]. Collagenase-3 is expressed in human osteoarthritic cartilage and degrades type II collagen more efficiently than collagenase-1 (49).

The massive lysis of intra-articular collagenous structures that typifies MSS strongly suggests collagen matrix-degrading metalloprotease activity. Collagenase and neutral protease activity was demonstrated in the synovial fluid from the shoulder joints of some, but not all, patients with MSS [5]. The neutral protease activity was likely due to stromelysin, but the presence of gelatinase was not evaluated. Similarly, Lohmander et al. (50) measured concentrations of stromelysin and collagenase-1 in a variety of joint disorders including OA and calcium pyrophosphate arthropathy. ELISAs were performed using monoclonal and polyclonal antibodies. Both proteins were detected in disease groups 15–45 times that of the control groups. The highest concentrations of both enzymes were found in pyrophosphate arthropathy (50).

Due to the association between synovial fluid BCP crystals and joint destruction, a hypothesis was formulated in which BCP crystals and possibly particulate collagens are endocytosed by synovial-lining cells. These cells are then stimulated to proliferate and secrete proteases. This hypothesis was tested in vitro by adding natural or synthetic BCP, CPPD, and other crystals to cultured human or canine synovium cells. Neutral protease and collagenase activity was augmented in a dose-related fashion approximately 5 to 8 times over control cultures incubated without crystals (51).

We recently expanded studies of metalloprotease induction and secretion using HFF proliferating in response to BCP crystals. We demonstrated the coordinate induction of collagenase-1, stromelysin, and 92 kD gelatinase messenger RNA (mRNA) accumulation in BCP crystal-stimulated cultures. This was followed by secretion of collagenase-1, stromelysin, and 92 kD gelatinase protein into conditioned media, identified by Western blot using specific antibodies. Activity of each enzyme was also confirmed (52,53). BCP crystals also caused collagenase-1 and collagenase-3 mRNA accumulation in adult porcine articular chondrocytes (54,55). This was followed by secretion of collagenase-1 (G.M. McCarthy, unpublished observation) and collagenase-3 protein into conditioned media.

It has been shown that the collagenase promoter contains a *cis* element, termed the 12-0-tetradecanoylphorbol 13-acetate (TPA) response element (TRE), which is involved in increased transcription in response to tumor necrosis factor alpha (TNFα) (56) and phorbol esters (57). Increased transcription modulated through the TRE depends on the transcription factor, activator protein-1 (AP-1), a heterodimer composed of the protein products of c-*fos* and c-*jun*, both primary response genes, which interact to stimulate transcription of AP-1 responsive genes (57). Synthesis of *fos* is essential for phorbol (TPA) induction of collagenase and also for the cells' response to interleukin-1 (IL-1), TNFα, and serum factors (46). Thus, inhibitors of protein synthesis such as cycloheximide would be expected to interfere with this mechanism of transcriptional activation. Cycloheximide blocks the response to IL-1β and TNFα which suggests that the response is dependent on the synthesis of *fos* and *jun*. Both c-*fos* and c-*jun* messenger RNA levels are increased by TNFα (56). Similarly, cycloheximide blocks BCP crystal induction of collagenase-1, stromelysin, and 92-kD gelatinase mRNA in human fibroblasts and also collagenase-3 mRNA in adult porcine articular chondrocytes (52,53,55). Since BCP crystals induce c-*fos* and c-*jun*, it is likely that the synthesis of a transcription factor containing *fos* and *jun* is also important in BCP crystal induction of metalloproteases (58).

The clinical features of calcium-containing crystal deposition disease suggest a prominent contribution of matrix metalloproteases. Current data suggests direct stimulation of MMP production by fibroblasts and chondrocytes upon contact with calcium-containing crystals.

C. Stimulation of Prostaglandin Synthesis

In addition to growth stimulation and enzyme production, calcium-containing crystals caused the release of prostaglandins from cultured mammalian cells, especially PGE_2 (51,59,60). All PGE_2 release occurred in the first hours after cells were exposed to crystals. Rothenberg (61) confirmed and extended this work. He demonstrated that phosphatidyl choline and phosphatidyl ethanolamine are the major sources of arachidonic acid for PGE_2 synthesis, confirming that the phospholipase A_2/cyclooxygenase pathway is the predominant route for PGE_2 production. BCP crystals appeared to stimulate synthesis of both phospholipase A_2 and cyclooxygenase (61).

Although PGE compounds are local mediators of inflammation, evidence from both in vitro and in vivo experiments indicates that they can suppress diverse effecter systems of inflammation. Both PGE_1 and PGE_2 also increase concentrations of cyclic AMP in human synovial cells in culture and suppress synovial cell proliferation (62,63). Since radioimmunoassays do not usually distinguish between PGE_1 and PGE_2 (64), PGE_1 may also have been released in response to BCP crystals. Whether the augmented PGE production induced by these crystals significantly downregulates their other biologic effects is an important question and may be one mechanism accounting for the clinical observation of accelerated articular damage in the presence of the cyclooxygenase inhibitor indomethacin (65).

We studied the effects of PGE_2, PGE_1, and its analog, the drug misoprostol, on the mitogenic response of human fibroblasts to BCP crystals. All three agents inhibited the mitogenic response to BCP crystals in a concentration-dependent manner. PGE_1 and misoprostol were more potent. PGE_1 and misoprostol, but not PGE_2, inhibited collagenase mRNA accumulation in response to BCP crystals (66,67).

Various classes of PG increase intracellular cAMP levels and increased cAMP levels inhibit mitogenesis in certain cell types. We explored the mechanism of inhibition of BCP crystal-mediated cell activation by PGE. We showed that PGE_1 is a more potent inducer of intracellular cAMP than PGE_2, and that PGE_1 inhibits BCP crystal-induced mitogenesis and MMP production through the cyclic AMP signal transduction pathway (67). It is possible that the augmented PGE production induced by BCP crystals downregulates their other biological effects (mitogenesis and MMP production) by a feedback mechanism.

V. CALCIUM-CONTAINING CRYSTAL-INDUCED INFLAMMATION

The chronic destructive arthropathies associated with CPPD or BCP crystals are probably much more important medically than are the dramatic acute inflammatory syndromes associated with neutrophilic phagocytosis (7,14). First, they are more common. Second, chronic joint destruction is irreversible whereas acute inflammatory events can be readily treated. Furthermore, repeated isolated inflammatory events over long periods of time are usually required before permanant joint damage ensues. The presence of calcium-containing crystals in osteoarthritic synovial fluids (SF) is common; however, associated episodes of acute inflammation with leukocytosis appear relatively uncommon clinically in OA and MMS. The phlogistic potential of crystals may be somewhat modified by intrasynovial inhibitory factors. Terkeltaub et al. have demonstrated the ability of serum and plasma to markedly suppress neutrophil responsiveness to BCP crystals (68). Factors causing such inhibition appeared to be crystal-bound proteins. Of the crystal-bound plasma proteins studied, α_2-HS glycoprotein (AHSG) appeared to be the most potent and specific inhibitor of neutrophil responsiveness to BCP crystals. AHSG is a liver-derived serum protein known to be greatly concentrated relative to other serum proteins in bone and mineralizing tissues (69). AHSG was present in noninflammatory synovial fluids and could be detected on native synovial fluid BCP crystals (68). The authors concluded that AHSG could modulate the inflammatory potential of BCP crystals in vivo. When the inflammatory potential of BCP crystals was evaluated using the rat air pouch model, variations in fluid volumes and white cell counts occurred according to specific surface area of the various crystal types tested and their calcium:phosphorus ratios (70). The authors postulate that BCP heterogeneity may be one explanation for their variable tolerance in human joints.

VI. ROLE OF CYTOKINES

Recently, there has been progress in understanding the mechanism of cartilage breakdown in osteoarthritis (71). The initial cleavage of cartilage matrix molecules is extracellular and is mediated primarily by proteases (46). The major proteases involved appear to be collagenase and stromelysin. Chondrocytes are capable of exhaustive degradation of their extracellular matrix (72). Interleukin-1, produced by synovial cells, polymorphonuclear leukocytes, and chondrocytes, has been suggested as the most potent stimulator of cartilage degradation (72). IL-1 stimulates increases in protease transcription, synthesis, and secretion by chondrocytes and synoviocytes while inhibiting matrix synthesis (71). Although it is possible that matrix degradation in calcium-containing crystal arthropathies is cytokine mediated, neither BCP nor CPPD crystals induced IL-1 production in vitro, unlike monosodium urate crystals (73). Current data strongly supports direct stimulation of MMP production by fibroblasts and chondrocytes upon contact with calcium-containing crystals.

VII. IMPLICATIONS FOR TREATMENT

There are no available drugs to inhibit deposition or effect reabsorption of the crystals (66). This contrasts with gout, where accumulation of urate crystals can be eliminated with hypouricemic therapy (74). Recently phosphocitrate, a potent inhibitor of hydroxyapatite crystal formation and a relatively nontoxic compound, was shown to inhibit the mitogenic effect of BCP crystals in a concentration-dependent manner. This inhibition appeared to be specific since the same concentrations of phosphocitrate had no impact on basal, PDGF-induced, or serum-induced (^{3}H)-thymidine incorporation (75). Phosphocitrate also blocked BCP crystal-induced proto-oncogene and collagenase transcription (58). Its mechanism of action is currently being explored, and recently it was shown to inhibit calcium-containing crystal induction of MAPK. This compound may ultimately prove useful in protecting articular tissues from the harmful biologic effects of calcium-containing crystals such as CPPD or BCP (44).

Others have shown that PGE_1 can have anti-inflammatory and tissue protective action (64). Misoprostol, a PGE_1 analog, is already approved for use in humans to prevent gastrointestinal damage induced by nonsteroidal inflammatory drugs (76). We have demonstrated the ability of these E-series prostaglandins to interfere with the biological effects of BCP crystals (66,67). These characteristics may also be of future therapeutic import.

Calcium-containing crystal deposition diseases and their role in cartilage damage remain poorly understood. Their importance in terms of morbidity will likely amplify as the aged population increases. Further studies of the mechanisms important for crystal deposition and for their biological effects are essential to rational prevention or reversal of the consequences of calcium-containing crystal deposition.

REFERENCES

1. H.R. Schumacher. Synovial inflammation, crystals, and osteoarthritis. *J Rheumatol (suppl 43) 22*:101–103 (1995).
2. D.J. McCarty, P.B. Halverson, G.F. Carrera, B.J. Brewer, and F.K. Kozin. Milwaukee shoulder: Association of microspheroids containing hydroxyapatite crystals, active collagenase, and neutral protease with rotator cuff defects, i: Clinical aspects, *Arthritis Rheum 24*:464–473 (1981).
3. C.S. Neer, E.V. Craig, and H. Fakuda. Cuff-tear arthropathy. *J Bone Joint Surg 65A*:1232–1244 (1983).
4. P.A. Dieppe, M. Doherty, D.G. Macfarlane, C.W. Hutton, J.W. Bradfield, and I. Watt. Apatite associated destructive arthritis. *Br J Rheumatol 23*:84–91 (1984).
5. P.B. Halverson, H.S. Cheung, D.J. McCarty, J. Garancis, and N. Mandel. Milwaukee Shoulder-association of microspheroids containing hydroxyapatite crystals, active collagenase, and neutral protease with rotator cuff defects. ii: Synovial fluid studies. *Arthritis Rheum 24*:474–483 (1981).
6. J.C. Garancis, H.S. Cheung, P.B. Halverson, and D.J. McCarty. Milwaukee shoulder: Association of microspheroids containing hydroxyapatite crystals, active collagenase and neutral protease with rotator cuff defects.iii. Morphologic and biochemical studies of an excised synovium showing chondromatosis. *Arthritis Rheum 24*:484–491 (1981).
7. P.B. Halverson and D.J. McCarty. Basic calcium phosphate (apatite, octacalcium phosphate, tricalcium phosphate) crystal deposition diseases; calcinosis. In: *Arthritis and allied conditions: A textbook of rheumatology*. (W. J. Koopman, Ed.), Williams and Wilkins, Baltimore, MD, 1997, p. 2127–2146.
8. P.A. Gibilisco, H.R. Schumacher, J.L. Hollander, and K.A. Soper. Synovial fluid crystals in osteoarthritis. *Arthritis Rheum 28*:511–515 (1985).
9. P.A. Dieppe, P.R. Crocker, C.F. Corke, D.V. Doyle, and D.A. Willoughby. Synovial fluid crystals. *Q J Med 192*:533–553 (1979).
10. A. Swan, B. Chapman, P. Heap, H. Seward, and P. Dieppe. Submicroscopic crystals in osteoarthritic synovial fluids. *Ann Rheum Dis 53*:467–470 (1994).
11. P.B. Halverson and D.J. McCarthy. Patterns of radiographic abnormalities associated with basic calcium phosphate and calcium pyrophosphate crystal deposition in the knee. *Ann Rheum Dis 45*:603–605 (1986).
12. G.J. Carroll, R.A. Stuart, J.A. Armstrong, P.D. Breidahl, and B.A. Laing. Hydroxyapatite crystals are a frequent finding in osteoarthritic synovial fluid, but are not related to increased concentrations of keratan sulfate or interleukin 1β. *J Rheumatol 18*:861–866 (1991).
13. H.R. Schumacher, J.L. Miller, C. Ludivico, and R.A. Jessar. Erosive arthritis associated with apatite crystal deposition. *Arthritis Rheum 24*:31–37 (1981).

14. L. Ryan and D. McCarty. Calcium pyrophosphate crystal deposition disease, pseudogout and articular chondrocalcinosis. In: *Arthritis and Allied Conditions*. (W. Koopman, Ed.), Williams and Wilkins, Baltimore, MD, 1997, p. 2103–2125.
15. J. Ledingham, M. Regan, A. Jones, and M. Doherty. Factors affecting radiographic progression of knee osteoarthritis. *Ann Rheum Dis 54*:53–58 (1995).
16. P. Dieppe, D. Doyle, E. Huskisson, D. Willoughby, and P. Crocker. Mixed crystal deposition and osteoarthritis. *Br Med J 1*:150 (1978).
17. D.J. McCarty, J.R. Lehr, and P.B. Halverson. Crystal populations in human synovial fluid. Identification of apatite, octacalcium phosphate and tricalcium phosphate. *Arthritis Rheum 26*:247–251 (1983).
18. P. Halverson and D. McCarty. Clinical aspects of basic calcium phosphate crystal deposition. *Rheum Dis North Am 14*:427–439 (1988).
19. D. McCarty. Crystal identification in human synovial fluids. *Rheum Dis Clin North Am 14*:253–267 (1988).
20. C.A. Scotchford and S.Y. Ali. Magnesium whitlockite deposition in articular cartilage: a study of 80 specimens from 70 patients. *Ann Rheum Dis 54*:339–344 (1995).
21. C. Scotchford and S. Ali. Association of magnesium whitlockite crystals with lipid components of the extracellular matrix in human articular cartilage. *Osteoarthritis Cart 5*:107–119 (1997).
22. H. Paul, A.J. Reginato, and H.R. Schumacher. Alizarin red S staining as a screening test to detect calcium compounds in synovial fluid. *Arthritis Rheum 26*:191–200 (1983).
23. P. Halverson and D.J. McCarty. Identification of hydroxyapatite crystals in synovial fluid. *Arthritis Rheum 22*:389–395 (1979).
24. A. Bjelle. Familial pyrophosphate arthropathy occurrence and crystal identification. *Scand J Rheumatol 24*:464–473 (1981).
25. M. Doherty, I. Watt, and P. Dieppe. Localized chondrocalcinosis in postmenisectomy knees. *Lancet 1*:1207–1210 (1982).
26. H. Schumacher. Pathology of crystal deposition diseases. *Rheum Dis Clin North Am 14*:269–288 (1988).
27. A.G. Fam, I. Morava-Protzner, C. Purcell, B.D. Young, P.S. Bunting, and A.J. Lewis. Acceleration of experimental lapine osteoarthritis by calcium pyrophosphate microcrystalline synovitis. *Arthritis Rheum 38*:201–210 (1995).
28. H.S. Cheung, M.T. Story, and D.J. McCarty. Mitogenic effects of hydroxyapatite and calcium pyrophosphate dihydrate crystals on cultured mammalian cells. *Arthritis Rheum 27*:668–674 (1984).
29. D. Barnes and S. Colowick. Stimulation of sugar uptake and thymidine incorporation in mouse 3T3 cells by calcium phosphate and other extracellular particles. *Proc Natl Acad Sci USA 74*:5593–5597 (1977).
30. H.S. Cheung and D.J. McCarty. Mitogenesis induced by calcium-containing crystals: role of intracellular dissolution. *Exp Cell Res 157*:63–70 (1985).
31. D. Bowen-Pope, and H. Rubin. Growth stimulatory precipitate of Ca^{++} and pyrophosphate. *J Cell Physiol 117*:51–61 (1983).
32. A. Borkowf, H.S. Cheung, and D.J. McCarty. Endocytosis is required for the mitogenic effect of basic calcium phosphate crystals. *Calcif Tiss Int 40*:173–176 (1987).

33. J. Owens, H. Cheung, and D. McCarty. Endocytosis precedes dissolution of basic calcium phosphate crystals by murine macrophages. *Calcif Tiss Int 36*:645–650 (1986).
34. G.M. McCarthy, H.S. Cheung, S.M. Abel, and L.M. Ryan. Basic calcium-phosphate crystal-induced collagenase production:role of crystal dissolution. *Osteoarthritis Cartilage* (in press).
35. H.S. Cheung, J.J. Van Wyk, W.E. Russell, and D.J. McCarty. Mitogenic activity of hydroxyapatite: Requirement for somatomedin C. *J Cell Physiol 128*:143–148 (1986).
36. P.G. Mitchell, W.J., Pledger, and H.S. Cheung. Molecular mechanism of basic calcium phosphate crystal-induced mitogenesis. Role of protein kinase C. *J Biol Chem 264*:14071–14077 (1989).
37. M. Berridge. Inosital phosphate and diacylglycerol: two interacting second messengers. *Annu Rev Biochem 56*:159–94 (1987).
38. H. Rasmussen. The calcium messenger system. Part II. *N Engl J Med 314*:1164–1170 (1986).
39. U. Kikkawa and Y. Nishizuka. The role of protein kinase C in transmembrane signalling. *Annu Rev Cell Biol 2*:149–178 (1986).
40. R. Rothenberg and H. Cheung. Rabbit synoviocyte inosital phosphate metabolism is stimulated by hydroxyapatite crystals. *Am J Physiol 254*:C554–C559 (1988).
41. B. Cochran, J. Zullo, I. Verma, and C. Stiles. Expression of c-fos and of a fos-related gene is stimulated by PDGF. *Science 226*:1080–1082 (1984).
42. K. Kelly, B. Cochran, C. Stiles, and P. Leder. Cell-specific regulation of the c-myc gene by lymphocyte mitogens and platelet-derived growth factor. *Cell 35*:603–610 (1983).
43. H.S. Cheung, P. Mitchell, and W.J. Pledger. Induction of expression of c-fos and c-myc proto-oncogenes by basic calcium phosphate crystals: effect of beta-interferon. *Cancer Res 49*:134–138 (1989).
44. D. Nair, R.P. Misra, J.D. Sallis, and H.S. Cheung. Phosphocitrate inhibits a basic calcium phosphate and calcium pyrophosphate dihydrate crystal-induced mitogen-activated protein kinase cascade signal transduction pathway. *J Biol Chem 272*:18920–18925 (1997).
45. G. McCarthy, P. Christopherson, A. Baldwin, and R. Scheinman. The mitogenic response to basic calcium phosphate (BCP) crystals is associated with induction of the trascription factor nuclear factor κB (NF-κB) in Balb-c/3T3 and human fibroblasts. *Arthritis Rheum 40*:S48 (1997).
46. J.F. Woessner. Matrix metalloproteinases and their inhibitors in connective tissue remodeling. *FASEB J 5*:2145–2154 (1991).
47. M. Fini, M. Karmilowicz, P. Ruby, A. Belman, K. Borges, and C. Brinckerhoff. Cloning of a complimentary DNA for rabbit proactivator. A metalloproteinase that activates synovial cell collagenase shares homology with stromelysin and transin and is co-ordinately regulated with collagenase. *Arthritis Rheum 30*:1254–1264 (1987).
48. M. Mohtai, R. Lane Smith, D.J. Schurman, T. Tsuji, F.M. Torti, N.I. Hutchinson, W.G. Stetler-Stevenson, and G.I. Goldberg. Expression of 92-kD type IV collagenase/

gelatinase (gelatinase B) in osteoarthritic cartilage and its induction in normal human articular cartilage by interleukin 1. *J Clin Invest 92*:179–185 (1993).

49. P. Mitchell, H. Magna, L. Reeves, L. Lopresti-Morrow, S. Yocum, P. Rosner, K. Geoghegan, and J. Hambor. Cloning, expression, and type II collagenolytic activity of matrix metalloproteinase-13 from human osteoarthritic cartilage. *J Clin Invest 97*:761–768 (1996).
50. L.S. Lohmander, L.A. Hoerrner, and M.W. Lark. Metalloproteinases, tissue inhibitor, and knee proteoglycan fragmants in knee synovial fluid in human osteoarthritis. *Arthritis Rheum 36*:181–189 (1993).
51. H. Cheung, P. Halverson, and D. McCarty. Release of collagenase, neutral protease, and prostaglandins from cultured mammalian synovial cells by hydroxyapatite and calcium pyrophosphate dihydrate crystals. *Arthritis Rheum 24*:1338–1344 (1981).
52. G.M. McCarthy, P.G. Mitchell, J.S. Struve, and H.S. Cheung. Basic calcium phosphate crystals cause co-ordinate induction and secretion of collagenase and stromelysin. *J Cell Physiol 153*:140–146 (1992).
53. G. McCarthy, A. Macius, P. Christopherson, L. Ryan, and T. Pourmotabbed. Basic calcium phosphate crystals induce synthesis and secretion of 92-kD gelatinase (matrix metalloproteinase 9/gelatinase B) in human fibroblasts. *Ann Rheum Dis* In press (1997).
54. P.G. Mitchell, J.A. Struve, G.M. McCarthy, and H.S. Cheung. Basic calcium phosphate crystals stimulate cell proliferation and collagenase message accumulation in cultured adult articular chondrocytes. *Arthritis Rheum 35*:343–350 (1992).
55. G. McCarthy, P. Christopherson, and P. Mitchell. Basic calcium phosphate crystals and tumor necrosis factor *a* induce matrix metalloprotease 13 (collagenase-3) in adult porcine articular chondrocytes. *Arthritis Rheum 40*:S127 (1997).
56. D. Brenner, M. O'Hara, P. Angel, M. Chojkier, and M. Karin. Prolonged activation of jun and collagenase genes by tumor necrosis factor a. *Nature 337*:661–663 (1989).
57. P. Angel, I. Baumann, B. Stein, H. Delius, H. Rahmsdorf, and P. Herrich. 12-O-tetradecanoyl-phorbol-13-acetate induction of the human collagenase gene is mediated by an inducible enhancer element located in the 5′-flanking region. *Mol Cell Biol 7*:2256–2266 (1987).
58. H. Cheung, J. Sallis, and J. Struve. Specific inhibition of basic calcium phosphate and calcium pyrophosphate crystal-induction of metalloproteinase synthesis by phosphocitrate. *Biochim Biophys Acta 1315*:105–111 (1996).
59. J.-M. Dayer, V. Evequoz, C. Zavadil-Grob, M.D. Grynpas, P.-T. Cheng, J. Schnyder, U. Trechsel, and H. Fleisch. Effect of synthetic calcium pyrophosphate and hydroxyapatite crystals on the interaction of human blood mononuclear cells with chondrocytes, synovial cels and fibroblasts. *Arthritis Rheum 30*:1372–1381 (1987).
60. D. McCarty, and H. Cheung. Prostaglandin (PG) E_2 generation by cultured canine synovial fibroblasts exposed to microcrystals containing calcium. *Ann Rheum Dis 44*:316–320 (1985).
61. R. Rothenberg. Modulation of prostaglandin E_2 synthesis in rabbit synoviocytes. *Arthritis Rheum 30*:266–274 (1987).
62. D. Baker, K. Krakauer, G. Tate, M. Laposata, and R. Zurier. Suppression of human

synovial cell proliferation by dihomo-γ-linoleic acid. *Arthritis Rheum 32*:1273–1281 (1989).
63. D. Newcombe, C. Ciosek, Y. Ishikawa, and J. Fahey. Human synoviocytes: activation and desensitization by prostaglandins and L-epinephrine. *Proc Natl Acad Sci USA 72*:3124–3128 (1975).
64. R. Zurier. Prostaglandin E_1: Is it useful? *J Rheumatol 17*:1439–1441 (1990).
65. S. Rashad, A. Hemingway, K. Rainsford, P. Revell, F. Low, and F. Walker. Effect of non-steroidal anti-inflammatory drugs on the course of osteoarthritis. *Lancet ii*:519–521 (1989).
66. G.M. McCarthy, P.G. Mitchell, and H.S. Cheung. Misoprostol, a prostaglandin E_1 analogue, inhibits basic calcium phosphate crystal-induced mitogenesis and collagenase accumulation in human fibroblasts. *Calcif Tissue Int 53*:434–437 (1993).
67. G. McCarthy, and H. Cheung. The role of cyclic-3′,5′-adenosine monophosphate in prostaglandin-mediated inhibition of basic calcium phosphate crystal-induced mitogenesis and collagenase induction in cultured human fibroblasts. *Biochim Biophys Acta 1226*:97–104 (1994).
68. R. Terkeltaub, D. Santoro, G. Mandel, and N. Mandel. Serum and plasma inhibit neutrophil stimulation by hydroxyapatite crystals. Evidence that serum α2-HS glycoprotein is a potent and specific crystal-bound inhibitor. *Arthritis Rheum 31*:1081–1089 (1988).
69. J. Triffit. Plasma disappearance of rabbit α2-HS glycoprotein and its uptake by bone tissue. *Calcif Tiss Res 26*:155–161 (1978).
70. F. Prudhommeaux, *et al.* Variation in the inflammatory properties of basic calcium phosphate crystals according to crystal type. *Arthritis Rheum 39*:1319–1326 (1996).
71. D. Hamerman. The biology of osteoarthritis. *N Engl J Med 320*:1322–1330 (1989).
72. A.R. Poole. Enzmatic degradation: Cartilage destruction. In: *Cartilage changes in osteoarthritis* (K. Brandt, Ed.), Indiana University School of Medicine, Indianapolis, IN, 1990.
73. S. Malawista, G. Duff, E. Atkins, H. Cheung, and D. McCarty. Crystal-induced endogenous pyrogen production. *Arthritis Rheum 28*:1039–1046 (1985).
74. G. McCarthy, C. Barthelemy, J. Veum, and R. Wortmann. Influence of anti-hyperuricemic therapy on the clinical and radiographic progression of gout. *Arthritis Rheum 34*:1489–1494 (1991).
75. H. Cheung, J. Sallis, P. Mitchell, and J. Struve. Inhibition of basic calcium phosphate crystal-induced mitogenesis by phosphocitrate. *Biochem Biophys Res Commun 171*:20–25 (1990).
76. R. Walt. Misoprostol for the treatment of peptic ulcer and anti-inflammatory drug-induced gastroduodenal ulceration. *N Engl J Med 327*:1575–1580 (1992).

5

Comparative Aspects of Nitrogen Excretion and Visceral and Articular Gout Deposition in Non-Human Species

Jeffrey H. Wimsatt
Colorado State University, Fort Collins, Colorado

Several excellent reviews have summarized what is known about urate disposition in nonmammalian vertebrates (1), nonhuman mammals (2), and the evolution of nitrogen excretion mechanisms (3,4). The comparative metabolism of nitrogen excretion has been reviewed as well (5,6). Finally, an extensive summary of the pharmacological basis for proposed renal mechanisms involved in urate excretion in mammals has been compiled (2). This chapter will highlight these and other findings in the context of what is known by taxonomic group for the animal kingdom and unique characteristics of species within those groups.

I. NITROGEN METABOLISM AND EXCRETION IN NONHUMAN SPECIES

A. Production and Packaging of Nitrogenous Waste

In general, ammonia, urea, and uric acid are nitrogen excreta produced in response to conditions of successively more restricted water availability (7). Each molecule of ammonia carries one Nitrogen, each molecule of urea 2, and uric acid 4 (8). Ammonia and urea are highly water soluble and require large amounts of water for excretion (1), in part because more molecules must be excreted. In contrast, uric acid is relatively insoluble in the free form or as a sodium monohydrate salt (9), and requires less water for elimination from the body because it has less aqueous tonicity and because cations readily complex to urates reducing the molecular number and balancing charge (10).

Uric acid production is metabolically costly. It requires 3.75–4.5 (the lower value is if pyrophosphorolysis occurs) ATP per N excreted, making it more costly to produce than urea, which may require as little as 2 ATP per N excreted (11). Thus, among many lower vertebrates lacking a developed facility to concentrate urine (e.g., lacking nephrons with a functional loop of Henle), with few exceptions, aquatic animals excrete proportionately more ammonia (4–80% for fish, some amphibians, and aquatic turtles), which is relatively neurotoxic when concentrated (1). This limitation to ammonia excretion may have been the primary impetus for a shift to urea employed by our aquatic vertebrate progenitors (4). Retaining nontoxic urea also benefitted many creatures by osmotically countering the saltwater environment where they lived (4,12). Modern examples of urea retention are found especially among the sharks known to accumulate high concentrations of urea (approximately 300–400 mosmol/L) to counter the hyperosmotic effects of seawater (13). In addition, to prevent detrimental protein solubilization at high urea concentrations, other ureaosmotic regulators including sarcosine, betaine, and trimethylamine oxide (14) are synthesized by them. Other examples exist among amphibians where in contrast to ammonia excretion, which remained constant, *Xenopus laevis* and *Bufo calamita* both accumulate urea in response to dehydration, which was released passively in the former and by active excretion in the latter once rehydrated (15). In general, semiaquatic species excrete predominantly nontoxic urea (e.g., 40–95% for most amphibians and pond and swamp turtles), and terrestrial species (except mammals) excrete primarily insoluble uric acid (e.g. 50–98% for land tortoises, snakes and lizards, and birds) (1,7). Yet, as an exception to the confinement of uricotely to arid settings, birds are uricotelic regardless of their habitat (1).

In contrast to uric acid excretion, virtually all vertebrates including squamate reptiles (snakes and lizards) (1), crocodiles (16), and ureotelic chelonians (17,18) and amphibians (19) eliminate varying amounts of ammonia containing excreta (1). Since pyrimidine (2 N) and purine bases (4+ N) are present in almost equimolar amounts in living organisms, and since pyrimidines are generally reduced to ammonia (whereas purines are oxidized), this may help to explain the regularity with which ammonia is produced in most species, albeit at lower levels than purine nitrogen metabolites (20,21). In addition, retention of ammonia for osmotic and ionic functions occurs in all vertebrates, and this should not be misconstrued as ammoniotely (22–25).

B. Precursors of Urate Production

The biochemical steps involved in nitrogen metabolism and excretion have been summarized in Figure 1. All living creatures employ pyrimidine (e.g., cytosine,

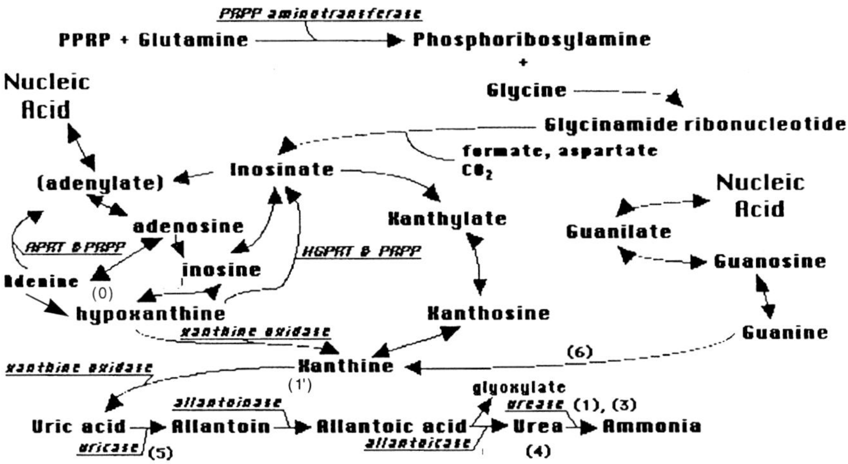

FIGURE 1 The addition, loss, and recovery of key enzymes leading to uric acid production are events responsible for many of the species differences of nitrogen excretion observed within the animal kingdom. Anodontia mussels, and leeches, are xanthine oxidase deficient. Humans emphasize the enzyme adenase (0) leading by successive steps to urea. Marine invertebrates and crustaceans emphasize guanase, xanthine oxidase, allantoinase, and allantoicase (I urease), producing urea and ammonia. Ureotelic mammals lack urease (1); and in selected species, allantoinase (1') is missing. Most teleost and elasmobranch fish are urease deficient (3). Some fish, including salmon (*Salmo* sp.), are allantoicase deficient (4). Most insects, uricotelic birds, squamate reptiles, and primates are uricase deficient (5). Piscivorous birds and spiders are guanase deficient (6). (Adapted from Ref. 30.)

thymine) and purine nucleic acids (e.g., adenine, guanine). The purine nucleotides adenine and guanine are both synthesized de novo and derived from dietary sources; dietary purine scavenging is not surprising since animals typically eat living things. Although preformed purine precursor amino acids (glycine, glutamate, and aspartate) may directly increase uric acid production as a result of proteolysis, the purine precursors aspartate and glutamate (ornithine-urea cycle), can be created by transamination from other amino acids (amino acid gluconeogenesis), linking protein catabolism directly to urate excretion. In nonmammalian uricotelic carnivores including raptorial birds, uric acid metabolism may result from both purine catabolism and from amino acid deamination, and the latter may represent a significant contribution (26). Purine nucleotide synthetic enzymes are also utilized in the synthesis of nitrogen metabolites. However, many uricotelic species tend to be hypoxanthine guanine phosphoribosyl transferase (HGPRT) and adenine phosphoribosyl transferase (APRT) deficient (Fig. 1), and purines would not be recycled (27). Urate synthesis requires three steps in addition (Fig. 1). Purine-derived inosinic acid (Inosinate) is converted to hypoxanthine, to xanthine, and finally to uric acid. The second step has at least two other alternative routes leading to xanthine. The second and third steps are catalyzed by xanthine dehydrogenase in birds and other nonmammalian vertebrates where other electron acceptors may serve the enzyme, and xanthine oxidase where oxygen (in most mammals) acts as the acceptor (28).* Urate-producing species often have increased activity of this enzyme in the liver and kidney (4,29).

In contrast, ureotelic mammals have two important mechanisms for nitrogen excretion (Fig. 2). On the one hand, they produce urea from amino acids (alpha amino groups) primarily by way of the ornithine-urea cycle (30). Possessing large amounts of arginase, usually in the liver, arginine is further degraded to urea regenerating ornithine in the process (Figure 2, II). Uric acid, on the other hand, is generated as an intermediate of purine catabolism, and in the absence of uricase, urate accumulates rather than becoming urea end product (30) (Figure 2, III).

In summary, the basic biochemical steps for the catabolism of the principal purine nucleic acids leading to a nitrogenous product excretion are surprisingly conserved among vertebrate species; therefore, the products formed in different species represent emphasis of a particular pathway or selected nitrogen metabolism enzyme deletions. In many lower vertebrates, the ornithine-urea pathway is present, but predominance of the glutamate transamination enzymes in uricotelic species favors uric acid synthesis over urea. Thus, allantoin is synthesized from urate when uricase is present, allantoic acid is the result of allantoinase activity, and allantoincase activity results in urea (7). In species where one or more enzymes are missing, intermediate nitrogen species are excreted instead, as depicted in Figure 1 (see numbers in parentheses).

C. Nitrogenous Waste Transport in the Blood

In most cases, uric acid, urea, or other nitrogen excretory precursors are transported from the site of synthesis, usually in the liver, to the kidneys for bulk excretion. Thus, it is generally assumed that an essential requirement for gout formation is that urates transported in the blood are in excess, leading to their deposition in tissues. However, many species avoid this dilemma in one of three ways: (1) by maintaining low urate levels and/or binding urates to circulating plasma proteins; (2) by excreting other metabolic end-products (such as allantoin, allantoic acid ammonia or urea); and (3) by transferring urate precursors in the blood to their final site of urate synthesis and excretion primarily in the kidneys.

Systematic study of those species presumed to make urates in the liver requiring transport (principally) to the kidneys is lacking, particularly as to evidence for gout preventive plasma protein binding. The bulk of comparative

*Overall, the terminology is somewhat arbitrary since both functions may reside in the same enzyme (28).

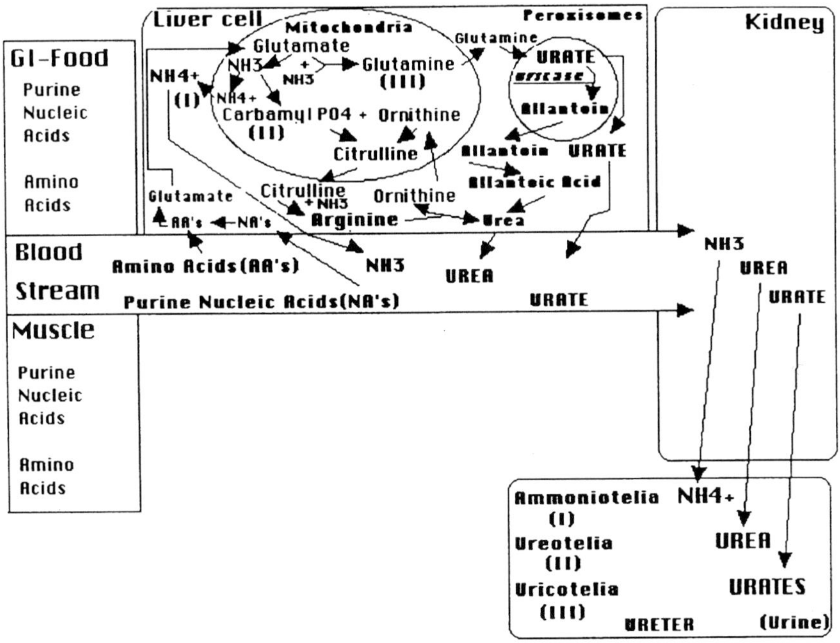

FIGURE 2 Nitrogen metabolism and nitrogenous waste excretion. Two basic sources of nitrogen precursors lead to urate production (uricotely) in the animal kingdom. The first, represented in all species and important in humans, is the catabolism of purine nucleic acids. These purines may make uric acid an intermediary or an endproduct. The second, more typical of protein gluconeogensis in lower vertebrates, involves the transamination of amino acids principally to glutamate, which is then utilized differently by ammoniotelic, ureotelic, and uricotelic species to make their respective endproducts for excretion. Glutamate is made in the cytosol of hepatocytes (principally) out of amino acids, and after transport to the mitochondria is packaged via one or more of three basic pathways, as shown: I, ammonia (ammoniotely); II, urea via citrulline (degradation to urea + ornithine by arginase), or III, into glutamine, and after transport to the peroxisomes, into urate for excretion. NH_4+ is the form transported from the mitochondria in ammoniotelic animals to preserve the electrochemical gradient. During the evolution of ureotely and uricotely, key enzymes initiating each path were sequestered inside mitochondria. Although the enzymes to make urates from amino acids were probably present in mitochondria of early vertebrates, peroxisomes may have taken on urate synthesis from purine metabolites. With the loss of allantoincase and allantoinase in early reptiles, allantoin became the primary product. Subsequent loss of uricase in the peroxisomes led to uricotely in primates and man. (Modified from Ref. 30.)

species information has come from a limited number of (primarily in vitro) equilibrium studies performed at low tonicity and at subnormal temperatures (31). In addition, the extent of plasma urate binding does not necessarily correlate with whether a particular species is uricotelic or not.

Originally, urate binding determinations were done at colder temperatures, typically 4°C. In frogs (*Anura* sp.), absence of protein binding was established and renal urate filtration appeared unimpeded (31). Among uricotelic reptiles, garter snakes (*Thamnophis* sp.) have been studied and exhibited little plasma protein binding (31). Among mammals, studies in canines indicated that neither the plasma proteins of dalmatians or mongrels bound urates (31). A similar finding was reported in the capuchin (*Cebus* sp.) monkey (31), a species known for high urate turnover and elevated plasma urate levels, comparable to hominid primates (2). At low temperatures, measurements yielded 26% binding in humans, 16% in rabbits, and 20% in rats (31). Similarly, studies in birds suggested 20% plasma urate binding at 4°C (31). It has been hypothesized that increased plasma urate binding at low temperatures, in those species where it occurs, would be adaptive to decrease the risk of urate deposition in the usually cooler extremities (32). This same mechanism could potentially protect exothermic vertebrates from urate deposition as well. This area remains controversial, especially since some early studies tested lithium urate, which appears to be more soluble at low temperatures (8). If, on the other hand, sodium urate solubility decreases with temperature (33), then plasma may well contain temperature-resistant solubilizing factors, and/or increased low-temperature binding protein sites, of considerable importance in uricotelic exotherms. Increased urate protein binding has been suggested at lower temperatures from dialysis binding studies (34). Indeed, even in human plasma, supersaturated levels of uric acid were maintained for extended periods without a crystal nidus to start precipitation (8); crystal lattice formation is endothermic, and requires exclusion of other molecular impurities, a state which may be difficult to obtain in plasma until extreme supersaturation occurs (7).

At warmer temperatures, human and rabbits exhibited ≤ 5% binding at 20°C (31), rats ≤ 5% at 37°C (34,36,37), and humans 7–8% at 37°C (34). In chicken blood, several investigators (38–41) showed that between 71 and 100% of urates were filterable, suggesting lower binding rates in vivo. These values belie the observation that avian species appear to have lower glomerular filtration rates than predicted from metabolic scaling as compared to similar-sized mammals (42). Two possible explanations for this disparity apply in birds. The first is that nephron filtration is more individualized in birds, particularly as applies to the population of urate-excreting "reptilian-like nephrons," and tubular secretion handles the bulk of urate excretion under normal conditions in birds anyway (1, 30).

Examples of nitrogen excretion other than urates utilized by different species has been summarized in Figure 1 (see numbers in parentheses). In selected species, soluble uric acid precursors (xanthine, hypoxanthine, etc.) have been shown to transit in the blood rather than urates; this variant has been well documented in birds (29, 43, 44). In the chicken, the relative renal contribution to urate production has been shown to vary with the composition and amount of protein—from 3% in fasted animals (45) to as much as 20% on a normal poultry diet (46). Infused hypoxanthine represented up to 50% of excreted urates in fasted chickens (45), suggesting in a large functional capacity. In the chicken, liver xanthine dehydrogenase was induced in response to increased dietary protein (i.e., 13-fold when the protein was increased from 5% to 75%) (47), and more so than the renal origin enzyme (47). In starved chicks, the enzyme was induced by inosine, but not by free purines (48), indicating that dietary protein rather than purines may be primarily responsible for "inducible" urate production in birds. Hypoxanthine was the preferred substrate in the pigeon, even though xanthine dehydrogenase was absent [thus, the pigeon served ideally in classic studies to deduce upstream intermediates (49)] from the liver, since it was present in the pancreas and kidneys (44, 50). Human xanthine oxidase is known to favor hypoxanthine as a substrate (51) as well, but the conditions appear to favor upstream ribonucleotide formation rather than downstream urate production (7). Unfortunately, avian xanthine dehydrogenase substrate specificity has not been evaluated systematically, although renal and liver isolates of the enzyme (present in these different locations at different developmental periods) appear to have very similar kinetic parameters (52). Levels from different tissues in various species are reported (53).

D. Physiological Urate Deposition

Whitish or silver appearing skin in some fishes derives its color (iridiphores) from physiological urate deposition often in combination with hypoxanthine and guanine (54). Guanine crystals are used in some fish species to limit gas leakage from the swim bladder (55, 56). Similarly, tapetal structures in dark adapted fish contain predominantly guanine or Ca guanate (guanin), a variation from analogous structures in invertebrates where uric acid is deposited for this purpose (57). In particular, primitive osteoglossiform fish, commonly called mooneyes (*Hiodon tergisus*) and goldeyes (*H. alosoides*) possess uric acid crystals in their tapeta lucida, a part of the retinal pigmented epithelium (58). Similar urate deposition has been observed in the outer choroidal layer of toadfishes (*Opsanus* sp.) (59). Understanding the physiological deposition of urates and the predisposition of certain tissues to accumulate urate deposits without inflammation may be significant in understanding pathological urate deposition in other species.

E. Lifestyle Changes and Nitrogen Excretion

A classic argument for the evolutionary development of urate excretion is the necessity of the cleidoic egg to evolving terrestrial vertebrates (60). However, the cleidoic egg may not have been the primary impetus for uricotely (3). Indeed, viviparous terrestrial species have evolved towards ureotelism, and a definitive placenta may be better able to deal with soluble nontoxid diffusible product(s). Moreover, even the embryos of dedicated urate producers, including birds (61), turtles (62), snakes (63), and others (see Ref. 62), have retained some ability to synthesize urea within the egg under humid conditions. Environmental conditions encountered by sessile eggs vary considerably. Changes in eggshell thickness can lead to varying rates of water loss, an adaptation apparently employed by arid climate lizards (64). Urate production has been shown to increase followed accentuated egg water losses in Japanese quail (*C. coturnix japonica*) (61). In addition, since available energy within the egg is necessarily limited, urea excretion may be advantageous, and the maintenance of both systems may be most adaptive (3).

A number of species have been documented to switch from one primary nitrogen excretion mechanism to another developmentally or in response to a changing environment. For example, tadpoles may be ammoniotelic and switch to ureotelism at metamorphosis when terrestrial life begins (65). Similarly, conversion of ammonia and urea to urates occurs in uricotelic tree frogs (*Phylomedusa* sp.) during metamorphosis (66).

Ammonia excretion in aquatic birds has been shown to increase in response to a hypotonic water environment (67). Sea turtles, primarily ammoniotelic in the ocean, become predominantly uricotelic on land (68). The dual ability of chelonians to produce either urea or uric acid, is thought to result from their direct lineage from primordial cotylosaurian reptiles (see Figure 3). Alligators may adapt in regard to the amount of ammonia versus uric acid excreted, depending on their hydration state (69). During dehydration, bladder sampling studies suggested Testudinid and other chelonians shifted toward urate production (70, 71). However, it was shown in terrestrial *(G. agassizii)* and semiaquatic turtles (e.g., *Pseudemys scripta*) that this effect is not seen using ureteral sampling (72, 73) suggesting that in bladder resorption of fluid was not considered in the earlier studies (1).

F. Renal Excretion of Nitrogenous Waste

The predominant renal mechanisms known to operate in different species for preformed uric acid excretion are summarized in Table 1. In most nonmammalian species, little work has been done to establish the extent to which uric acid is freely filtered; it is generally assumed that, without significant blood binding in vivo, filtration occurs unfettered. Even in species where preferential tubular secretion is evident, urate filtration may act to supplement this effect; this has been suggested in birds (1, 74). In a wide range of species, the most important site of renal urate tubular secretion appears to be the proximal tubule (75); the straight, convoluted, and more distal segments of the proximal tubules have all been shown to be involved in the different vertebrates examined (1, 2) (Table 1). In some species, such as the rabbit, secretory and resorption transporters appear to intermix within the same segment (30), suggesting that a tem-

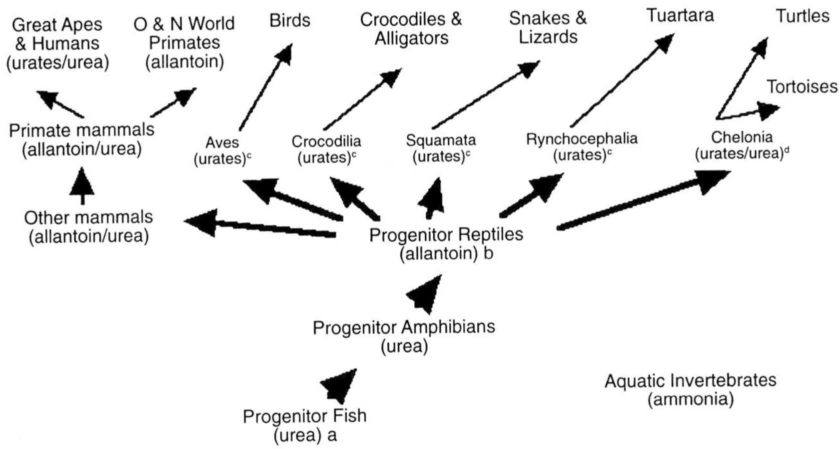

FIGURE 3 A plausible scheme for the evolution of uricotely has been proposed (3,4). Progenitor vertebrates were believed to be ammoniotelic, but a subset of these leading to terrestrial vertebrates become ureotelic. As animals developed an increasingly terrestrial existence, the synthesis of allantoin and finally uric acid became important. Of these animals, some groups including mammals developed increased renal concentrating ability via long looped nephrons in lieu of uric acid production. In the great apes and humans, up to 10% uric acid synthesis occurs out of the available excretory nitrogen pool. Gout is most common in hominoid primates and uricotelic vertebrates (especially squamate reptiles and birds) descended from terrestrial progenitors. (Adapted from Ref. 30.) a = progeniter urea producers; b = progeniter reptiles switch to allantoin excretion; c = the reptiles avian lineage became predominantly urate producers while the lineage leading to mammals and ultimately primates continued to produce allantoin and urea, and primates and man have secondarily developed some uric acid producing capability.

peral or functional separation between the inflow and outflow pumps may be important.

II. AMMONIOTELIC AND UREOTELIC SPECIES

A. Fish

In the safety of an aquatic environment, fish excrete large amounts of ammonia, which diffuse out through the gills [as was established in classic experiments in carp *(C. carpio)* and goldfish *(C. auratus)* 76)]. The skin is an important excretory organ in marine species such as the dab *L. limanda)* (77), and the kidneys have a secondary nitrogen excretory role (13). Ammonia can exert charge, a

TABLE 1 Summary of Urinary Urate Excretion in Nonhuman Species

Species	Free filtration	T. secretion	T. resorption
Amphibians			
Salamander (*Necturus* sp.)	yes	yes	yes (> secr)
Leopard frog *(R. pipiens)*[a]	yes	yes	yes
S. Am. Hylid frog (30°C) *(P. sauvagei)*	likely (≥ 5%)	yes (< 95%)	?
Reptiles			
Snakes			
Garter (*Thamnophis* spp.)	yes	pt 10: dt 1	?
Brown (*Storeria* spp.)	yes		
Water (*Natrix* spp., at 28°C)	likely	yes	no
Chelonians			
Yellow-bellief turtle	*(P. scripta)*	yes	? (< secr)
Desert tortoise	*(G. agassizii)*	yes	? (< secr)
Avians			
Chicken (cortical nephrons)	71% (plasma bind?)	yes (cn)	no/yes
Duck *(A. platyrhynchos)*	?	yes	no
Mourning dove (Z. macroura)	?	yes	no
Mammals			
Rabbit *(O. cunniculus)*	>95%	yes (st pt)	yes[b] (< secr)
Dog (mongrel)	likely	yes (pt < Dalmat.[c])	yes
Dalmatian	likely	yes (pt)	yes
Rat	likely	yes (pct)	yes (pct)
Goats[a]	likely	yes	yes (< secr)
Calves[a]	likely	yes	yes (< secr)
Cat	likely	?	yes
Guinea pig	likely	?	yes
Rat	≥ 90%	yes (mid pt)	yes (early pt, pr, < secr)
Primate			
Many N. W. monkeys *(Cebus)* sp.	likely	yes	yes (> secr)
Red howler *(A. semiculus)*	likely	yes	yes (< secr)
Moustached tam. *(S. mystax)*	likely	yes	yes (< secr)
Squirrel monkey *(S. sciureus)*	likely	yes	yes (< secr)
Many O. W. monkeys	likely	yes	yes (< secr)
Bushbaby *(G. Crassicaudatus)*	likely	yes	yes (> secr)
Olive baboon *(P. anubis)*	likely	yes	yes (< secr)

TABLE I Continued

Species	Free filtration	T. secretion	T. resorption
Hominoid primates			
Chimpanzee *(P. troglodytes)*	likely	yes	yes (> secr)
Human	yes?	yes	yes (> secr)

[a]Uric acid infusion studies.
[b]Under urate load, net resorbers became net secretors
[c]The increased secretion of urate in dalmatians is generally accepted to be a functional response to higher levels of urates in the plasma rather than a difference in renal transporters.
pr = pars recta; pt = proximal tubule; pct = proximal convoluted tubule; st pt = straight proximal tubule; dt = distal tubule; cn = cortical "reptilian-like" nephrons (only); ? = unknown.

gaseous partial pressure, and pH, whereas urea is relatively inert at physiological concentrations (78). The enzymatic conversion of urea to ammonia requires urease, which is not produced by vertebrates (13); therefore ammonia is most likely produced by means other than either uricolysis or arginolysis (as discussed above; see Fig. 3, I).

Some marine chondrichthyians (shark relatives), a few teleosts, the primitive coelacanth, and aestivating dipnoans (lungfish) are predominantly ureotelic (13). Urea is usually created by three potential pathways. The first is the gamma-guanidino urea hydrolase pathway, which has been documented in carp *(C. Carpio),* although its significance is unclear (79). The second pathway is via arginolysis (Fig. 3, II) of dietary arginine, and has been well documented in certain osteichthyian ("boney") and agnathan fishes (13). Possession of arginase appears to be widespread among fish (80–82) and is shared with higher vertebrates. Urea synthetic enzymes were found predominantly in the liver of those species examined; arginolysis appeared to involve several different organs, including the kidneys (83), but was highest in the liver in several freshwater species that appeared capable of ureotely (82). Third, in some fish, synthesized and subsequently uric acid is converted to allantoin by the action of uricase; allantoin is further catabolized to allantoic acid and urea. The location of uricase, allantoinase, and allantoicase have been shown to be located in the liver of several marine fish (85,86), principally in the peroxisomes (86).

Uricolytic enzymes were found only in the liver (82). Many species, including carp [or Lampreys (87)], depend on the uricolytic pathway to produce urea (82,88). Thus, these species could become susceptible to gout if hepatic uricase enzyme activity was compromised and uric acid production continued unabated. Gout has infrequently been reported in fish (89).

B. Ureotelic Amphibians

Most amphibians preferentially excrete ammonia and urea via their kidneys, although small amounts of uric acid may be excreted also (90,91). It has been postulated that ancestral amphibians developed ureotelism to detoxify ammonia, and further loss of the peroxisomal enzymes allantoinase and allantoincase in descendent reptiles led predominantly to allantoin product; higher vertebrates probably followed this path (4).

In modern amphibians, degrading enzymes allantoinase and allantoicase suggest considerable conservation as compared to the fish enzymes; however, unlike the situation reported in fish, the two are joined together as one enzyme in amphibians (86,92). Hepatic uricolytic enzymes have been shown to change during development in *Rana catesbiana,* and appear to be present in a salamander *(Necturus maculosus)* (88).

Limited information on nitrogenous waste oxidation enzymes is available in amphibians, but uricolysis may be important for urea synthesis. Xanthine dehydrogenase was below detectable levels in liver, but detectable in the kidneys (at moderate levels) in two representative species of ureotelic frogs (*Bufo arenarum* and *L. chaquensis*) (93). Uricase levels in the liver and kidney were highest in ureotelic species as compared to uricotelic frogs or in a uricotelic lizard *(Diplosaurus dorsalis).* Therefore, renal synthesis of urates appears to be converted to urea in the kidneys and elsewhere. Arginase activity was higher in the liver but was detectable in the kidneys of uricotelic and ureotelic frogs, whereas levels were low in both tissues in a uricotelic lizard *(D. dorsalis).* Thus, frogs, regardless of what they excrete, appeared to retain the arginolytic and uricolytic pathways (93). Amphibians exhibit considerable developmental and across-species variation in arginase levels (94).

Early experiments evaluating the disposition of that suggested infused uric acid plasma binding and tubular secretion in leopard frogs *(Rana pipiens)* were both minimal; thus, filtration appeared to be a primary means of handling uric acid excretion in a ureotelic species (95). However, tubular secretion was demonstrated in another study when the portal vein was perfused with uric acid (96).

C. Ureotelic Reptiles

Turtles and tortoises (Order chelonia) appear to have retained the primitive reptilian plan of mixed uricotelism and ureotelism as assumed to be possessed by their cotylosaurian ancestors; species use urea or urate excretion depending on water availability. Thus, aquatic species may produce equal amounts of ammonia and urea, with only a small fraction as uric acid. Terrestrial species such as xeric testudinid tortoises (17, 18) produce mainly uric acid (97); these tortoises also produce urea at levels above those encountered in squamate reptiles (98). Xerophilic desert tortoises

(G. agassizii) are primarily ureotelic (72). Mature sea turtles, normally living in a free water–deprived oceanic environment, had serum urea values of 20–80 mg/dl (99), and turtles maintained up to 3 days out of water had ammonia values < 5% of total nitrogen excretion, while urea and urates were excreted in large amounts (100).

D. Ureotely in Mammals

1. Introduction

Therapsid reptiles, progenitors of the evolutionary line leading to mammals, developed in the direction of ureotely, as is universal to modern mammals. Hepatic arginase levels in representative mammals reflect this development (94). Even primitive mammals are ureotelic (101). However, purines are catabolized to allantoin (30).

One of the highest circulating blood levels of urea encountered under physiological conditions occurs in the common vampire bat *(D. rotundus),* an exclusively sanguinivorous species that consumes a very high protein (85.5%), and low fat (1%) and carbohydrate (1.7%) diet, where peak urea levels were demonstrated to reach 343 mg/dl (57 mmol/L) following a blood meal (102). Urea concentrating ability may be highly developed in desert-adapted species such as the Australian hopping mouse (*Notomysalexis*), which produce highly concentrated urine following the generation of a large urea gradient in the kidneys (94).

Even in arid climate–adapted species, urate levels in mammals ranged from 1 to 2% of total nitrogen excretion (74). In lower mammals, the presence of uricase converts what uric acid is produced to allantoin for renal excretion (103).

Domestic animals, including ruminants, elaborate primarily urea and allantoin, except the pig, which is reported to produce significant amounts of guanine (104). However, although early studies reported guanine crystalline deposits in pigs with limb weakness and polyuria (105–107), more recent studies argue against a functional guanase deficiency in pigs (108, 109).

De novo synthesis of urate has been demonstrated in the kidneys (110–112), lungs, and spleen of rats (111). The demonstration of renal urate degradation in the kidney was less convincing (30).

The role of ions in renal urate transport in the rat (113–117) and in the dog (118, 119) indicate these ions may primarily serve to balance charge. Thus, cations do not appear to serve as obligatory cotransporters.

In dogs, free glomerular filtration auric acid has been inferred from a lack of protein binding (30). The dalmatian has increased uric acid clearance compared to nondalmatians; reduced renal resorption rather than accentuated secretion has been implicated (119–122). There is little evidence to suggest the renal differences are anything but compensatory (121), although other possibilities exist (2). Also, generous amounts of uricase were found in canine hepatic tissue samples (123).

An established mechanism for why dalmations have higher circulating urate concentrations and for their predisposition to develop urate stones is an inability of urates to enter uricase containing hepatocytes and red cells (124). Other dogs (124) and humans (125, 126) appear to perform this important step more readily. Ureteral ligation in canines caused noticeable increases in allantoin production, indicating uricase was intact (127).

2. Ureotelic Primates and Uricotely

Primates are considered ureotelic. However, in many species uric acid is produced in significant amounts. Capuchin monkeys, members of the new world platyrrhine primates, have been considered one of the best models of human urate transport (128, 129). While capuchins *(C. albifrons)* maintain urate levels comparable to chimpanzees and humans, their liver contains higher uricase levels than hominoid primates, and as a result it has been surmised that they turnover larger amounts of uric acid than other simian primates. A loss of functional uricase has arisen in the higher primates (i.e., the anthropoid primates—apes and man). (130)

III. URICOTELY

Although the overall need to conserve water is reflected in the lifestyles of uricotelic species, other adaptations to arid environments arose. For example, functional avian kidney mass is smaller in those species employing salt glands (131). The maximum attainable osmolarity of representative amphibians is essentially isosthenuria, in reptiles it is that of plasma, and in birds it is approximately twice that of plasma (1, 132). Thus, to conserve water in a terrestrial environment, two strategies were developed. The first was a urea gradient concentrating kidney, as evolved in mammals and to a minor degree in other species, and the second was the switch to mainly urate excretion.

It has been argued that the renal anatomical constraints involved in the ultimate development of renal mechanisms for urate concentration became a major impetus for ureotely, explaining, for example, the short nephrons of lower vertebrates (30). This argument is teleologically suspect, in that lower ureotelic species have simple nephrons and some uricotelic vertebrates have developed ways of concentrating urine laden with urates (132, 133). Evolution toward a terrestrial existence, particularly among the ancestral sauropsids, is believed to have led to a dual ureotelic/uricotelic system, as exhibited in the primitive tuatara (*Splenodon punctatus,* order Rynchocephalia) (134, 135). A more likely proposal suggests this basic distinction represents a turning point in vertebrate evolution, because urea could undergo renal tubular concentration, and renal tubules with long concentration segments (loops of Henle) could be counterproductive to significant urate excretion (74). According to this view, significant conversion to uricote would most likely clog mammalian nephrons and the countercurrent exchange system upon which these progenitors depended for conserving water during excretion; thus, renal structural changes that evolved along the line of ureotelic progenitors to current mammals may have destined them to develop urea-concentratng mechanisms to the exclusion of significant urate synthesis (3).

Uricotely is more efficient for water conservation than other means of nitrogenous waste excretion (74,132). Therefore, a 16 to 20-fold reduction in osmotic pressure results from reduced solubility, excretion of larger molecules of a smaller number, and binding of cations to the free acid (211). The concentration of uric acid is 0.1–1.0 M in bird urine, well above the solubility limit, and urine in birds and other uricotelic species is a urate colloidal suspension.

A. Uricotely, Diet, and Nutrition

In carnivorous lizards and snakes, physiological hyperuricemia (50–300+% increases) occurred followed feeding, and peaked 24 hours after feeding when whole mice were fed (136). After feeding, residual plasma urate elevations may be seen for days in exothermic species (137), and appear to be dose-related (138). Carnivorous birds (raptors), including turkey vultures, excrete 75–85% of their nitrogen as urates. On a high-protein diet these birds excreted 4.8 times more N/ml of urine than fasted birds, which was preferentially excreted as urates (26). Similar, protein catabolic effects have been observed in other raptors, including peregrine falcons (139).

Increasing the protein intake in gramnivorous species appeared to have a less remarkable effect. For example, in domestic fowl urate synthetic capacity in the liver increased (140), but the relative proportion of urate excretion in the urine fraction appeared minimally affected (141–143).

High-purine-containing diets have been reported to predispose to gout in susceptible species, including humans (144–146). Increasing dietary protein intake also increased the rate-limiting enzyme amidophosphoribosyl transferase in other species, (140); however, this effect is probably minor, unless the diet contains high purine levels. Increased purines in the diet induced liver xanthine dehydrogenase in the chicken (152). Similarly, rat xanthine oxidase activity increased fivefold when the dietary protein content increased from 8% to 23% (153). Other urea cycle enzymes also increased in response to protein changes in the diet, while still others did not (154).

Amino acid–deficient diets (147–149) and pyridoxine deficiency led to dramatically increased urate excretion in insects (tenfold), because pyridoxine is a modulating cofactor for aminotransferase function. Similarly, free amino acid shifts during vitamin B_6 deficiency in insects have been observed in rats (150, 151), suggesting the possibility of such an effect in other vertebrates as well.

Vitamin E deficiency (antioxidant) increased xanthine oxidase activity in rabbits (155), most likely nonspecifically, by decreasing reactive oxygen intermediates. Arginase is believed to require manganese, and its activity increased in response to high protein diets or essential amino acid deficiency (9). Iron and molybdenum are components of xanthine oxidase, and diets deficient in these elements decreased hepatic enzyme activity in experimental animals (156).

B. Uricotely in Invertebrates

Invertebrates are strikingly similar to vertebrates in regard to the synthesis of nitrogenous endproducts of nitrogen metabolism; the importance of uricotely in insects has recently been reviewed (157). Uricolysis has been well documented in invertebrates, and requisite enzymes have been identified in the hepatopancreas (7). In aquatic invertebrates, including molluscs, the primary endproduct of purine metabolism is ammonia, while in spiders it is guanine (7,158).

Invertebrates have developed unique uses for nitrogen products for environmental adaptation, as chemical messengers, in nutrient storage, and even as a currency for paternal investment in egg production.

Periwinkles are partially uricotelic littoral gastropods in contrast to most ammoniotelic marine species. Longer submersion in higher salinity surroundings has been shown to increase urate storage in several organs, especially the nephridium, requiring stored urate to be converted to ammonia first (159). The fresh water snail *(Bellamya bengalensis)* (160) and the slug *(Semperula muculata)* (161) appear to accumulate uric acid in various tissues in response to environmental (temperature, season, etc.) changes, suggesting that organ urate storage rather than urate excretion may be more important for water and nitrogen conservation. The storage of uric acid principally in the fat body of American cockroach nymphs *(Periplaneta americana)* during dietary protein excess, suggests this organ may serve as a nitrogen reservoir during leaner times, again obviating urate excretion (162). The stored urate crystals appear spherical and contain large amounts of bound potassium, and may provide a means for conserving this electrolyte as well (163, 164). In the tropical cockroach *(Xestoblatta hamata),* males ingest urates and eat high protein diets in order to provide their mates with urates as a paternal investment; females transfer the urates to maturing oocytes (165). In the British crayfish *(Austropotamobius pallipes),* uric acid (i.e., circulating urate ion) and other circulating purines appear to increase hemocyanin oxygen affinity (166). Whether a similar relationship exists in vertebrates could have implications for changes in plasma levels in vertebrates. Uric acid and urea accumulation in the growth medium has been shown to arrest larval development in response to overcrowding (167).

C. Uricotelic Fish and Amphibians

In contrast to most amphibian species, members of the tree frog genuses *Chiromantis (C. xerampelina)* (168) and *Phyllomedusa* (e.g., *P. sauvagei* 80%, *P. pailona* and *P. iherengi* 45% and *P. hypochondrialis* 24% urate nitrogen) (66, 169, 170) appear to be primarily uricotelic as adults. The shift to uricotely occurred around the time of larval metamorphosis in *P. sauvagei* from the more primordial larval condition of ammonia and urea excretion (66).

Based on clearance studies, renal urate synthesis appears unlikely in this species (93). *Phyllomedusa* species also exhibited high liver and measurable kidney levels of xanthine dehydrogenase (66); whereas, arginase and uricase activities were lower than in (typically) ureotelic anurans (66, 171). Urate clearance in *P. sauvagei* closely paralleled that of PAH, suggesting that secretion was the primary mode of elimination (93). Levels of urea cycle enzymes were lower in the liver of the uricotelic South African tree frog species *Chiromantis xerampelina,* although xanthine dehydrogenase was not appreciably different as compared to other amphibians. Some enzymes levels examined appeared to change in response to increased environmental humidity, while others did not (172).

D. Uricotelic Reptiles

Sauropsid cotylosaurs developed along a lepidosauran (tuataras and squamate reptiles) line distinct from the archosaurs (birds and crocodilians, see below) already mentioned. This line further split into uricotelic/ureotelic tuataras as well as uricotelic snakes and lizards. Uricotelic reptiles, particularly those consuming high protein diets, including most lizards and snakes, excrete 80–90% of their nitrogen as uric acid. Although semiaquatic, crocodilians are carnivorous and appear to excrete predominantly uric acid as well (16).

In an early study, iguanas *(Iguana iguana)* appeared to filter only 5% of the uric acid cleared (173). Blood urea levels in primarily uricotelic reptiles are < 10 mg/dl (174). From single nephron studies in the garter snake (*Thamnophis* sp.), proximal tubules appear to be most actively involved in urate excretion, although the distal tubules and collecting ducts appeared involved in renal excretion to a much lesser extent (175, 176). Active urate excretion was demonstrated throughout the proximal tubules, whereas active PAH excretion occurred only in the distal proximal tubule segment, suggesting independent mechanisms (30). Active renal tubular urate transport in garter snakes (*Thamnophis* sp.) appears to depend on the presence of potassium (177) and sodium (175). Gentamicin toxicity induced both proximal tubular damage and visceral gout in gopher snakes *(P. melanoleucus catenifer)* (178).

Few studies have examined the uric acid synthetic enzymes and their distribution in reptiles. Selected tissues of an arid climate adapted lizard species

(Diplosaurus dorsalis) were examined for uricase, arginase, and xanthine dehydrogenase in the kidneys (66). Arginase activity was measurable but low in the kidneys and very low in the liver (66). It may be this idiosyncratic enzyme distribution is peculiar to this species, and other sites make arginase or other pathways dominate. Indeed, arginase is reported at high levels in tissues from nine other lizard species (179). Xanthine dehydrogenase was not detected in the liver but renal activity was unusually high (66). Uricase activity was moderate in the kidneys and liver (66). Thus, kidneys appear to make uric acid by the ornithine-urea and arginase pathways in many cases, and the ability to make urea from uric acid catabolism is probably retained in many species (66). Crocodilians and squamate reptiles have essentially lost key hepatic ureotelic enzymes (except arginase) resident in tuataras, and little or no urea excretion occurs as a result (74,180). As in birds, many squamate (snake and lizard) reptile species form urate spherules, apparently to ease renal tubular excretion (181).

E. Uricotelic Birds

Sauropsid cotylosaur ancestors leading to birds (Fig. 2) developed along one line into archosaurs (crocodilians and birds), which emphasized uricotely. Birds possess both reptilian- and mammalian-type nephrons: The former nephrons primarily in the renal cortex excrete urates, and the latter (more medullary) nephrons are capable of building a countercurrent urea gradient for urine concentration to some degree (10). Exquisite filtering control appears in birds to induct the correct nephron population when needed. Renal portal blood flow goes primarily to the reptile-like nephrons and urate excretion. The ability to turn nephron filtration on and off appears in arid adapted mammals possessing two distinct nephron types as well (74). Avian species appear to possess a majority of "reptilian-type" simple nephrons that appear most involved in urate excretion.

Although birds typically produce predominantly uric acid, guanine, ammonia, and urea may be excreted, depending in large measure upon the ecological niche of the species and the nature of the diet consumed (182). For example, fish scales have a high guanine concentration, and many marine piscivorous birds excrete guanine (especially from fish scales: "guano") without further metabolic packaging (7).

Clinically, prerenal azotemia (BUN elevations $\leq$ ten- to 15-fold) is caused by dehydration in birds; and in the dehydrated pigeon, concurrent uric acid elevations in the same period were typically two-fold or less (183). Thus, it appears that urate excretion is relatively resistant to dehydration, and this may be the result of differential nephron functioning and perfusion (184). Thus, the renal portal blood flow that primarily perfuses these "reptilian nephrons" may be more resistant to dehydration, but appears to be adaptive; it is also stress hormone responsive (10,184). In addition, most birds can accumulate urea and create a partial urea concentrating gradient in times of dehydration using their second population of "mammalian-type" nephrons, often comprising 10–30% of the total nephron number (184). In birds where mammalian and reptilian nephrons are both present, arid adapted species may possess more reptilian-type urate excreting nephrons (e.g., 85% or more) (131). Avian species also package their urates into 0.5 to 13μm composite spheres (60% uric acid) making urates less prone to plug the renal tubules (185).

In avians, visceral gout has been described as gout resulting from renal disease, whereas articular gout is believed to result more from genetic factors. Based on gross morphology, the two diseases are probably indistinguishable (186, 187). Siller has argued that visceral gout (under ideal conditions) is usually precipitous and causes little cellular reaction (i.e., tophi); this is recognizable histopathologically (186). A genetic chicken model (HUA, gout prone strain) or impaired renal excretion or uric acid has been characterized (188). Experiments with normal chickens (LUA) suggested the existence of (at least) a cation pump–dependent (responsive to Na, K, and ouabain) pathway of urate uptake, and a ouabain-independent one as well. LUA birds were rendered equivalent in renal urate excretion function to HUA birds in response to ouabain, suggesting that it may be the ouabain-dependent pump that fails to function properly in the HUA-impaired renal excretion strain (189). Moreover, p-aminohippuric acid (PAH) infusion at lower (0.4 μmol/min) and higher (50.0 μmol/min) concentrations caused decreased uric acid transport in both strains, but was most noticeable in the HUA strain. PAH may compete with uric acid for renal transport during tubular secretion in some instances (190). However, in others it appears to be independent (191). This effect may in part reflect how much is given. Finally, obstructive gout refers to gout resulting from a renal outflow obstruction, and as has been documented following experimental ureter ligation, during urolithiasis (192) and following renal tubule cellular metaplasia resulting from Vitamin A deficiency (187).

As in many species, birds have arginase activity, and avian kidney tissue generally has greater arginase activity than liver tissue (9). However, the levels are typically lower than encountered in ureotelic species (97). The necessity of the avian liver for uric acid production is doubtful in certain avian species. For example, in geese a rapid rise in blood ammonia occurs in response to complete hepatectomy; infused ammonia induces uric acid rise in the blood (97).

Stress-induced elevations in plasma uric acid and urea reported in wintering green-winged teal could be explained by increased endogenous protein catabolism, increased food consumption to meet energy needs, or relative dehydration (193). Similar trends have been reported in premigratory hyperphagic geese (194). Molt-related hyperuricemia has been attributed to endogenous utilization of protein stores as well (186). Fasting also led to elevated plasma uric acid and urea elevations in common buzzards *(Buteo buteo),* although accompanying dehydration may have contributed to the result. Fasting appeared to have a similar effect in gramnivores (195). Parasitic infestation leading to a protein-losing enteropathy, and secondarily in endogenous protein catabolism and dehydration, caused hyperuricemia in experimentally infected Egyptian herons (196). Experimental heavy metal intoxication caused gout in turkeys (197) and excess nitrates/nitrites in poultry food induced gout. In fasting king penguins, uric acid levels did not elevate, suggesting that fat catabolism coupled with metabolic water production may have minimized protein catabolism and dehydration-induced plasma increases in urates (198).

In the domestic fowl, radio-labelling studies suggest that renal excretion is the most important. Yet, uric acid in the avian is produced in the liver, kidney (50), and the pancreas, depending on the species (50). Uric acid precursors, hypoxanthine and xanthine also released from the latter organs (along with uric acid), may be further converted to uric acid to some degree in adipose and muscular tissues (41). Species differences exist in the distribution of the key synthetic enzymes. For example, xanthine dehydrogenase is found in the liver of domestic fowl, but not in the liver of pigeons (43,199). Thus, most of the final conversion to uric acid in pigeons occurs in the kidneys prior to excretion.

Significant renal damage, particularly to the proximal tubules, of "reptilian-type" nephrons would in theory cause hyperuricemia due to loss of renal excretory function. For example, red-tailed hawks experimentally intoxicated with gentamicin had proximal tubular lesions and high plasma uric acids levels (200); however, little work has been done in birds to specifically characterize the renal tubular mechanisms directly responsible for urate excretion in most species.

Before gout occurs, compensatory mechanisms to correct hyperuricemia would operate. For example, induction of all urate secreting nephrons, allowing less blood to bypass the kidney, increased PAH clearance ten- to 20-fold (and presumably would do the same for urate clearance) (201). Skahauge reviewed urate clearance in the domestic fowl. Under normal conditions, 80–90% of tubular secretion accounts for urate excretion (182). Renal portal blood flow accounted for just over half of renal urate excretion, and renal portal blood flow changes dramatically affected urate excretion (182). In addition, when urate secretory overload occurs in a pro-gout state, urate filtration has been shown to help compensate for increased levels (10). Active renal tubular urate transport in chickens appears to depend on the presence of potassium, that may serve as a cotransporter (177).

Gout in birds is relatively common (186, 187). Experimentally, allopurinol is reported to inhibit avian xanthine dehydrogenase, just as it inhibits the homologous enzyme xanthine oxidase in mammals (46, 61). The potential for this drug to cause toxic metabolites (oxypurinol, etc.) or xanthine crystal deposits in the kidneys may help to explain the empirical observation that allopurinol was questionably effective or even toxic for the treatment of gout in avian carnivores (202). However, others report clinical improvement and tophi reduction when allopurinol is combined with colchicine during gout treatment in graminivorous psittacines (203).

F. Mammals

As a group, mammals are considered to be ureotelic. However, small amounts of uric acid are produced in most species as a product of purine breakdown, and, at least in the rat, conservation via reabsorption of urate occurs in the loop of Henle at low flow rates (204), but not in the proximal tubules (37).

G. Primates

Overall, there is a trend toward high circulating urate levels in moving from lower primates to higher primates and man. For example, relatively primitive proscimian primates (lemurs, etc.) are similar to rats in their circulating levels of uric acid (e.g., 0.5 mg/kg) (205). An apparent exception to this trend appears in New World capuchin *(Cebus albifrons)* (206) and woolly (*Lagothrix* sp.) monkeys (207), which exhibit higher urate levels than many of their Old or New World primate counterparts; this suggests they possess a higher turnover rate, as compared to a decreased catabolism typical of humans (206). Like humans, cebid monkeys undergo net tubular resorption, exhibit minimal plasma protein binding (discussed above) (206, 208), and uricase activities (as for other New World platyrhine primates) appear lower (at least in some cases) than values found in various Old World (nonape catarrhine primates) monkey species examined (209,210). In contrast, white-fronted capuchin monkeys *(Cebus albifrons)* have a high uricase activity (206).

Thus, the overall level of plasma uric acid in primates across species is inversely related to uricase levels in that species and the net uric acid resorption performed by the kidneys. In humans more than 90% of uric acid is resorbed by the kidneys (221). Similarly, the great apes and humans do not produce uricase and 2–5% of nitrogen excretion in humans is uric acid; this is in contrast to many other primate and nonprimate mammals where uric acid would be further catabolized to allantoin and eventually excreted as urea (186). Uricase production has been reported to be to be less consistent among lower simian (Old World) primates (205). Uricase isolated from Old World primates (compared to proscimian enzyme) appears to be labile and easily inactivated in vitro (209,210), potentially leading to differing reported values in the past. In vivo radioisotope disposition studics suggcst that thc Humboldt's woolly monkcy *(Lagothrix lagotrichia)* has a diminished uricase activity as compared to other New World monkeys, although extrarenal sites of urate disposition may be operating (207). Uricase appears to be active in several tissues when found, but was not detected in the rhesus monkey *(M. mulatta)* kidney (212).

It has been hypothesized that uric acid acts as an important antioxidant and free radical scavenger and this evolutionary development within the primate order corresponds to the loss of endogenous ascorbic acid synthesis (213,214). If so, this might help to explain why some primates appear to undergo net resorption, and why the rhesus monkey appears to bind 20% of circulating urate while possessing a high uricase activity. Similarly, New World species, although they lack significant plasma binding, still appear to maintain high circulating levels. Hominoid primates appear to lack uricase altogether, allowing urate levels to rise to half or more of the precipitation concentration in the blood (2). Coincidentally, the loss of the ability to make ascorbate, a potent antioxidant, occurred during the evolution from proscimians to simian primates (215). Thus we expect that circulating uric acid levels in proscimians should be lower. Unfortunately very little work has been done in proscimians, but the Galago *(Galago crassicaudatus)* appears to be a net urate resorber with moderate urate levels; this could have more to due with their unique diet (216).

As in humans, hereditary hyperuricemia, due to one of three known inborn defects in metabolism, would be expected to occur in nonhuman primates, and arise clinically, particularly pet monkeys fed human foods in large proportion. However, such a model has yet to be characterized. Similarly, as in humans, higher incidences are expected in males and postmenopausal females (217). However, although nonhuman primates have not been systematically studied in this regard, no gender-related predisposition has been recognized in lower vertebrates that have been examined (187,218,219).

IV. URATE METABOLISM IN OTHER TISSUES AND AT OTHER SITES

Blood values likely reflect a dynamic equilibrium among all urate synthetic and excretory tissues, including the liver and kidneys. However, the ability to make uric acid within other tissues cannot be discounted as a contribution to this circulating pool. Moreover, numerous tissues were capable of urate production yet only low levels were found in the various tissues examined; thus, urates may be rapidly removed and production levels closely regulated from secondary synthetic sites (111). In a carefully conducted rat study, lung, spleen, and kidney tissue had low measurable urate levels, and numerous tissues (excluding brain and muscle) appeared capable of urate synthesis. White cells and other tissues may perform uricolysis as well, as has been demonstrated in the rat (220), although these other sources are poorly defined in nonhuman species. The importance of these tissues is likely to increase when excretion mechanisms fail, as is the case in humans (221,222). If urates are entering the circulation from all tissues, then studies examining tissue synthesis of uric acid might provide a clearer picture of whole body urate balance in health and disease than plasma levels per se. Metabolic differences could help to explain the tissue distribution of lesions associated with visceral gout in animals.

The role of reno-enteric recycling to nitrogen recovery in birds has been reviewed (223). Radiolabeled uric acid instillation directly into the cecum in willow ptarmigan *(Lagopus lagopus lagopus)* resulted in an output of 45% of radiolabeled CO_2 in the first hour suggesting rapid urate breakdown and utilization (224). Uricolysis of extrarenal uric acid passing into the gut in saliva, digestive secretions, and bile has been attributed to account for up to one-third of urate excretion in man, particularly when renal mechanisms are compromised (222); however, little nitrogen is generally found in the stool (221). High activity of xanthine dehydrogenase in the pancrease of pigeons; may indicate another mode of excretion used in avian species as well (44,50).

After the action of various bacterial origin nitrogen-splitting enzymes, resorbed ammonia passing back to the liver could thus contribute to the overall uric acid pool. The role of bacteria in this process has been investigated, and few bacteria involved were obligate nitrogen splitters (225–228). Urate nitrogen resorption accounted for up to 49% of urate nitrogen produced and occurred predominantly in the cecum, rather than in the ileum and colon (229). Cecal injection of radiolabeled nitrogen-uric acid into fowl led to a 77% disappearance of the uric acid and a 28% conversion to labeled ammonia (230). Uricolysis of urate with resultant ammonia production and reabsorption has been shown to occur in humans as well, where as much as one-third of the uric acid was turned over in this way each day (221,222). Some amino acid (and thus nitrogen) recovery may also occur at that site (231). Concomitantly, the loss of ions joined together to the urates would lead to a negative ion balance if resorption of these elements did not also occur in the lower intestine. (185,232) Water is also resorbed during this process. Finally, the carbon components of the uric acid are converted to volatile fatty acids, and their resorption would likely facilitate ion transport as well (233).

V. EXPERIMENTAL AND SPONTANEOUS HYPERURICEMIA AND GOUT DEVELOPMENT IN ANIMALS

A. Physiological Hyperuricemia

Hyperuricemia is recognized based on plasma urate elevations above normal values for that species. Physiological or benign elevations occur in reptiles (138) and birds (discussed above) postprandially. In avian species, elevations have been documented in response to breeding stress (194) and in association with fasting (198, 234), molting (194), and premigratory hyperphagia (194). Precipitation of uric acid occurs at 10–12 mg/dl, even considering high Na concentrations, and higher body temperatures typical in birds (139, 186). These normal events complicate the clinical recognition of gout predisposing elevations in the plasma. Clinical gout has been seen in an alligator with 70 mg/dl in serum (a carnivore), a debilitated king penguin with 100 mg/dl (a piscivore), chickens with plasma uric acid levels of 22.3 mg/dl, and the levels of 25 mg/dl in the parakeet (gramnivores) (235). Experimental ureteral ligation caused urate elevations to peak at 304 mg/dl in ducks (236) and at 284 mg/dl in chickens (39). Because birds typically exceed the precipitation concentration of uric acid, plasma binding or other mechanism(s) appear to be protective. In agreement with this view is the observation that urate crystal deposition in avian visceral gout does not typically occur in blood vessels (187).

B. Gout in Lower Vertebrates

A gout-like condition has been reported in association with cultured catfish *(Parasilurus asotus)* fed an artificial diet composed in large part of eel. Articular and visceral lesions and a granulomatous response were reported (237). Urate deposition in the viscera and renal tubules has been reported in association with an infection with *Corynebacterium* sp. (238, 239). Hepatorenal syndrome in turbot was characterized by urate deposits (240). Cultured fish appear to be most commonly reported with urate deposits, so it is unclear whether environmental effects including diet may be responsible (237, 240, 241).

C. Gout in Reptiles

The incidence of clinical visceral gout at one zoological institution was found to be 2.8% among reptiles (242); where dehydration and high protein diets were most commonly implicated (243). Clinical gout, with renal, periarticular, and disseminated urate deposits, has been reported in crocodilians (304) and appeared to have the highest incidence in male hatchlings (244). Crocodiles that developed visceral gout in a pathological survey were thought to be overfed protein or had metabolic depression associated with temperature decreases to < 20–25°C, dehydration, or renal failure (247). In alligators, dehydration per se had a less significant effect on renal urate excretion than low temperatures, which depressed renal tubular function (248). Articular gout also occurred in the joints of the extremities of crocodiles (247), as in other species. Reports of gout in chelonian species have been documented (245,246).

Soft tissue urate deposition is a commonly reported occurrence in herbivorous reptiles with a high protein diet and/or dehydration induced renal failure, and in association with suboptimal management practices in captive reptiles

(249). A poor response to treatment has been noted in reptiles, perhaps because of the often advanced progression and severity of the disease before it is diagnosed (243, 250). Unilateral nephrectomy has been advocated when urate deposits can be demonstrated to reside predominately in only one kidney (251).

Gout was linked to high mortality rates in one study of exothermic reptiles, including 12.3% in snakes and 11.7% in lizards; in chelonians, which are typically more ureotelic, the rate was 3.9% (252). In nonendothermic species, the active secretion of uric acid in the renal tubules diminishes in response to decreased ambient temperatures. Low ambient temperatures may further reduce urate solubility in the blood, but liver production and protein metabolism also probably decrease.

D. Gout in Avians

Although genetically prone gout strains have been characterized, it is interesting that high protein diets are usually required in these birds to develop clinical disease (253). In commercial flocks, gout has been shown to occur on lower protein diets (254). Other factors may play a role. Visceral gout has been associated with ochratoxicosis in chickens (255); this nephrotoxin is widespread in nature, and chickens were more susceptible than turkeys or quail (256). Similarly, oosporein toxicity caused severe visceral and articular gout. Gout was observed in rooks *(Corvus frugilegus)* and pheasants *(Phasianus colchicus)* undergoing toxicity studies with 3-chloro-4-methyl-benzamine HC1, a putative avicide (303). Urate deposits in the kidneys were unimpressive. Both liver and renal proximal tubular necrosis were evident in both species, although the rooks appeared more susceptible. Alloxan induced hyperglycemia, hyperuricemia, and urate deposition in pigeons (258). In eight spontaneous gout cases seen in aviary birds received from a zoo for necropsy, all had renal urate deposits, 67% had superficial heart associated deposits, and only 50% had articular lesions. The cranes examined in this series had high protein diets, and vitamin A deficiency and cold temperatures were considered as contributing factors in gout development (259). Pre-formed Vitamin A is required by some species, such as raptorial birds (260), so the form in which it is given may be important. Hyperuricemia is a late sign, after significant pathology has occurred (261). Conversely, drugs that compete for renal tubular secretion, such as p-aminohippuric acid in birds (262), lead to hyperuricemia and gout. Therefore, methods of early gout detection may be of more value than treatment. Visceral gout induction occurred in pigeons fed a 16% (on a dry matter basis) complete psittacine diet within a few days when water intake was kept at maintenance levels. However, reducing the protein content to 8% and supplying maintenance water did not cause disease over the next 10 days of study (Wimsatt, 1995 unpublished data). Monosodium glutamate caused rapid gout signs in chickens, and part of this effect was believed to be due to the administration of a urate precursor (263).

In a retrospective study, urinary failure induced gout had an incidence of ≈6% in commercial poultry operations over a 9-year period (264). Certain strains of infectious bursal disease appear to preferentially attack the urinary system and predispose to gout (265). Gout has been attributed to decreased water intake, toxins (261,263), infection (266,267), increased (e.g., dietary) bicarbonate (261,268), and Vitamin A deficiency in poultry (265,269,270). The origin of secondary gout could result from overt urinary obstruction rather than renal parenchymal damage (265), as occurs in nephrolithiasis or in Vitamin A deficiency when the ureters plug (187).

A causal relationship between renal dysfunction and visceral gout has been suggested (265) (186). Experimental avian influenza inoculations of waterfowl strains into chickens caused renal gout in 78% of the birds that died; epicardial and pericardial urate deposits were present in some cases (267). Visceral gout associated with inexperienced handlers was reported in chicks during sexing (271). Stress induced corticosterone elevations and adrenal hypertrophy leading to visceral gout lesions were thought to be reversed by estradiol and/or progresterone in castrated roosters following ureter cannulation surgery (272). Other inciting agents reported include avian influenza (267) eimeria infection led to transient hyperuricemia in a susceptible chicken strain (273). *Clostridium perfringins* type A toxin injections induced nephritis and uric acid diathesis in captive willow ptarmigan (274). Supplying grass mix rather than just lowering dietary protein content of the concentrate to better match the low protein density and fiber of the natural diet in early winter greatly reduced the incidence of gout associated with clostridial toxemia (275). Seasonal shifts in the incidence of gout were not related to changes in liver xanthine dehydrogenase levels (276).

Of some confusion is the fact that synovial urate deposits have been observed in association with visceral lesions (187). Siller (187) has noted that renal gout leads a to rapid death, and that the synovial lesions accompanying visceral gout have little or no inflammation associated with them as a result. In addition, since birds do not make Hageman's factor, kinin release by this mechanism seems unlikely.

Articular gout in poultry is rarer than renal gout and appears to have a genetic basis (188). Articular gout has a predisposition for the extremities (metatarsal-phalangeal and interphalangeal) joints as in man. The wing and vertebral joints have been reported to be involved infrequently, the latter having connections to the air sacs may maintain a lower temperature, more like the extremities. The wattle contained deposits in some cases, thus synovial tissue trophism alone appears to be an unlikely explanation in birds (187).

E. Gout in Mammals

Gout in dalmations presents most commonly as a urinary obstruction resulting from renal, ureteral, or cystic stone development. The stones are composed primarily of sodium urate, lending credence to a precipitating metabolic defect and secondary renal urinary compromise (277). Experimental models of acute gout-associated attacks have been developed in the canine, and were caused using intra-articular injection of urate (278–284), or by instilling endotoxin absorbed urate crystals into the joints (285). Similar studies involving intra-articular sodium urate injections have been reported in the rabbit (286) and rat (287). Hyperuricemic nephropathy was induced in rats fed uric acid and/or oxonic acid (288–290). Stavric and Nera reviewed the use of the rat (especially uricase inhibition) to study gout (291).

Hyperuricemia in humans does not cause gout in all individuals, yet hyperuricemia is usually required for gout to occur. Under normal conditions, the liver's capacity to produce uric acid can exceed the capacity of excretory mechanisms. Gout can be seen as the result of conditions or disease states leading to increased production of uric acid, decreased blood carrying capacity, or reduced excretion. Therefore, species that do not produce uric acid in any amount are less prone to develop gout. However, species apparently at low risk for developing gout have been documented to do so, indicating that even at low levels of production, clinical gout can still arise and can respond to standard gout treatment (262).

Chronic renal disease induced calcium gout *(calcinosis circumstripta)*, having a predilection for the lower legs in dogs; this condition could be mistaken for gout (89) except that predisposing hypercalcemia and hyperphosphatemia were characteristic (292) rather than uricemia (299) as documented in true gout. Overproduction with adequate renal compensatory capacity may lead to hyperuricosuric calcium oxalate nephrolithiasis, especially at urine pHs below 5.47 (293). In this setting, urates may serve as a nidus of calcium oxalate precipitation (294). Similarly, dalmation specific hyperuricemia typically presents as urate nephrolithiasis. Although uric acid may be produced as a metabolic intermediate in the production of other nitrogenous endproducts, and accumulation of urates due to an innate error of urate metabolism is reported in humans (295,296), specific metabolic defects in urate synthesis have not been identified in nonhuman species as yet. Drugs that compete for renal tubular secretion, such as probenecid in dogs (297), can lead to hyperuricemia, ultimately precipitating acute gout.

Diet was suggested as a potential cause of cutaneous urate deposits in a hyperuricemic Amazon river dolphin *(Inia geoffrensis)*, because little is known of their blood parameters or habits in the wild. This animal responded to allupurinol therapy (298). Similarly, a hyperuricemic lame painful dog responded to colchicine (299). Chemotherapy, myeloproliferative disease, and sickle-cell-like disorders would be expected to induce increased uric acid synthesis although not characterized in animals to date.

Finally, decreased renal excretion of preformed uric acid can occur for many reasons. In addition to renal excretory dysfunction such as is seen in chronic renal disease, urate excretion is aggravated by the therapeutic use of aspirin and thiazide diuretics. Hyperuricemia occurs in response to the toxic effects of nephrotoxins such as lead, secondary to imbibing alcohol, or during lactic acidosis and ketoacidosis, which acidify the urine. Likewise, species producing predominantly uric acid, are more prone to develop gout in response to a metabolic imbalance than ureotelic species.

Excessive dietary sources of purines and protein, such as may be fed to nonmammalian noncarnivorous species in captivity, could predispose to gout, especially with water restriction, although diet per se is not always shown to be directly responsible (300). Purine-free diets caused a 35% decrease in uric acid levels in the healthy male volunteers, whereas addition of RNA to the diet increased uric acid levels in the blood (211). Oddly, the role of purines in non-human gout has not been studied.

Hyperuricemia was a salient feature of experimental *Clostridia dificile* toxin injections in young macaques (301), resulted from handling stress, and appeared to follow a circadian rhythm in Capaebian monkeys (*Capella*) (35). Hyperuricemia was observed in baboons that had their renal arteries partially clamped during pregnancy to create a model of pregnancy-induced hypertension (302). Essential hypertension is associated with hyperuricemia in humans, and insulin resistance may be a common link relating these disorders. If fetal demand for increased nitrogen metabolism could also explain this phenomenon, hyperuricemia would then result during pregnancy and be expected to be higher with twins. Moreover, renal load during pregnancy is increased and the excretion of uric acid could therefore be less efficient. Finally, an attractive hypothesis for uric acid elevation that may explain increases associated with exercise, lead poisoning, alcohol overindulgence, and obesity that is inclusive of renal mechanisms, is that compensatory uric acid synthesis occurs. Hyperuremia might thus act as a physiological antioxidant to meet increased oxidative stress during periods when lipids peroxidative damage is likely (213). Uric acid has been shown to be protective in vitro in protecting against red cell lysis and peroxidation (214), and may be particularly important as an antioxidant in newborns, who maintain higher blood urate levels (214).

REFERENCES

1. W. H. Dantzler, Chapter 8: Urate excretion in nonmammalian vertebrates, In: W. N. Kelley and I. M. Weiner, eds., Uric Acid, Springer-Verlag, New York, N.Y., 1978: 185–210.
2. F. Roch-Ramel and G. Peters, Chapter 9: Urinary excretion of uric acid in nonhuman mammalian species, In: W. N. Kelley and I. M. Weiner, eds., Uric Acid, Springer-Verlag, New York, N.Y., 1978: 211–255.
3. J. W. Campbell, J. E. Vorhaben, and D. D. Smith Jr., Uricoteley: its nature and origin during the evolution of tetrapod vertebrates, *J Exp Zool 243:*349–363 (1987).
4. J. B. Balinsky, Phylogenetic aspects of purine metabolism, *S Afr Med J 46:*993–997 (1972).

5. J. W. Campbell, L. Goldstein, Nitrogen metabolism and the environment. J. W. Campbell, ed., New York, NY: Academic Press, 1970.
6. J. W. Campbell, The vertebrates, In: J. W. Campbell, ed., Comparative biochemistry of nitrogen metabolism, Vol 2 Academic Press, New York, N. Y., 1970 pp. 796–887.
7. G. H. Hitchings, Chapter 1: Uric acid: chemistry and synthesis, In: W. N. Kelley and I. M. Weiner, eds., Uric Acid, Springer-Verlag, New York, N. Y., 1978: 1–20.
8. J. B. Wyngaarden and W. N. Kelley, Gout and hyperuricemia, Grune and Stratton, New York, N. Y., 1976: 53–66.
9. L. Stevens, Chapter 5: Protein and amino acid metabolism, *Avian Biochemistry and Molecular Biology,* L. Stevens, ed., Cambridge University Press, Cambridge, England (1996).
10. P. D. Sturkie, Chapter 16. Kidneys, exrarenal salt excretion and urine, In: P. D. Sturkie, *Avian Physiology,* 4th Ed., Springer-Verlag, New York, N. Y., 359–382 (1986).
11. J. P. Mapes, H. A. Krebs Rate-limiting factors in urate synthesis and gluconeogenesis in avian liver, *Biochem J 172:*193–203 (1978).
12. P. A. King, L. Goldstein, Renal excretion of nitrogenous compounds in vertebrates, *Renal Physiol 8:*261–278 (1985).
13. C. M. Wood, Chapter 13: Ammonia and urea metabolism and excretion, In: D. H. Evans, ed., The Physiology of Fishes, CRC Publishers, Boca Raton, Fla., 379–426 (1993).
14. P. H. Yancey, G. N. Somero, Counteraction of urea destabilization of protein structure by methylamine osmoregulatory compounds of elasmobranch fishes, *Biochem J 183:*317 (1979).
15. J. B. Balinsky, M. M. Cragg, E. Baldwin, The adaptation of amphibian waste nitrogen excretion to dehydration, *Comp Biochem Physiol 3:*236–244 (1961).
16. F. Khalil, G. Haggag, Nitrogenous excretion in crocodiles, *J Exp Biol 35:*552–555 (1958).
17. V. Moyle, Nitrogenous excretion in chelonian reptiles, *Biochem J 44:*581–584 (1949).
18. W. B. Baze, F. R. Horn, Ureogenesis in chelonia, *Comp Biochem Physiol 34:*91–100 (1970).
19. A. F. Munro, The ammonia and urea excretion of different amphibia during their development and morphogenesis, *Biochem J 54:*29–36 (1953).
20. M. P. Schulman, Purines and pyrimidines, In: D. M. Greenberg, ed., Metabolic Pathways, Vol. II, Academic Press, New York, N. Y., 389–457 (1961).
21. J. F. Henderson, A. R. P. Paterson, Nucleotide Metabolism, An Introduction, Academic Press, New York, N. Y. (1973). pp 304.
22. K. Simkiss, Sex differences in the acid-base balance of adult and immature fowl, *Comp Biochem Physiol 34:*777–778 (1970).
23. R. A. Coulson, T. Hernandez, Kidney. *Comp Biochem Physiol 74b:*143–175 (1983).
24. J. Maetz, Interaction of salt and ammonia transport in aquatic organisms, In: J. W. Campbell and L. Goldstein, eds., Nitrogen Metabolism and the Environment, Academic Press, New York, N. Y., 105–154 (1972).

25. R. F. Pitts, Chapter 15. Production and excretion of ammonia in relation to acid-base regulation, In: J Orloff, ed., Handbook of Physiology, Section 8, Renal Physiology, American Physiology Society, Bethesda, Md. (1973).
26. F. M. A. McNabb, R. A. McNabb, I. D. Prather, R. N. Conner, C. S. Adkisson, Nitrogen excretion by turkey vultures, *Condor 82:*219–223 (1980).
27. B. Lipstein, P. Boer, O. Sperling, Regulation of de novo purine synthesis in chick liver. Role of phosphoribosylpyrophosphate availability and of salvage purine nucleotide synthesis, *Biochim Biophys Acta 521:*45–54 (1978).
28. I. H. Fox, Chapter 5. Degradation of purine nucleotides, In: Uric Acid, Handbook of Experimental Pharmacology, Vol 51, N. Kelley and I. M. Weiner, eds., Springer-Verlag, New York, N. Y., 106–108 (1978).
29. E. J. Morgan, Distribution of xanthine oxidase, *Biochem J 20:*1282–1291 (1926).
30 R. G. Abramson, M. S. Lipkowitz, Evolution of the uric acid transport mechanisms in vertebrate kidney, *Comp Physiol 3:*115–153 (1990).
31. P. A. Simkin, Uric acid binding to serum proteins: differences among species, *Proc Soc Exp Biol Med 139:*604–606 (1972).
32. R. Greger, F. Lang, P. Deetjen, Renal excretion of purine metabolites, urate and allantoin, by the mammalian kidney, In: K. Thuran, ed., Kidney and Urinary Tract Physiology, Vol. 2, University Park Press, Baltimore, Md., 257–281 (1976).
33. J. N. Loeb, Influence of temperature on the solubility of monosodium urate, *Arthritis Rheum 15:*189–191 (1972).
34. R. Greger, F. Lang, F. Puls, P. Deetjen, Urate interaction with plasma proteins and erythrocytes: possible mechanism for urate resorption in the kidney medulla, *Pflügers Arch 352:*121–133 (1974).
35. T. Shinosaki, H. Inagaki, T. Nakai, T. Yammashita, Y. Yonetani. Circadian Rhythm of plasmauric acid and handling stress-induced Hyperuricemia in conscious cebus monkeys. *Jap J Pharmacol 58*: 443–450 (1992)..
36. F. Lang, Parameters and mechanisms of urate transport in the rat kidney, Amino acid transport and uric acid transport, S. Silbernagl, F. Lang, R. Gregor, eds., Conference Proceedings, 1975, 217–227.
37. R. Greger, F. Lang, P. Deetjen, Handling of uric acid by the rat kidney. I. microanalysis of uric acid in the proximal tubular fluid, *Pflügers Arch 324:*279–287 (1971).
38. E. B. Marys, Secretion as a factor in elimination by the bird kidney, *J Physiol (Lond.) 58:*276–287 (1924).
39. R. Levine, W. Q. Wolfson, R. Lenel, Concentration and transport of true urate in the plasma of the azotemic chicken, *Am J Physiol 151:*186–191 (1947).
40. J. A. Shannon, The excretion of uric acid by the chicken, *J Cell Comp Physiol 11:*135–148 (1938).
41. L. Martindale, Renal urate synthesis in the fowl *(Gallus domesticus), Comp Biochem Physiol A 53:*389–391 (1976).
42. V. H. Shoemaker, Osmoregulation and excretion in birds In: D. S. Farner, J. R. King, K. C. Parker, eds., Avian Biology, Vol. II, Academic Press, New York, N. Y. 533–536 (1972).
43. E. J. Landon, C. E. Carter, The preparation properties and inhibition of hypoxanthine dehydrogenase of avian kidney, *J Biol Chem 235:*819–824 (1960).

44. N. L. Edson, H. A. Krebs, A. Model, The synthesis of uric acid in the avian organism: hypoxanthine as an intermediary metabolite, *Pflügers Arch 360:*1–6 (1975).
45. T. Y. Chin, A. J. Quebbeman, Quantitation of renal uric acid synthesis in the chicken, *Am J Physiol 234:*F446–F451 (1978).
46. A. J. Quebbeman, Renal synthesis of uric acid, *Am J Physiol 224:*1398–1402 (1973).
47. R. Itoh, K. Tsushima, Comparisons of adaptations to diet of enzymes involved in uric acid production from IMP in chickens and rats, *J Biochem (Toyko) 75:*715–721 (1974).
48. F. Stirpe, E. Della Corte, Regulation of xanthine dehydrogenase in chicken liver. Effect of starvation and of oral administration of purines and purine nucleotides, *Biochem J 94:*309–313 (1965).
49. G. R. Greenberg, Incorporation of carbon-labeled formic acid and carbon dioxide into hypoxanthine in the pigeon liver homogenastes, *Arch Biochem Biophys 19:*337–339 (1948).
50. N. L. Edson, H. Krebs, A. Model, The synthesis of uric acid in the avian organism: hypoxantine as an intermediate metabolite, *Biochem J 30:*1380–1385 (1936).
51. T. A. Krenitsky, R. Papionannou, G. B. Elion, Human hypoxanthine phosphoribosyltransferase I. Purification, properties and specificity, *J Biol Chem 244:*1263–1270 (1969).
52. C. F. Strittmatter, Studies on avian dehydrogenase, *J Biol Chem 240:*2557–2564 (1965).
53. D. A. Richert, W. W. Westerfield, Xanthine oxidases in different species, *Proc Soc Exp Biol Med 76:*252–254 (1951).
54. R. Fujii, Cytophysiology of fish chromatophores, *Int Rev. Cytol 143:*191 (1993).
55. G. N. Lapennas, K. Schmidt-Nielsen, Swim bladder permeability to oxygen, *J Exp Biol 67:*175 (1977).
56. E. J. Denton, J. D. Liddicoat, D. W. Taylor, Impermeable "silvery" layers in fishes, *J Physiol 207:*64P (1970).
57. G. L. Walls, The Vertebrate Eye, Cranbrook Institute of Science, Brookfield Hills, Mich., Bulletin No. 9 pp. 235–244 (1942).
58. E. S. Zyznar, F. B. Cross, J. A. C. Nicol, Uric acid in the tapetum lucidum of mooneyes Hiodon (Hiodontidae Teleostei), *Proc R Soc Lond B 201:*1–6 (1978).
59. J. A. C. Nicol, Uric in the stratum argenteum of toadfishes opsanus, *Can J Zool 58:*492–496 (1980).
60. J. Needham, Biochemistry and morphogenesis, Cambridge University Press, Cambridge, England pp. 505–523 (1942).
61. P. M. Bradfield, G. Baggott, Effect of water loss upon urate, urea and ammonia content of the egg of the Japanese Quail (Coturnix coturnix japonica), *Comp Biochem Physiol 106A:*187–193 (1993).
62. G. C. Packard, M. J. Packard, Patterns of nitrogen excretion by embryonic softshell turtles *(Trionyx spiniferus)* developing in cleidoic eggs., *Science 221:*1049–1050 (1983).
63. M. Tomita, Beiträge zur embryo chemie der reptilien, *J Biochem 10:*351–356 (1929).
64. W. A. Dunson, C. R. Bramham, Evaporative water loss and oxygen consumption

of three small lizards from the Florida Keys: *Sphaerodactylus cinerus, S. notatus,* and *Anolis sagrei, Physiol Zool 54:*253–259 (1981).
65. P. P. Cohen, G. W. Brown, Ammonia metabolism and urea biosynthesis, In: M. Florkin and M. S. Mason, eds., *Comparative Biochemistry,* Vol. 2, Academic Press, New York, N. Y. (1960).
66. V. H. Shoemaker, L. L. McClanahan, Enzymatic correlates and ontogeny of uricotelism in tree frogs of the genus Phyllomedusa, *J Exp Zool 220:*163–169 (1982).
67. D. J. Stewart, W. N. Holmes, G. Fletcher, The renal excretion of nitogenous compounds by the duck *(Anas platyrhynchos)* maintained in fresh water and on hypertonic saline, *J Exp Biol 50:*527–539 (1969).
68. C. L. Prosser, Comparative animal physiology, W. B. Saunders, Philadelphia, PA, p. 888 (1950).
69. J. D. Wallach, Feeding and nutritional diseases, In: M. E. Fowler, ed., Zoo and Wild Animal Medicine, W. B. Saunders, Philadelphia, Pa., 123–128 (1978).
70. F. Khalil, G. Haggag, Ureotelism and uricotelism in tortoises, *J Exp Zool 130:*423–432 (1955).
71. L. J. Robers, The nitrogen excretion of Chelonia longicollis under conditions of hydration and dehydration, *Comp Biochem Physiol 18:*249–260 (1966).
72. W. H. Dantzler, B. Schmidt-Nielsen, Excretion in fresh-water turtle *(Pseudemys scripta)* and desert tortoise *(Gopherus agassizii), Am J Physiol 210:*198–210 (1966).
73. P. J. Bentley, Osmorgulation in reptiles, In: C. Gans, ed., Biology of the Reptilia, Academic Press, New York, N. Y. Vol. V (1976).
74. W. H. Dantzler, Renal adaptations of desert vertebrates, *Bioscience 32:*108–113 (1982).
75. A. B. Gutman, Significance of uric acid as a nitrogenous waste in vertebrate evolution, *Arthritis Rheum 8:*614–620 (1965).
76. H. W. Smith, Excretion of ammonia and urea by the gills of fish, *J Biol Chem 81:*727 (1929).
77. M. D. J. Sayer, J. Davenport, The relative importance of the gills to ammonia and urea excretion in five seawater and one teleost species, *J Fish Biol 31:*561 (1987).
78. R. R. Smith, G. L. Rumsey, Nutrient utilization by fish, Firstt Int. Symp., Feed Composition, Animal Nutrient Requirements, and Computerization of diets, Utah State University, Utah Argricultural Experiment Station, Logan, Utah, 320 (1976).
79. F. Vellas, A. Sefaty, L'ammoniaque et l' urée chez un Téléosteen d'eau douce: la Carpe *(Cyprinus carpio L.), J Physiol (Paris) 68:*591 (1974).
80. L. J. Read, A study of ammonia and urea production and excretion in the freshwater-adapted form of the Pacific lamprey *(Entosphenus tridentatus), Comp Biochem Physiol 26:*455 (1968).
81. N. Saha, B. K. Ratha, Comparative study of ureogenesis in freshwater air-breathing teleosts, *J Exp Zool 252:*1 (1989).
82. V. A Cvancara, Studies on tissue arginase and ureogenesis in freshwater teleosts, *Comp Biochem Physiol 30:*489–496 (1969).
83. N. Saha, B. K. Ratha, Comparative study of ureogenesis in freshwater air-breathing teleosts, *J Exp Zool 252:*1 (1989).
84. D. R. Watson, Gout in a dog. *Vet Rec 104:*129 (1979).

85. T. Noguchi, Y. Takada, S. Fujiwara, Degradation of uric acid to urea and glyoxylate in peroxisomes, *J Biol Chem 254:*5272–5275 (1979).
86. S. Hayashi, S. Fujiwara, T. Noguchi, Degradation of uric acid in fish liver peroxisomes. Intraperoxisomal localization of hepatic allantoicase and purification of its peroxisomal membrane-bound form, *J Biol Chem 264:*3211–3215 (1989).
87. L. J. Read, Absence of ureogenic pathways in the liver of the hagfish *(Bdellostoma cirrhatum), Comp Biochem Physiol 51B:*139 (1975).
88. L. Goldstein, R. P. Forster, The role of uricolysis in the production of urea by fishes and other aquatic invertebrates, *J Comp Biochem Physiol 14:*567 (1965).
89. R. Connes, M. Granie Prie, J. P. Diaz, J. Paris, Ultrastructure des bourgeons du gout du teleosteen marin Dicentrarchus labrax L, *Can J Zool 66:*2133–2142 (1988).
90. P. C. Withers, S. S. Hillman, R. C. Drewes, O. M. Sokol, Water loss and nitrogen excretion in sharp-nosed reed frogs (Hyperolius nasutus: Anura, Hyperoliidae), *J Exp Biol 97:*335–343 (1982).
91. A. Salibian, L. A. Fichera, Excretion nitrogenada urinaria de Bufo Arenarum, *Bolet Fisiol Animal (Sao Paulo) 8:*109–118 (1984).
92. T. Noguchi, S. Fujiwara, S. Hayashi, Cudution of allantoinase and allantoicase involved in urate degradation in liver peroxisomes, A rapid purification of amphibian allantoinase and comparison with fish allantoinase and allantoincase. *J Biol Chem 261:*4221–4223 (1986).
93. V. H. Shoemaker, P. E. Bickler, Kidney and bladder function in the uricotelic treefrog *(Phylomedussa sauvagei), J Comp Physiol 133:*211–218 (1979).
94. G. W. Brown, P. P. Cohen, Comparative biochemistry of urea synthesis, *Biochem J 75:*82–91 (1960).
95. J. Bordley, A. N. J. Richards, Quantitative studies of the composition of glomerular urine, *J Biol Chem 101:*193–221 (1933).
96. B. Lueken, *Arch Ges Physiol 229:*557 (1932).
97. E. Baldwin, Chapter 13: Excretory metabolism of proteins and amino-acids, (5th edn ed.) Dynamic Aspects of Biochemistry, 5th Ed., Cambridge University Press, Cambridge, England, 263–289 (1967).
98. E. R. Jacobson, J. M. Gaskin, M. B. Brown, Chronic upper respiratory disease in free-ranging desert tortoises *(Xerobates agassizii), J Wildl Dis 27:*296 (1990).
99. T. W. Campbell, Chapter 57. Sea turtle rehabilitation, In: D. M. Mader, ed., *Reptile Medicine and Surgery,* W. B. Saunders, Philadelphia, Pa., 427–436 (1996).
100. K. A. Bjorndal, Urine concentrations of ammonia, urea and uric acid in the green turtle, *Chelonia mydas, Compar Biochem Physiol a Compar Physiol 63:*509–510 (1979).
101. D. A. Denton, M. Reich, Ureotelism of echidna and platypus, *Science 139:*1225 (1963).
102. W. N. McFarland, W. A. Wimsatt, Renal function and its relation to the ecology of the vampire bat, *Desmodus rotundus, Comp Biochem Physiol 28:*985–1006 (1969).
103. M. Florkin, G. Duchateau, Les formes du systéme enzymatique de L'uricolyse et l'evolution du catabolisme purique chez les animaux, *Arch Int Physiol 53:*267–307 (1943).
104. H. A. Simmonds, P. J. Hatfield, J. S. Cameron, *Biochem Pharmacol 20:*2553–2563 (1973).

105. J. Ewing, *Proc N Y Path Soc* (1895).
106. R. Verchow, *Arch Path Anat Physiol 35:*358 (1866).
107. R. Verchow, *Arch Path Anat Physiol 36:*147 (1866).
108. D. A. Farebrother, P. J. Hatfield, H. A. Simonds, J. S. Cameron, A. S. Jones, A. Cadenhead, Acute intratubular crystal deposition causing permanent renal damage in the pig. *Adv Exp Med Biol 41:*523–534 (1974).
109. P. J. Hatfield, H. A. Simmonds, D. A. Farebrother, A. S. Jones, Acute intratubular crystal deposition causing permanent renal damage in the pig, *Ann Rheum Dis 32:*393 (1973).
110. A. J. Quebbeman, Renal synthesis of uric acid, *Am J Physiol 224:*1398–1402 (1973).
111. M. Friedman, S. O. Byers, Distribution of uric acid in rat tissues and its production in tissue homogenates, *Am J Physiol 172:*29–32 (1953).
112. T. Y. Chin, W. Cacini, M. J. Zmuda, A. J. Quebbemann, Quanitification of renal uric acid synthesis in the rat, *Am J Physiol 238:*F481–F487 (1980).
113. E. J. Weinman, S. C. Sansom, D. A. Steplock, A. U. Sheth, T. F. Knight, H. O. Senekjian, Secretion of urate in the proximal tubule of the rat, *Am J Physiol:*F383–F387 (1980).
114. A. M. Kahn, S. Branham, E. J. Weinman, Mechanism of urate and p-aminohippurate transport in rat renal microvillus membrane vesicles, *Am J Physiol 245:*F151–F158 (1983).
115. A. M. Kahn, H. Shelat, E. J. Weinman, Urate and p-aminohippurate transport in rat renal basolateral vesicles, *Am J Physiol 249:*F654–F661 (1985).
116. R. G. Abramson, V. F. King, M. C. Reif, E. Leal-Pinto, S. B. Baruch, Urate uptake in membrane vesicles of rat renal cortex. Effect of copper, *Am J Physiol 242:*F158–F170 (1982).
117. R. G. Abramson, M. S. Lipowitz, Carrier-mediate concentrative urate transport in rat renal membrane vesicles, *Am J Physiol 248:*F574–F584 (1985).
118. A. M. Kahn, P. S. Aronson, Urate transport via anion exchange in dog renal microvillus membrane vesicles, *Am J Physiol 244:*F56–F63 (1983).
119. W. Lathem, B. B. Davis, G. P. Rodnan, Renal tubular secretion of uric acid in the mongrel dog, *Am J Physiol 199:*9–12 (1960).
120. M. Friedman, S. O. Byers, Observations concerning the causes of the excess excretion of uric acid in the dalmation dog (1948). *J Biol Chem 175:*727–735.
121. R. H. Kessler, K. Hierholzer, R. S. Gurd, Localization of urate transport in the nephron of mongrel and Dalmation dog kidney, *Am J Physiol 1959:*601–603 (1959).
122. T. F. Yu, L. Berger, S. Kupfer, A. B. Gutman, Tubular secretion of urate in the dog, *Am J Physiol 199:*1199–1204 (1960).
123. F. W. Klemperer, H. Trimble, A. B. Hastings, Uricase of dogs including the Dalmation, *J Biol Chem 125:*445–449 (1938).
124. A. M. Harvey, H. N. Christensen, Uric acid transport system: apparent absence in erythrocytes of the Dalmation coach hound, *Science 145:*826–827 (1964).
125. K. Overgaard-Hansen, U. V. Lassen, Active transport of uric acid through the human erythrocyte membrane, *Nature (Lond.) 184:*553–554 (1959).
126. B. Lucas-Heron, C. Fontenaille, Uric acid transport characteristics in human red blood cells, *J Clin Chem Clin Biochem 14:* Abst. 307 (1976).

127. C. Bishop, J. H. Talbott, Uric acid: its role in biological processes and the influence upon it of physiological, pathological and pharmacological agents, *Pharmacol Rev 5:*231–274 (1953).
128. M. D. Skeith, L. A. Healey, Urate clearance in Cebus monkeys, *Am J Physiol 214:*582–584 (1968).
129. R. Bluestone, I. Kippen, J. R. Klinenberg, M. W. Whitehouse, Effect of some uricosuric and anti-inflammatory drugs on the binding of uric acid to human serum albumin in vitro, *J Lab Clin Med 76:*85–91 (1970).
130. I. M. Weiner, G. M. Fanelli, Renal urate excretion in animal models, *Nephron 14:* 33–47 (1975).
131. D. I. Frazier, M. P. Jones, S. E. Orosz, Pharmacokinetic considerations of the renal system in birds: Part I. Anatomic and physiologic principles of allometric scaling, *J Av Med Surg 9:*92–103 (1995).
132. W. H. Dantzler, E. J. Braun, Comparative nephron function in reptiles, birds, and mammals, *Am J Physiol 239:*R197–R213 (1980).
133. W. H. Dantzler, The role of the kidneys and bladder in the handling of water and solutes in the fresh water turtle (Pseudemys scripta and the desert tortoise) *(Gopherus agassizii),* Ph.D. thesis, Duke University, Durham, N. C., (1964).
134. L. Hill, W. H. Dawbin, Nitrogen excretion in the tuatara, *Splenodon punctatus, Comp Biochem Physiol 31:*453–468 (1969).
135. B. Schmidt-Nielsen, D. Schmidt, Renal function of *Splenodon punctatum, Comp Biochem Physiol 44A:*121–129 (1973).
136. J. M. Maixner, E. C. Ramsay, L. H. Arp, Effects of feeding on serum uric acid in captive reptiles, *J Zoo Anim Med 18:*62–65 (1987).
137. P. Zwart, Chapter 11: Urogenital system, In: *Manual of Reptiles,* Brit. Small Animal Veterinary Association. Cheltenham, England. 117–127 (1992).
138. J. M. Smeller, K. Slickers, M. Bush, Effect of feeding on plasma uric acid levels in snakes, *Am J Vet Res 39:*1556–1557 (1978).
139. J. T. Lumeij, J. D. Remple, Plasma urea, creatinine and uric acid concentrations in relation to feeding in peregrine falcons *(Falco peregrınus), Av Pathol 20:*79–83 (1991).
140. D. Wiggins, P. Lund, H. A. Krebs, Adaptation of urate synthesis in the chicken liver, *Comp Biochem Physiol 72B:*565–568 (1982).
141. F. M. A. McNabb, R. A. McNabb, Proportions of ammonia, urea, urate, and total nitrogen in avian urine and quantitative methods for their analysis on a single urine sample, *Poultry Sci 54:*1498–1505 (1975).
142. I. Tasaki, J. Okumura, Effect of protein level of diet on nitrogen excretion in fowls, *J Nutr 83:*34–38 (1964).
143. R. A. Teekill, C. E. Richardson, A. B. Watts, Dietary protein effects on urinary nitrogen components in the hen, *Poultry Sci. 47:*1260–1266 (1968).
144. O. Frank, Nutritional state and purine metabolism, *Adv Exp Med Biol:*0065–2598 (1977).
145. N. Zollner, A Griebsch, Diet and gout, *Adv Exp Med Biol 41:*435–442 (1974).
146. P. Hevia, R. H. Shaffer, W. C. Weir, A. J. Clifford, Plasma uric acid and hepatic purine enzyme levels in gouty chicks, *Fedn Proc 35:*282 (1976).
147. Y. Horie, K. Watanabe, Effects of dietary pyridoxine on larval growth, free amino acid pattern in haemolymph and uric acid excretion in the silkworm, Bombyx mori, *Insect Biochem 13:*205–212 (1983).

148. Y. Horie, T. Inokuchi, Protein synthesis and uric acid excretion in the absence of essential amino acids in the silkworm, Bombyx mori, *Insect Biochem 8:*251–254 (1978).
149. Y. Horie, K. Watanabe, Effect of various kinds of dietary protein and supplementation with limiting amino acids on growth, haemolymph components and uric acid excretion in the silkworm, Bombyx mori, *J Insect Physiol 29:*187–199 (1983).
150. O. H. Okada, K. Suzuki, Amino acid metabolism in rats fed a high protein diet without pyridoxine, *J Nutr 104:*287–293 (1974).
151. D. J. Kurtz, H. Levy, J. N. Kanfer, Cerebral lipids and amino acids in the vitamin-B6-deficient, *J Nutr 102:*291–298 (1972).
152. N. D. Woodward, P. C. Lee, N. W. Delapp, J. R. Fisher, Induction of chicken liver xantine dehydrogenase by purines, *Arch Biochem Biophys 153:*537–542 (1972).
153. P. B. Rowe, J. B. Wyngaarden, The mechanism of dietary alterations in rat hepatic xanthine oxidase levels, *J Biol Chem 241:*5571–5576 (1966).
154. R. T. Schimke, Adaptive characteristics of urea cycle enzymes in the rat, *J Biol Chem 237:*459–468 (1962).
155. G. L. Catignani, F. Chytil, W. J., Darby, Vitamin E deficiency: immunochemical evidence for increased accumulation of liver xanthine oxidase, *Proc Nat Acad Sci (USA) 71:*1966–1968 (1974).
156. R. C. Bray, Xanthine oxidase, (P. Boyer HL, K. Myrbach, eds., The Enzymes, 2nd ed., Academic Press Inc., New York, N.Y., 533 (1963).
157. K. V. Lazar, U. V. K. Mohamed, Uricotelism in insects, In: O. P. Agrawal, ed., Perspectives in Entomological Research, Scientific Publishers, Jodpur, pp. 1–13.
158. A. L. Lehninger, Chapter 24: The biosynthesis of amino acids; nitrogen fixation, In: Biochemistry, Worth Publishers, Inc., New York, N. Y., 557 (1970).
159 D. Eichelberg, K. P. Heil, Studies on the significance of the uric acid formation in the periwinkle Littorina littorea (L. 1758), *Medio Ambiente 10:*69–76 (1989).
160. K. M. Kulkarni, D. Q. Baramatiwala, Uric acid storage during season and temperature acclimation stress in snails Bellamya bengalensis, *Environment and Ecology (Kalyani) 4*(1):151–152 (1986).
161. K. M. Kulkarni, D. Q. Baramatiwala, S. S. Tankar, Thermal relations in the slug, Semperula maculata (Semper: 1885) 7. Uric acid contents, *J Curr Biosc 4*(1):5–7 (1987).
162. D. G. Cochran, Uric acid accumulation in young American cockroach nymphs, *Entomologia Experimentalis Et Applicata 25*(2):153–157 (1979).
163. D. E. Mullins, Isolation and partial characterization of uric acid crystals obtained from cockroach tissues *(Dictyoptera), JNY Entomol Soc 85:*192 (1978).
164. D. E. Mullins, Isolation and partial characterization of uric acid spherules obtained from cockroach tissues *(Dictyoptera), Com Biochem Physiol A: Comp Physiol 62:*699–705 (1979).
165. C. Schal, W. J. Bell, Ecological correlates of paternal investment of urates in a tropical cockroach, *Science 218:*170–173 (1982).
166. S. Morris, C. R. Bridges, M. K. Grieshaber, A new role for uric acid: modulator of haemocyanin oxygen affinity in crustaceans, *J Exp Zool 235:*135–139 (1985).
167. L. M. Botella, A. Moya, M. C. Gonzalez, J. L. Mensua, Larval stop, delayed devel-

opment and survival in overcrowded cultures of Drosophila melanogaster: effect of urea and uric acid, *Journal Of Insect Physiology 31*(3):179–185 (1985).

168. J. P. Loveridge, Observations on nitrogenous excretiona and water relations of Chiromantis xerampelina (Amphibia, Anura), *Arnoldia (Rhodesia) 5:*1–6 (1970).
169. V. H. Shoemaker, D. Balding, R. Ruibal, L. L. McClanahan, Uricotelism and low evaporative water loss in a South American frog, *Science 175:*1018–1020 (1972).
170. V. H. Showmaker, L. L. McClanahan, Evaporative water loss, nitrogen excretion and osmoregulation in phylomedusine frogs, *J Comp Physiol 100:*331–345 (1975).
171. N. J. Carlisky, V. Botbol, C. A. Garcia Argiz, A. Barrio, V. L. Lew, Properties and subcellular distribution of ornithine cycle enzymes in amphibian kidney, *Comp Biochem Physiol 25:*835–848 (1968).
172. J. B. Balinsky, S. M. Chemaly, A. E. Currin, A. R. Lee, R. L. Thompson, D. R. Van der Westhuizen, A comparative study of enzymes of urea and uric acid metabolism in different species of amphibia, and the adaptation to the environment of the tree frog *Chiromantis xerampelina, Comp Biochem Physiol 54B:*549–555 (1976).
173. E. K. Marshall, Kidney secretion in reptiles. *Proc Soc Exp Biol Med 29:*971–973 (1932).
174. T. W. Campbell, Chapter 22: Clinical pathology, In: D. M. Mader, ed., Reptile Medicine and Surgery, W. B. Saunders, Philadelphia, Pa., 248–257 (1996).
175. W. H. Dantzler, S. K. Bentley, Low sodium effects on PAH transport and permeabilities in isolated snake renal tubules, *Am J Physiol 230:*256–262 (1976).
176. W. H. Dantzler, Characteristics of urate transport by isolated perfused snake proximal renal tubules, *Am J Physiol 224:*445–453 (1973).
177. W. H. Dantzler, Effects of K, Na, and ouabain on urate and PAH uptake by snake and chicken kidney slices, *Am J Physiol 217:*1510–1519 (1969).
178. R. J. Montali, M. Bush, J. M. Smeller, The pathology of nephrotoxicity of gentamicin in snakes. A model for reptilian gout, *Vet Pathol 16:*108–115 (1979).
179. T. G. Baby, S. C. Goel, S. R. R. Reddy, A comparative study of arginase activity in lizards, *Physiol Zool 49:*286–291 (1976).
180. J. E. Vorhaben, J. W. Campbell, Glutamine synthetase: a mitochondrial enzyme in uricotelic species, *J Biol Chem 247:*2763–2767 (1972).
181. J. E. Minnich, P. A. Piehl, Spherical precipitates in the urine of reptiles, *Comp Biochem Physiol A 41:*551–554 (1972).
182. E. Skadhauge, Formation and composition of urine, Physiology and Biochemistry of Domestic Fowl, B. M. Freeman, ed., Academic Press, London, England, Vol. 4, 108–135 (1983).
183. J. T. Lumeij, Plasma urea, creatinine and uric acid concentrations in response to dehydration in racing pigeons *(Columbia livia domestica), Av Pathol 16:*377–382 (1987).
184. D. I. Frazier, M. P. Jones, S. E. Orosz, Pharmacokinetic considerations of the renal system in birds: Part II. Review of drugs ecreted by renal pathways, *J Av Med Surg 9:*104–121 (1995).
185. E. J. Braun, Renal response of the starling (Srurnus vulgaris) to an intravenous salt load, *Am J Physiol 234:*F270–F278 (1978).
186. W. G. Siller, Avian nephritis and visceral gout, *Lab Invest 8:*1319–1346 (1959).

187. W. G. Siller, Renal pathology of the fowl—a review, *Avian Pathology 10:*187–262 (1981).
188. R. K. Cole, R. E. Austic, Hereditary uricemia and articular gout in chickens, *Poult Sci 59:*951–975 (1980).
189. R. E. Austic, R. K. Cole, Hereditary variation in uric acid transport by avian kidney slices, *Am J Physiol 231:*1147–1151 (1976).
190 I. M. Weiner, G. H. Mudge, Renal tubular mechanisms for excretion of organic bases and acids, *Am J Med 36:*743–762 (1964).
191. M. J. Zmuda, A. J. Quebbemann, Localization of renal tubular uric acid transport defect in gouty chickens, *Am J Physiol 229:*820–825 (1975).
192. S. H. Fitz-Coy, S. A. Edgar, F. J. Hoerr, An outbreak of urolithiasis in single-comb white Leghorn pullets, *Avian Dis 32:*563–566 (1988).
193. J. W. Bennett, E. G. Bolen, Stress response in wintering freen-winged teal, *J Wildl Manage 42:*81–86 (1978).
194. J. G. Mori, J. C. George, Seasonal changes in serum levels of certain metabolites, uric acid and calcium in the migratory Canada goose (Branta canadensis interior). *Comp Biochem Physiol 59B:*263–269 (1978).
195. J. I. Okamura, I. Tasaki, Effect of fasting, in feeding and dietary protein level on uric acid and ammonia content of blood, liver and kidney in chickens, *J Nutr 92*:316–320 (1969).
196 M. A. Mansour, M. A. M. Hegazi, H. E. El Sheikh, Effect of Nephrostomum ranosum and Apharyngostrigea ibis on serum, proteins and uric acid of the Egyptian heron, *J Egyptian Soc Parasitol 14*(1):275–281 (1984).
197. J. L. Bollman, C. F. Schlotthauer, Experimental gout in turkeys, *Am J Dig Dis Nutr* 483–488 (1936).
198. Y. Cherel, Y. le Maho, Changes in body mass and plasma metabolites during short-term fasting in the king penguin, *Condor 90:*257–258 (1988).
199. N. Nagahara, T. Nishino, M. Kanisawa, K. Tsuhima, Effect of protein on purine nucleoside phosphorylase and xanthine dehydrogenase activities of liver and kidney in chicken and pigeon, *Comp Biochem Physiol 88B:*589–593 (1987).
200. J. E. Bird, M. M. Walser, G. E. Duke, Toxicity of gentamicin in red-tailed hawks, *J Am Vet Med Assoc 44:*1289–1291 (1983).
201. R. Blackburn, D. Prasad, The avian renal portal system: a model for studying nephrotoxicity of xenobiotics, *Toxicol Lett 53:*219–221 (1990).
202. J. T. Lumeij, P. T. Redig, Hyperuricaemia and visceral gout induced by allopurinol in red-tailed hawks *(Buteo jamaicensis), VIII. Tagung der Fachgruppe "Geflugelkrankheiten", Munchen 5:*265–269 (1992).
203. K. Quesenberry, Disorders of the musculoskeletal system, In: R. B. Altman SLC, G M Dorrestein & K. Quesenberry, ed., Avian Medicine and Surgery, W. B. Saunders Co., Philadelphia, Pa., 532–533 (1997).
204. R. Gerger, F. Lang, P. Deetjen, Urate handling by the rat kidney, *Pflügers Arch 352:*115–120 (1974).
205. F. Roch-Ramel, G. Peters, Urinary excretion of uric acid in nonhuman mammalian species. In: W. N. Kelley and I. M. Weiner, eds., Uric Acid, Handbook of Experimental Pharmacology Series, Springer-Verlag New York, N. Y., Vol. 51, 211–255, (1978).

206. P. A. Simkin, Uric acid metabolism in *Cebus* Monkeys, *Am J Physiol 221:*1105–1109 (1971).
207. D. C. Logan, D. E. Wilson, C. M. Flowers, P. J. Sparks, F. H. Tyler, Uric acid catabolism in the woolly monkey, *Metabolism 25:*517–522 (1976).
208. G. M. Fanelli, D. Bohn, S. Stafford, Functional characteristics of urate transport in the *Cebus* monkey, *Am J Physiol 218:*627–636 (1970).
209. P. Christen, W. C. Peacock, A. E. Christen, W. E. C. Wacker, Urate oxidase in primate phylogenesis, *Eur J Biochem 12:*3–5 (1970).
210. P. Christen, W. C. Peacock, A. E. Christen, W. E. C. Wacker, Urate oxidase in primates, *Folia Primatol (Basel) 13:*35–39 (1970).
211. Circulation, respiration, and fluid balance Volume 2 of Physiology and Biophysics Series. 20th ed. T. C. Ruch and H. D. Patton, eds., W. B. Saunders Co. 1973.
212. C. C. Tisher, R. M. Finkel, S. Rosen, E. M. Kendig, Renal microbodies in the Rhesus monkey, *Lab Invest 19:*1–6 (1968).
213. B. N. Ames, R. Cathcart, E. Schwiers, P. Hochstein, Uric acid provides an antioxidant defense in humans against oxidant- and radical-caused aging and cancer: a hypothesis, *Proc Natl Acad Sci 78:*6858–6862 (1981).
214. H. M. Berger, D. van Zoeren, J. Karsdon, The anti-oxidant capacity of uric acid and adaptation to a terrestrial environment, *Speculat Sci Techn 9:*83–84 (1986).
215. Y. Nakajima, T. R. Shanthra, G. H. Bourne, Histochemical detection of L-gulonolactone: phenazine methosulfate oxidoreductase activity in several mammals with special reference to synthesis of vitamin C in primates, *Histochemie 18:*293–301 (1969).
216. R. M. Nowak, J. L. Paradiso, The Primates, In: *Walker's Mammals of the World*, Johns Hopkins University Press, Baltimore, MD., 358–366 (1983).
217. I. Machtey, A. Meer, On the problem of hyperuricemia in certain physiological stress conditions, *Adv Exp Med Biol 41B:*419–21 (1974).
218. D. W. Knox, R. J. Montali, G. Migaki, Gout in reptiles and birds, with observations on a comparable syndrome in man, In: *The Comparative Pathology of Zoo Animals*, R. J. Montali and G. Migaki, eds., Smithsonian Institution Press, Washington, D. C., 137–141 (1980).
219. D. C. McFarland, S. G. Kenzy, C. N. Coon, A micromethod for plasma uric acid determinations in companion birds, *Av Dis 23:*772–774 (1979).
220. E. S. Canellakis, A. L. Tuttle, P. P. Cohen, A comparative study of the end-products of uric acid oxidation by peroxidases, *J. Biol Chem 213:*397–404 (1955).
221. J. B. Wyngaarden, W. N. Kelley, Gout and hyperuricemia, Grune and Stratton, New York, N. Y., 111–117 (1976).
222. L. B. Sorensen, D. J. Levinson, origin and extrarenal elimination of uric acid in man, *Nephron 14:*7–20 (1975).
223. E. J. Braun, C. E. Campbell, Uric acid decomposition in the lower gastrointestinal tract, *J Exp Zool, Suppl 3:*70–74 (1989).
224. A. Mortensen, A. R. Tindall, Caecal decomposition of uric acid in captive and free-ranging willow ptarmigan *(Lagopus lagopus lagopus), Acta Physiol Scand 111:*129–133 (1981).
225. E. M. Barnes, C. S. Impey, The occurrence and properties of uric acid decomposing anaerobic bacteria in the avian caecum, *J Appl Bacteriol 37:*393–409 (1974).

226. E. M. Barnes, C. S. Impey, Some properties of the nonspore forming anaerobes from poultry caeca, *J Appl Bacteriol 37:*393–409 (1972).
227. E. M. Barnes, Ecological concepts of the anaerobic flora in the avian intestine, *Am J Clin Nutr 30:*1793–1798 (1977).
228. E. M. Barnes, The avian intestinal flora with particular reference to the possible ecological significance of the cecal anaerobic bacteria, *Am J Clin Nutr 25:*1475–1479 (1972).
229. C. E. Campbell, E. J. Braun, Cecal degradation of uric acid in Gambel quail, *Am J Physiol 251 251:*R59–R62 (1986).
230. Y. Karasawa, M. Okamoto, H. Kawai, Ammonia production from uric acid and its absorption from the caecum of the cockerel, *Br Poultr Sci 29:*119–124 (1988).
231. J. Lind, B. G. Munck, O. Olsen, E. Skadhauge, Effects of sugars, amino acids and inhibitors on electrolyte transport across hen colon at different sodium chloride intakes, *J Physiol 305:*315–325 (1980).
232. E. J. Braun, P. R. Reimer, M. M. Pacelli, The nature of uric acid in avian urine, *Physiologist 30:*120 (1987).
233. G. E. Rice, E. Skadhauge, Caecal water and electrolyte absorption and the effects of acetate and glucose, in dehydrated, low-NaCl diet hens, *J Comp Physiol 147:*61–64 (1982).
234. Y. Cherel, J. C. Stahl, Y. le Maho, Ecology and physiology of fasting in king penguin chicks, *Auk 104:*254–262 (1987).
235. H. G. Schlumberger, Snovial gout in a parakeet, *Lab Invest 8:*1304–1318 (1959).
236. M. L. Petrak, Diseases of case and aviary birds, Lea & Febiger, Philadelphia, Pa., 492–497 (1982).
237. C. H. Chien, T. C. Yu, Histopathological study on systemic granuloma in catfish *(Parasilurus asotus), Nat Sci Counc Sympos Ser 7:*10–14 (1983).
238. R. L. Herman, Visceral granuloma and nephrocalcinosis, *US Bur. Sport Fish Wildl Fish Dis Leafl 32* (1971).
239. C. E. Dunbar, R. L. Herman, Visceral granuloma in brook trout *(Salvelinus fontinalis), J Nutr 101:*1445–1451 (1971).
240. C. D. Anderson, R. J. Robert, J. Macjebzuem, A. H. MacVicar, The hepato-renal syndrome in cultured turbot *(Scophthalmus maximus* L.), *J Fish Biol 8:*331–341 (1976).
241. H. I. Paperna, J. G. Harrison, G. W. Kissil, Pathology and histopathology of a systemic granuloma in sparus aurats (L) cultured in the Gulf of Aqabe, *J Fish Dis 3:*213–221 (1980).
242. J. D. Wallach, C. Hoessle, Visceral gout in captive reptiles, *J Am Vet Med Assoc 151:*897–899 (1967).
243. F. L. Frye, Reptile medicine and husbandry, *Vet Clin North Am Small Anim Pract 9:*415–428 (1979).
244. G. N. Buenviaje, P. W. Ladds, L. Melville, S. C. Manolis, Disease-husbandry associations in farmed crocodiles in Queensland and the Northern Territory, *Aust Vet J 71:*165–173 (1994).
245. F. L. Frye, F. R. Dutra, Articular pseudogout in a turtle *(Chrysemys s. elegans), Vet Med Sm An Clin 71:*658–659 (1976).

246. F. L. Frye, Nutritional disorders in reptiles, In: (G L G. L. Hoff FLF and E. R. Jacobson, eds.) Diseases of Amphibians and Reptiles, Plenum Press, New York, N. Y., 633–659 (1984).
247. P. Youngprapakorn, L. Ousavaplangchai, S. Kanchanapangka, A Color Atlas of the Diseases of the Crocodile, Crocodile Wildlife Breeding Research Center, Samutprakan Crocodile Farm and Zoo, Samutprakan Style Creative House, Thailand p. 76 (1995).
248. H. C. Dessauer, Chapter 1: Blood chemistry of reptiles, In: C. Gans, ed., *Biology of the Reptilia,* Academic Press, New York, N. Y. 1–72 (1970).
249. D. R. Mader, Gout, In: DRM, ed., *Reptile Medicine and Surgery,* W. B. Saunders Co., Philadelphia, Pa., 374–379 (1996).
250. K. Wright, Use of oral allopurinol and saline dialysis in management of hyperuricemia in a Chilean tortoise, *Bull Assoc Amphib Rept Vet 2:*7 (1992).
251. B. L. Raphael, Diagnosis and management of renal gout in captive snakes, *Am Associ Zoo Vet Proceed,* 1984, 53.
252. R. Ippen, H.-D. Schröder, Zu den Erkrankungren der reptilien, Verhandlungsbericht des 19th Internationalen Symposiums über die Erkrankungen der Zoo and Wildtiere, Akademie-Verlag, Berlin, Germany, 187–196 (1977).
253. D. W. Peterson, W. H. Hamilton, A. L. Lilyblade, Hereditary susceptibility to dietary induction of gout in selected lines of chickens, *J Nutr 101:*347–354 (1971).
254. G. H. Snoeyenbos, I. M. Reynolds, T. Tzianabos, Articular gout in turkeys-case report, *Av Dis 6:*32–36 (1962).
255. M. G. Prior, C. S. Sisodia, J. B. O'Neil, Acute oral ochratoxicosis in day-old white leghorns, turkeys and Japanese quail, *Poult Sci 55:*786–90 (1976).
256. K. B. Raper, D. I. Fennell, The Genus *Aspergillus,* Williams & Wilkins, Baltimore, Md., p. 380 (1965).
257. R. A. Pegram, R. D. Wyatt, T. L. Smith, Oosporein-toxicosis in the turkey poult, *Avian Dis 26:*47–59 (1982).
258. M. G. Goldner, G. Gomori, Effect of alloxan on carbohydrate and uric acid metab olism of the pigeon, *Proc Soc Exp Biol Med 58:*31–32 (1945).
259. S. Damodaran, S. Viswanathan, P. Mahalingma, Gout in cage and aviary birds, *Ind Vet J 55:*193–194 (1978).
260. W. H. Halliwell, Diseases of birds of prey, *Vet Clin North Am Small Anim Pract 9:*541–568 (1979).
261. J. Bokori, Gout in Poultry. III. Production of gout by chemical damage to the kidneys, *Acta Vet Scient Hungar 16:*273–286 (1966).
262. A. H. Sykes, The renal clearance of uric acid and P-aminohippurate in the fowl, *Res Vet Sci 1:*308–314 (1960).
263. T. Shimizu, R. Hirohata, Y. Nomura, K. Aibara, K. Miyaki, Nephrotoxic effect of MSG (monsodium glutamate) in the chicken, *Jap J Med Sci Biol 24:*271–279 (1971).
264. F. J. Dudley, N. Dubson, R. F. Gordon, Mortality in egg-laying trials in Great Britain during the period 1927–1937, *Vet Rec 53:*323–330 (1941).
265. R. Ernst, D. McMartin, Gout in layers, *Poultry Adviser 28:*73–75 (1995).

266. M. Chandra, Occurrence and pathology of nephritis in poultry, *Acta Veterinaria Yugoslavia 35:*5–6 (1985).
267. R. D. Slemons, L. N. Locke, M. G. Sheerar, R. M. Duncan, V. S. Hinshaw, B. C. Easterday, Kidney lesions associated with mortality in chickens inoculated with waterfowl influenza viruses, *Avian Dis 34:*120–128 (1990).
268. S. Davison, R. F. Wideman, Excess sodium bicarbonate in the diet and its effect on Leghorn chickens, *Br Poult Sci 33:*859–870 (1992).
269. J. Bokori, Studies on nutritional gout in poultry II. The aetiological role of A-avitaminosis in poultry gout, *Acta Vet Scient Hungar 15:*421–440 (1965).
270. A. Minbay, H. Camas, H. Erdinc, Study on the pathology, biochemistry and treatment of gout in laying hens, *Veteriner Fakultesi Dergisi Ankara Universitesi 32:*493–506 (1985).
271. D. P. Shaw, D. A. Halvorson, Early chick mortality associated with rupture of the yolk sac, *Avian Dis 37:*720–723 (1993).
272. J. D. Moore, The effects of estrdiol-17B and/or progesterone on nitrogen balance values in studies on the castrated rooster, *Gen Compar Endocrinol 7:*430–444 (1966).
273. Y. C. Su, C. I. Chao, Comparison of resistance ability and alteration of iron, copper, and zinc concentrations to Eimeria tenella among country chickens, white leghorn and broiler, *J Clin Soc Vet Sci 19:*228–242 (1993).
274. I. Hanssen, Clostridium perfringens type A toxins in relation to nephritis and uric acid diathesis in captive willow ptarmigan *(Lagopus l. lagopus), Acta Vet Scand 23:*466–467 (1982).
275. I. Hanssen, Nephritis and uric acid diathesis in captive willow ptarmigan *(Lagopus l. lagopus).* Effect of feed protein concentration and grass meal admixture, *Acta Vet Scand 23:*446–455 (1982).
276. Y. Karasawa, R. Tsubota, C. Sakiyama, M. Maeda, M. Yamaguchi, T. Maruyama, Incidence of gout in broiler chickens during the early life in midsummer and late-autumn, *Japanese Poultry Sci 28:*278–283 (1991).
277. J. D. Hoskins, Appendix 2: Congenital defects of the dog, In: S. J. Ettinger, ed., Veterinary Int Med, Vol. 2, W. B. Saunders and Co., Philadelphia, PA, 2115–2129 (1995).
278. P. Phelps, Appearance of chemotactic activity following intra-articular injection of monsodium urate crystals: effect of colchicine, *J Clin Lab Med 76:*622–631 (1970).
279. Y.-H. Change, E. J. Gralla, Suppression of urate-induced canine joint inflammation by heterologous Anti-polymorphonuclear leukocyte serum, *Arth Rheum 11:*145–150 (1968).
280. M. E. Rosenthale, J. Kassarich, F. Schneider, Effect of anti-inflammatory agents on acute experimental synovitis in dogs, *Proc Soc Exp Biol Med 122:*693–696 (1966).
281. P. Phelps, D. J. McCarty, Crystal-induced inflammation in canine joints. II. The importance of polymorphonuclear leukocytes, *J Exp Med 124:*115–125 (1996).
282. D. J. McCarty, P. Phelps, J. Pyenson, Crystal-induced inflammation in canine joints. I. An experimental model with quantification of the host reponse, *J Exp Med 124:*99–114 (1966).

283. J. S. Faires, D. J. McCarty, Acute arthritis in man and dog after intrasynovial injection of sodium urate crystals, *Lancet,* 682–684 (1962).
284. H. R. Schumacher, P. Phelps, C. A. Agudelo, Urate crystal induced inflammation in dog joints: Sequence of synovial changes, *J Rheumatol 1:*102–113 (1974).
285. C. G. Van Arman, R. P. Carlson, P. J. Kling, D. J. Allen, J. V. Bondi, Experimental gouty synovitis caused by bacterial endotoxin adsorbed onto urate crystals, *Arth Rheum 17:*439–449 (1974).
286. J. Ripault, M. Benoist, D. Nguyen-Huy, H. Bloch-Michel, Synovite proliférative apr´ injections intr-articulaires de micro-cristaux D'urate de sodium chez le lapin note préliminair e, *Expansion Scientifique Francaise 36:*435–440 (1969).
287. M. E. Webster, H. M. Maling, M. H. Zweig, M. A. Williams, W. Anderson, Jr., Urate crystal induced inflammation in the rat: Evidence for the combined actions of kinins, histamine and components of complement, *Immunol Commun 1:*185–198 (1972).
288. J. Waisman, L. M. Mwasi, R. Bluestone, J. R. Klinenberg, Acute hyperuricemic nephropathy in rats: An electron microscopic study, *Am J Pathol 81:*367–378 (1975).
289. J. Waisman, R. Bluestone, J. R. Klinenberg, A preliminary report of nephropathy in hyperuricemic rats, *Lab-Invest 30:*716–722 (1974).
290. R. Bluestone, J. R. Klinenberg, J. Waisman, L. S. Goldberg, Experimental hyperuricemia in rats, *Adv Exp Med Biol 41:*551–554 (1974).
291. B. Stavric, E. A. Nera, Use of the uricase-inhibited rat as an animal model in toxicology, *Clin Toxicol 13:*47–74 (1978).
292. N. Kowalewich, E. C. Hawkins, Calcinosis circumscripta involving the metatarsal region in a dog with chronic renal failure, *Can Veterinary J 33:*465–466 (1992).
293. C. Y. C. Pak, O. Waters, L. E. A. Arnold, Mechanism for calcium urolithiasis among patients with hyperuricosuria: Supersaturation of urine with respect to monsodium urate, *J Clin Invest 59:*426–432 (1977).
294. C. Y. C. Pak, D. E. Barilla, K. E. A. Holt, Effect of oral purine load and allopurinol on the crystallization of calcium salts in urine of patients with hyperuricosuric calcium urolithiasis, *Am J Med 65:*593–599 (1978).
295. M. A. Becker, J. E. Seegmiller, Genetic aspects of gout, *Annu Rev Med 25:*15–28 (1974).
296. E. A. Mateos, J. G. Puig, Purine metabolism in Lesch-Nyhan syndrome versus Kelley-Seegmiller syndrome, *J Inherit Metab Dis 17:*138–142 (1994).
297. W. Lathem, B. B. Davis, G. P. Rodnan, Renal tubular secretion of uric acid, *Am J Physiol 199:*9–12 (1960).
298. R. H. Garman, M. J. Nuzzi, J. N. Geraci, Cutaneous gout in an Amazon dolphin, *J Am Vet Med Assoc 183:*1292–1294 (1983).
299. R. M. Miller, R. E. Kind, A gout-like syndrome in a dog, *Vet Med Sm An Clin, 61*:237–240 (1996).
300. L. Karstad, L. Sileo, Causes of death in captive waterfowl in the Kortright Waterfowl Park, 1967–1970, *J Wildl Dis 7:*236–241 (1971).
301. S. S. Arnon, D. C. Mills, P. A. Day, R. V. Henrickson, N. M. Sullivan, T. D. Wilkins, Rapid death of infant rhesus monkeys injected with clostridium difficile toxins A and B: physiological and pathological basis, *J Pediatr 104:*34–40 (1984).

302. D. Cavanagh, P. S. Rao, R. A. Knuppel, U. Desai, J. U. Balis, Pregnancy-induced hypertension: development of a model in the pregnant primate *(Papio anubis), Am J Obstet Gynecol 151:*987–999 (1985).
303. E. Nikodemusz, R. Imre, Pathological features of 3-chloro-4-methylbenzamine HCl toxicity in rooks (*Corvus fragilegus L.*) and pheasants (*Phasianus colchicus L.*) *Gegenbaurs Morphol Jahrb 128*:753–761 (1982).
304. P. W. Ladds, H. Mangunwirjo, D. Sebayang, P. W. Daniels, Diseases in young farmed crocodiles in Irian Jaya [Indonesia] *Vet Rec 136*:121–124 (1995).

6
Introduction to Gout and Hyperuricemia

DANIEL J. MCCARTY
Medical College of Wisconsin, Milwaukee, Wisconsin

I am privileged to write this introduction because it is an opportunity to commemorate our senior editor, Charley Smyth, Charley never lacked energy and vision in his long and productive life; it is most unfortunate that he did not live to see the completion of his final project.

A book on gout is literally a book on history, not only because of the many historically important persons who suffered from it through the ages, but because the disease itself is history (1). It can be diagnosed with 100% certainty by specific crystal identification and treated with exquisite precision. None should now suffer from this disease. It is a paradigm of the conquest of a disease based on a scientific understanding of its etiopathogenesis. It is so well understood that, in my opinion, it is now poorly taught at both the medical student and resident level. Such widespread disinterest may represent what Eugene Garfield of Current Contents calls the "extinction phenomenon." The diagnosis of gout is often wrongly based on the coincidence of joint pains and hyperuricemia. Lifelong therapy with allopurinol is often prescribed without much thought. Liang and Fries estimated that this drug is overprescribed by a factor of 7 (2). The ensuing chapters are mostly authored by older clinical scientists who have made highly significant past contributions to the study of gout and/or purine metabolism. Hopefully, this volume will rekindle interest in the appropriate teaching of the pathophysiology of gout at all levels.

Unlike the monosodium urate (MSU) crystals of gout, calcium pyrophosphate dihydrate and basic (apatitic) calcium phosphate crystals remain a subject of lively interest. Like MSU, these particles have important biological activities that relate both to joint inflammation and joint tissue degeneration. Knowledge of etiopathogenesis remains incomplete, and there is presently no effective way to remove these crystals or to prevent their formation. As the mean age of the populations of most countries is increasing, these relatively insoluble crystals will become an ever-greater health problem.

Gaps remain in our knowledge of gout. Why some hyperuricemic patients nucleate and grow MSU crystals and others do not is simply not known. As MSU crystal solubility is strikingly temperature-dependent, everyone is probably saturated with respect to sodium urate in the cooler joints of the forefeet (solubility 4.5 mg/dl at 30°C), and the temperature in a normal first metatarsophalangeal joint was 32.8°C (3). Why don't we all take the gout? This consideration is important when using drugs to lower serum uric acid and reverse the process of MSU crystal deposition in tissues. One should strive to achieve steady state levels of less than 4 mg/dl. The possible importance of MSU crystal deposition in renal parenchyma to long-term renal function and to associated hypertension has long been of concern. Talbott and Terplan showed MSU crystals in the interstitium of nearly all of 200 gouty kidneys obtained at necropsy before the age of effective drug therapy for hyperuricemia (4). These deposits were associated with nephrosclerosis and with a sterile pyelonephritis at a time when the phlogistic properties of MSU crystals were not appreciated. About a fifth of their subjects had developed chronic renal failure. Current thinking holds that kidney damage in gout is due to the associated hypertension and age, however, and not to crystal deposition (discussed below). Lastly, the striking negative association of gout with seropositive rheumatoid arthritis remains unexplained.

Problems with treatment also remain. Hypersensitivity to allopurinol in patients with decreased renal function is not a rare problem to consultant rheumatologists. Acute gouty attacks in patients with organ transplants and renal tubular damage secondary to immunosuppression with cyclosporine often start in central joints such as hips and the sacroiliac, structures rarely affected in gout associated with hyperuricemia due to other causes (5). In such cases, septic arthritis must be ruled out by needle aspiration done under direct vision with an image intensifier.

The most dramatic aspect of gout—the acute attack—can be terminated promptly by oral nonsteroidal antiinflammatory drugs (NSAIDs) or by 1 mg colchicine, given intravenously. (There is now no reason to give colchicine orally for this purpose.) An NSAID can be safely combined with IV colchicine, but the latter should never be given to patients taking it prophylactically, because the body burden of the drug, which is concentrated intracellularly by binding to a specific site on tubulin dimers, is completely unknown. Failure to follow this dictum has led to lethal consequences and misguided pleas to have the drug removed from hospital pharmacies (6).

The mechanism of action of colchicine is discussed in this book by Cronstein and his colleagues. They have discovered that it inhibits expression of an adhesion molecule needed for neutrophils to leave the postcapillary venules. Although trendy, such a mechanism hardly explains the relative specificity of colchicine on MSU or other forms of crystal-induced inflammation. The work of Paulding Phelps, who discovered a cell-derived chemotactic factor (CCF), a 12,500 MW glycoprotein, released by neutrophils after MSU (or other) crystal endocytosis (7), and of Spilberg, who subsequently showed a specific cell surface receptor for CCF (8), has been virtually ignored. CCF release is inhibited by ambient colchicine concentrations of 10^{-10}M, one ten-thousandth of the levels needed for other drug effects on neutrophils. In my opinion, this effect of the drug is the best explanation for its action because (1) it requires the presence of the specific particulate, not only an interacting cell, and (2) the generation and release of CCF in response to particulate is exquisitely and uniquely sensitive to the drug.

Modern medicine owes much to its clinical scientists—peculiar individuals with one foot in the clinic, one foot in the laboratory, and their seat in the library. The natural history of the study of a disease includes times where activity in one of these three arenas dominates the others. Gout is now largely in the third arena. Diseases associated with crystals containing calcium are presently in the second arena. Drs. Smyth and Holers deserve our thanks for their vision and perseverance in the development of a multiauthored authoritative treatise on the fascinating and important medical conditions associated with the deposition of microcrystals.

REFERENCES

1. Seegmiller JE. *The Conquest of Gouty Arthritis in Landmark Advances in Rheumatology* (DJ McCarty, ed., Contact Associates International Ltd. for the American Rheumatism Association, 89–101 (1985).
2. Liang MH, Fries JF. Asymptomatic hyperuricemia: the case for conservative management. Ann Intern Med 1978; 88:666–670.
3. McCarty DJ. Gout without hyperuricemia. JAMA 1994; 271:302–303.
4. Talbott JH, Terplan KH. The kidney in gout. Medicine (Balt) 1960; 39:405–468.
5. Cohen MR, Cohen EP. Transplantation arthritis: enthesopathies and sacroilitiis following kidney transplantation. Arthritis Rheum 1992; 35:S130 (abstr).
6. Roberts WM, Liang MH, Stern SH. Colchicine in acute gout. JAMA 1987; 257:1920–1921.
7. Phelps P. Polymorphonuclear leukocyte motility in vitro. IV. Colchicine inhibition of chemotactic activity formation after phagocytosis of urate crystals. Arthritis Rheum 1970; 131:1–9.
8. Spilberg I, Mehta J. Demonstration of a specific neutrophil receptor for a cell-derived chemotactic factor. J Clin Invest 1979; 63:85–88.

7

The Epidemiology of Hyperuricemia and Gout

William M. Mikkelsen
The University of Michigan Medical School, Ann Arbor, Michigan

I. INTRODUCTION

Epidemiology explores the nature of a particular disease in populations rather than in individuals. It aims at elucidation of those factors that may play a role in disease causation or indicate an increased risk of development of the disease under study in order that more effective therapies or preventive programs may be be developed. This approach has been difficult to apply to the study of rheumatic diseases for a number of reasons, including the lack of definitive diagnostic criteria in many cases and the relative rarity of most of the rheumatic diseases. In the field of gout, however, population studies have achieved useful results, which this chapter will attempt to summarize.

II. POPULATION STUDIES

Several studies have described the distribution of serum uric acid (SUA) levels and the prevalence of gout in well-defined population groups (1–4). Together they have done much to clarify the effects of age and sex on SUA levels, to emphasize the arbitrary nature of any definition of hyperuricemia, and to provide estimates of the relative risks for development of clinical gout and other potential consequences of hyperuricemia.

A. Frequency Distribution of Serum Uric Acid Levels: Effects of Age and Sex

In the Tecumseh, Michigan study in which 6000 subjects 4 years of age and over had SUA measurements obtained using an automated enzymatic spectrophotometric method, the mean value for all subjects was 4.5 ± 1.3 SD mg/dl (1). For all males the mean value was 4.9 ± 1.4 SD and for all females 4.2 ± 1.2 SD. The sex-specific distribution curve for males was broad with slight skewing toward higher values, while that for females was narrower, peaking sharply at a value well below the peak in the male curve, and showing a greater degree of skewing at the higher end of the scale (Figure 1). Somewhat higher values were reported in other studies, reflecting in large part the older age distribution of participants (2–4). All studies agreed in showing a unimodal distribution curve with skewing toward the higher values.

The Tecumseh data well illustrate the effect of both age and sex on SUA level (1). Childhood levels were quite low in comparison to those of adults, and were approximately equal in male and female subjects (Figure 2). Mean values rose slowly until about the time of puberty, when male values rose sharply to peak in the 20–24 year age group. Thereafter male values declined slightly and showed little subsequent variation. The pubertal rise in females was much more modest, and in the age range 20–39 years showed little variation. They then began to rise, reaching highest levels in the 50–64 year age group and declining slightly thereafter, but remaining lower than male levels throughout the age span. A similar rise in female values at about the time of the menopause was observed in the Sudbury study, in which premenopausal subjects age 15 years and

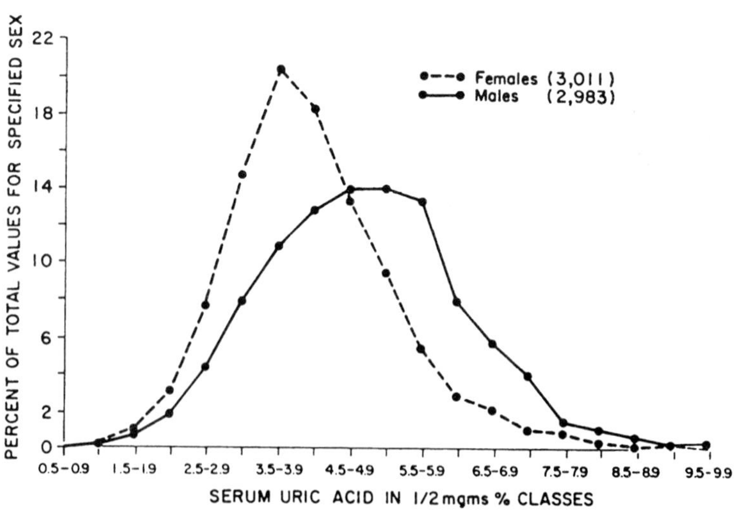

FIGURE 1 Distribution of serum uric acid values, Tecumseh, Michigan, 1959–1960. Reprinted by permission of the publisher from Ref. 1, Copyright 1965 by Excerpta Medica Inc.

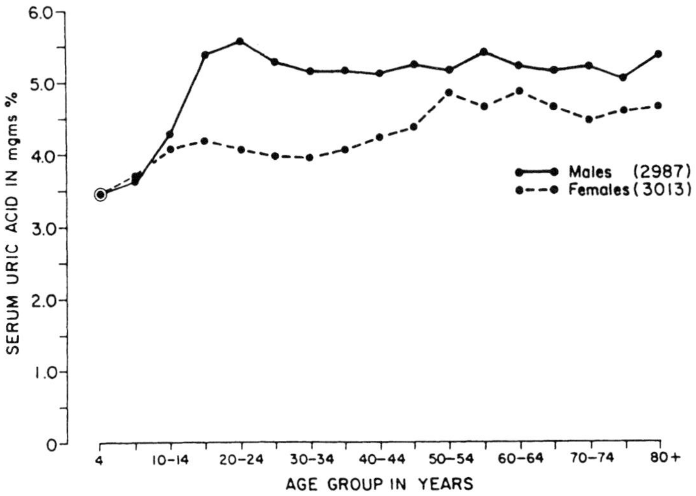

FIGURE 2 Age-sex specific mean serum uric acid values, Tecumseh, Michigan, 1959–1960. Reprinted by permission of the publisher from Ref. 1, Copyright 1965 by Excerpta Medica Inc.

over had mean levels of 4.15 mg/dl, as contrasted to mean levels of 4.47 for menopausal, and 5.01 for postmenopausal subjects (4), and in the Framingham study (2).

These observations strongly suggest hormonal influences on SUA levels. An androgenic effect is suggested by the finding that mean levels are quite low and without gender difference in the prepubertal subjects, and that male levels rise markedly beginning at puberty so that in the age range 15–39 years they remain about 1.0 mg/dl above those of females. An estrogenic effect is suggested by the gradual increase in female values during the years associated with menopause. It is also of interest that in the Tecumseh study the 68 women who were pregnant at the time of examination had SUA levels that were significantly lower than nonpregnant women of the same age (1).

B. The "Normal Range" of Serum Uric Acid Distribution

Population studies have shown that the distribution of SUA levels is unimodal, with some skewing toward higher levels. It has not been possible to demonstrate the existence of two populations, one normouricemic and one hyperuricemic. Neither has it been possible to identify any cutting point above which clinical complications develop and below which they do not. As a result any definition of hyperuricemia must be considered arbitrary.

Based on statistical evidence from population studies as well as clinical experience, the upper limit of normal for measurements by the enzymatic spectrophotometric method has been set at about 7.0 mg/dl for males and 6.0 mg/dl for females. These upper limits have considerable physiologic significance since they closely approach the theoretical solubility limit for monosodium urate in serum, especially in males. Since the major clinical consequences of hyperuricemia, acute gouty arthritis and tophus formation, clearly result from the local precipitation of urate crystals, it seems logical to consider a single definition of hyperuricemia for the two sexes based on urate solubility. Laboratory investigation indicates that this is about 7.0 mg/dl (5). Since female urate levels are lower than those of males at all ages this perspective helps explain the observed sex ratio in gout.

In population studies it is difficult to characterize subjects as normouricemic or hyperuricemic, especially if more than one examination is performed. In addition to the many problems inherent in the collection and handling of the samples and in the technical aspects of the determination, large individual variations (6) as well as diurnal and seasonal variations (7,8) have been reported. Despite these concerns, population studies have clarified the association of hyperuricemia with gout and some of its correlates.

1. Acute Gouty Arthritis

Despite its characteristic clinical features and invariable association with hyperuricemia in clinical settings, it is often difficult to confirm the diagnosis of gout in epidemiologic settings. Several sets of diagnostic criteria have been proposed, but none have proved satisfactory. It is unfortunate that the ultimate diagnostic criterion—the demonstration of urate crystals—is not feasible in population studies. Even hyperuricemia, so useful in clinical settings, has proved to be a poor criterion in population studies since in most of the cases of gout have been present in normouricemic subjects. This should not be interpreted to mean that hyperuricemia is not a necessary precondition for the development of gout in view of the measurement considerations that have been noted.

One of the clearest demonstrations of the risk of acute gouty arthritis among hyperuricemic subjects comes from the Normative Aging Study, in which a cohort of 2046 initially healthy men were followed for 14.9 years with serial examinations and SUA measurements (9). Among those with prior SUA levels of 9.0 mg/dl or more, the annual incidence of gout was 4.9%, compared with a rate of 0.5 for those with levels of 7.0 to 8.9 mg/dl and 0.1 for those with levels below 7.0 mg/dl. The cumulative incidence rate among those with urate levels of 9.0 mg/dl or greater reached 22% after 5 years, as compared to a rate of only 3% for those with levels of 7.0 to 8.9 mg/dl.

These results confirm and extend the findings of the Framingham study, in which subjects were examined an average of 7 times over a period of 12 years (2). In that study, the cumulative incidence of acute gouty arthritis rose progressively with increasing degrees of hyperuricemia, occurring in 1.8% of those with maximal levels of 6.0–6.9, 11.8% for those with values of 7.0–7.9, and 36% of those with values greater than 8 mg/dl. These figures, which represent total prevalence rather than annual incidence of gout, actually are in close agreement with the Normative Aging Study findings. When expressed as cases per human-years of observation, they represent about 2.4 cases per 1000 years of observation, as compared to 2.8 for the Normative Aging Study. Both figures correspond well with the reported prevalence of 2.6 cases per 1000 for Great Britain as of December 31, 1975 (10). Annual incidence figures during the years 1971–1975 varied from 0.25 to 0.35 per 1000.

In the Framingham study, it appeared that in males the greater the degree of hyperuricemia the earlier the onset of gout (2). By the time the adult population had reached an average age of 58 years, 1.5% had experienced at least one attack of acute gouty arthritis. The incidence of new attacks appeared to increase up to a mean age of 47 years, after which it declined even though only one-third of those with maximal SUA levels of 8.0 mg/dl or more had developed gout. This observation suggested that gout might not be a function of hyperuricemia and time alone, but that other factors might also be involved.

In the Sudbury study, a prevalence estimate of 3.7 gout cases per 1000 was reported (4). The authors stressed the very important role played by diagnostic criteria in arriving at a diagnosis of gout, indicating the need for caution in comparing prevalence and incidence rates from different studies.

In the 1983–1985 National Health Interview Survey (NHIS), gout was self-reported by 990/100,000 participants, 1360/100,000 males and 640/100,000 females (11). Frequency increased with age and was greatest in those age 65 and over. It was noted that over time these surveys had revealed an increase in the frequency of self-reported gout, an observation paralleled by an apparent secular trend for increasing serum uric acid levels noted by others (2,9).

An investigation and questionnaire of black and white male physicians since medical school revealed a two fold increased risk for the development of gout among the black men (12). This excess risk appeared to be related to a greater incidence of hypertension among the black subjects. It was not possible to dissociate the effect of antihypertensive treatment from that of hypertension alone. In the Evans County, Georgia, study, there was no significant difference between SUA levels of black and white males, or between those of black and white females (23). The study did not identify gouty subjects.

Other investigators have reported on the SUA levels and prevalence of gout in a variety of differing ethnic and geographic populations. However, the many methodologic problems relating to SUA measurements make it difficult to make direct comparisons between different studies.

2. Tophi

Tophi have rarely been observed in population studies. In addition, it is not feasible in such studies to demonstrate the presence of urate crystals to confirm their composition.

In the Sudbury study, 5 of the 22 subjects (22.7%) with a clinical diagnosis of gout were thought to have tophi (4). In the Framingham study, five men and one woman were thought to have tophi (2). All but one man had had acute gouty arthritis. Only 7% of those with a diagnosis of gout had tophi, confirming the clinical impression that tophi are a late manifestation of gout, but also raising the possibility that gout as it occurs in the general population may be a milder disease than that encountered in hospital settings.

3. Uric Acid Nephrolithiasis

Epidemiologic studies have demonstrated a relationship between SUA levels and urinary calculi (chemical composition not known). In the Framingham study, of male subjects with a maximal SUA level of 7.0 mg/dl or more, 12.7% had a history of urolithiasis; of those with levels of 8.0 or more, 22% gave such a history; and for those with levels of 9.0 or greater the figure rose to 40% (2). Of all gouty subjects, 13.3% had a history of renal stones, virtually the same figure as for those with maximal urate levels of 7.0 mg/dl or more. In the Sudbury study, 22.7% of those diagnosed with gout had a history of kidney stones, as compared with 2.8% for the remaining population (4).

Among males enrolled in the Kaiser-Permanente Health Plan, the risk of urolithiasis was 1 in 852 per year in normouricemic subjects, 1 in 295 per year among those with asymptomatic hyperuricemia, and 1 in 114 for those with established gout (13). From this and other studies, it appears that the annual risk of urolithiasis among those with gout or asymptomatic hyperuricemia is about 1%.

Despite this relationship, most patients with uric acid stones do not have gout or hyperuricemia. A persistently acidic urine urine appears to be a major risk factor and, in some geographic areas, dehydration and low urinary volume may also play an important role.

4. Urate Nephropathy

In clinical settings, renal disease, usually nephrosclerosis, commonly occurs in gouty patients, but is usually associated with hypertension, which is assumed to be the true culprit. In epidemiologic studies, gout and/or hyperuricemia are often found in association with renal disease and hypertension, but it is seldom possible to determine the sequence of events.

In the Framingham study, 12 of the 240 subjects with one or more SUA levels above 7.0 mg/dl developed clinical evidence of renal disease (2). However, in only 4 was it considered that hyperuricemia might possibly have been a contributing cause, since 5 subjects had preexisting renal disease and possible alternative causes were usually found in the others.

In the Kaiser-Permanente study, azotemia, when it occurred in association with asymptomatic hyperuricemia or gout, was generally mild and of little clinical significance (13,14). No deaths from renal disease that could be attributed to hyperuricemia occurred among 1356 men, age 60–69 when SUA was measured, who were followed for 10 years. Projecting creatinine levels of subjects age 20–29 four decades into the future suggested that initial SUA levels 3 SD above the mean would have only a minor effect on renal function as reflected by serum creatinine, and that even with initial urate levels 6 SD above the mean (approximately 10 mg/dl in women and 13 mg/dl in men), creatinine levels at age 60–69 would reach only 2.0 mg/dl in females and 2.6 mg/dl in males (13). A cross-sectional view of the same subjects in 10-year age groupings confirmed the impression that a substantial increase in SUA level was associated with only a slight rise in serum creatinine (14).

Only 11 of 1658 males followed for 14.9 years in the Normative Aging Study were found to have serum creatinine levels of 2.0 mg/dl or more at last examination (9). Of these, 10 had other conditions explaining the decline in renal function.

Thus, results of these and other epidemiologic studies do not support the view that hyperuricemia by itself is a significant risk factor for kidney disease, and have led some authors to question the existence of urate nephropathy as a distinct entity (15,16). This view is in accord with an extensive clinical study in which renal insufficiency, when present in gouty patients, tended to be associated with hypertension, ischemic heart disease, or preexisting renal disease (17).

Some cases with gout, renal failure, and hypertension have been attributed to chronic lead intoxication (18,19) and others to a syndrome of familial hyperuricemia, gout, and renal failure (20).

C. Associated Conditions

While various population studies have suggested correlations between SUA and a number of other conditions, the relationships are extremely complex and difficult to unravel. Further, it should be cautioned that apparently "significant" correlations do not prove a causal relationship, and should be interpreted with great care.

1. Obesity and Nutrition

In population studies, the most convincing association of SUA level has been with with some measure of obesity or body mass (1,2,21–26). In one study it appeared that nonadipose weight, presumably muscle mass, was the important correlate of SUA (14). In several studies, when measures of body fat were held constant, the significance of the correlation of other variables was largely lost (27,28). This association of SUA with body mass is so strong that the authors of one report were led to state that "weight and relative-weight indices are the only variables that predict SUA levels beyond a negligible degree" (26).

Although anecdotal, the observation is very pertinent that in Europe the incidence of acute gouty arthritis during the two world wars was quite low, but rose after each as protein became available and nutritional status improved (29,30). Weight loss has been shown to be significantly associated with decrease in serum urate levels (31). The great importance of obesity was further demonstrated in the case report of an obese, gouty subject in whom weight loss reduced the serum urate to normal levels (32). Metabolic studies showed an increase in renal excretion of urate and a decreased rate of urate production, both of which had been shown to be abnormal initially. An association has been demonstrated between SUA and alcoholic intake (21,25), and a negative correlation was shown with cigarette smoking (26).

2. Diabetes Mellitus

Several studies have shown that hyperuricemia has predictive value for the future development of diabetes mellitus (33,34). However, subjects with established diabetes have consistently shown lower SUA levels than nondiabetic subjects, presumably as the result of the uricosuric effect of hyperglycemia (1,22,26,33,35). Except for these observations, epidemiological studies have shown no association between SUA and blood sugar levels (2,36), or between clinically diagnosed gout and diabetes (2).

3. Hyperlipidemia

Population studies have shown a significant correlation of SUA levels with triglyceride levels (24,34) but not with cholesterol (22,36). Patients whose gout is secondary to chronic lead nephropathy do not share the hypertriglyceridemia of primary gout patients, indicating that this is not the direct consequence of hyperuricemia alone (18). In addition, the first-degree relatives of gouty subjects do not have hypertriglyceridemia, suggesting that environmental factors such as excess caloric and alcohol intake are responsible rather than genetic factors (37). A significant but small negative correlation of SUA with HDL cholesterol was observed in one study (26).

4. Hypertension

A number of associations between hyperuricemia and hypertension have been recognized. Hypertension resulting from chronic renal disease is frequently accompanied by hyperuricemia, and antihypertensive therapy often produces hyperuricemia. Clinical studies have indicated an increased frequency of hyperuricemia in untreated hypertensive subjects. Some population studies have shown a significant association of hyperuricemia with hypertension (22,23,25,26,34,35), although in most cases this correlation lost significance when other variables, especially weight, were taken into consideration (22,25,26,35).

5. Psychosocial Factors

A number of studies have suggested relationships between SUA and various social and psychological factors, including social class, occupation, intelligence, psychological or physiological stresses, and behavioral characteristics such as drive, achievement, and leadership, although their significance has generally remained obscure.

6. Coronary Heart Disease

In a 5-year study involving 10,000 Israeli men, no association was observed between SUA and the development of angina pectoris (38). In this same population, although subjects with diagnosed myocardial infarction or angina pectoris had elevated SUA levels, SUA proved to have no predictive value for the later development of incident cases of coronary heart disease (CHD) (26). In another study, no increase in mortality from coronary artery or cerebrovascular disease could be demonstrated in male or female gouty subjects or their first-degree relatives, suggesting that in the absence of other risk factors hyperuricemia and gout alone did not entail a serious risk for the development of vascular disease (39). Among 5421 participants in the first National Health and Nutrition Survey, on whom baseline data were collected in 1971–1975 and who were followed through 1987, SUA level was predictive of mortality from all causes and from ischemic heart disease in women, although no association was observed in men (40). In the Evans County, Georgia, study, an apparent association of hyperuricemia and CHD became insignificant when other variables were controlled for (23). Review of data from the fourth through the thirteenth biennial examinations of subjects in the original Framingham cohort indicated that SUA was significantly related to the incidence of CHD in general, and myocardial infarction in particular, in both sexes (34). However, on multivariate analysis, including age, systolic blood pressure, relative weight, cigarette smoking, and serum cholesterol, SUA did not contribute independently to the prediction of CHD. Thus, at present it appears that hyperuricemia itself is not a significant independent risk factor for coronary heart disease, but that it is significantly associated with more important risk factors, such as obesity, hypertension, and hyperlipidemia.

D. Genetic Aspects of Population Studies

Early family studies of gouty patients were interpreted to indicate that hyperuricemia was the result of action of a single dominant gene on the basis of an apparently bimodal distribution of SUA levels among family members. Later investigators found the evidence for bimodality to be unconvincing, and suggested that a multifactorial inheritance was at least as tenable. Population studies have shown that SUA levels display a unimodal distribution, without evidence of two groups, one normouricemic and the other hyperuricemic, a finding compatible with polygenic inheritance (1,24). Estimates of heritability were found to be relatively low (24,40), and it was concluded that the SUA phenotype results from the interaction of multifactorial inheritance with environmental factors. Those specific genetic errors that have been found to result in hyperuricemia and gout are of such rarity that they have not demonstrated their presence in epidemiologic studies.

E. Preventive Programs

By providing reliable estimates of certain risks associated with hyperuricemia, population studies have established a rationale for consideration of programs aimed at the prevention of gout and its tophaceous complications. However, our knowledge of the natural history of gout argues against such measures. Individuals with hyperuricemia may remain asymptomatic for many years, and indeed many never develop gout. Clinical experience suggests that chronic arthritic changes and/or tophaceous changes do not precede the appearance of acute gouty arthritis but develop many years later and therefore do not warrant institution of therapy prior to the onset of acute gout. The risk of urolithiasis is sufficiently low that preventive therapy has not been considered to be indicated prior to appearance of a stone. Available evidence suggests that moderate hyperuricemia does not result in significant renal damage (9,13), again supporting a conservative approach. The relationships between uric acid and other disorders, such as hypertension, diabetes, hyperlipidemia, and heart disease, are poorly understood and there is little evidence that correction of hyperuricemia by itself would directly influence any of these conditions.

In managing individuals found to have asymptomatic hyperuricemia, a conservative approach thus seems indicated. The finding of an elevated SUA level should be verified, preferably by an enzymatic method. Consideration should be given to medications or underlying diseases to which the hyperuricemia might be attributable. It is advisable to screen for the major risk factors for coronary artery disease, because of their frequent association with hyperuricemia, and to initiate appropriate treatment when indicated. If the patient is significantly overweight, a program of weight reduction may help to normalize the SUA level. The patient should be educated regarding the potential risks of hyperuricemia and advised to seek prompt medical attention should acute arthritis develop. If a uric acid stone forms, SUA and 24-hour urinary uric acid excretion should be measured. If urinary uric acid excretion is high (greater than 1 gm/24 hours), allopurinol therapy may be considered, although in many cases maintenance of an adequate fluid intake and an alkaline urine may be sufficient. Although prophylactic allopurinol therapy has been suggested for those with urate levels persistently above 10 mg/dl, especially if they are urate hyperexcreters (42), presumably to minimize the risk of urate nephropathy, such levels are relatively uncommon in uncomplicated primary gout, and epidemiologic studies provide little in the way of a rationale for such an approach. The risks and benefits of therapy should be carefully reviewed with the patient. In general, the fact that the patient is asymptomatic and likely to remain so, coupled with considerations of cost, problems with compliance, and potential hazards of therapy, will mitigate against a decision to initiate treatment.

REFERENCES

1. W. M. Mikkelsen, H. J. Dodge, H. A. Valkenburg, and S. Himes. The distribution of serum uric acid values in a population unselected as to gout or hyperuricemia, Tecumseh, Michigan, 1959–1960, *Am J Med 39*:242 (1965).
2. A. P. Hall, P. E. Barry, T. R. Dawber, and P. M. McNamara. Epidemiology of gout and hyperuricemia; a long-term population study, *Am J Med 42*:27 (1967).
3. H. A. Isomaki and H. Takkunen. Gout and hyperuricemia in a Finnish rural population, *Acta Rheumato Scand 15*:112 (1969).
4. J. B. O'Sullivan. Gout in a New England town. A prevalence study in Sudbury, Massachusetts, *Ann Rheum Dis 31*:166 (1972).
5. J. E. Seegmiller. The acute attack of gouty arthritis, *Arthritis Rheum 8*:714 (1965).
6. E. K. Harris, P. Kanofsky, G. Shakarji, and E. Cotlove. Biological and analytic components of variation in long-term studies of serum constituents in normal subjects. II. Estimating biological components of variation, *Clin Chem 16*:1022 (1979).
7. M. S. Devgun and H. S. Dhillon. Importance of diurnal variations on clinical value and interpretation of serum urate measurements, *J. Clin Pathol 45*:110 (1992).
8. R. A. Goldstein, K. L., Becker, and C. F. Moore. Serum urate in healthy men—intermittent elevations and seasonal effect, *N Engl J Med 287*:649 (1972).
9. E. W. Campion, R. J. Glynn, and L. O. DeLabry. Asymptomatic hyperuricemia. Risks and consequences in the Normative Aging Study, *Am J Med 82*:421 (1987).
10. W. J. C. Currie. Prevalence and incidence of the diagnosis of gout in Great Britain, *Ann Rheum Dis 38*:101 (1979).
11. R. C. Lawrence, M. C. Hochberg, J. L. Kelsey, F. W. McDuffie, T. A. Medsger, W. R. Fields, and L. E. Shulman. Estimates of the prevalence of selected arthritic and musculoskeletaal diseases in the United States, *J Rheumatol 16*:427 (1989).

12. M. C. Hochberg, J. Thomas, D. J. Thomas, L. Mead, D. M. Levine, and M. J. Klag. Racial differences in the incidence of gout. The role of hypertension, *Arthritis Rheum 38*:628 (1995).
13. W. J. Fessel. Renal outcomes in gout and hyperuricemia, *Am J Med 67*:74 (1979).
14. W. J. Fessel and G. D. Barr. Uric acid, lean body weight, and creatinine interactions. Results from regression analyses of 78 variables, *Semin Arthritis Rheum 7*:115 (1970).
15. R. J. Foley and E. J. Weinman. Review: urate nephropathy, *Am J Med Sci 288*:208 (1984).
16. L. H. Beck. Requiem for gouty nephropathy, *Kidney Int 30*:280 (1986).
17. T.-F. Yu and L. Berger. Impaired renal function in gout, *Am J Med 72*:95 (1982).
18. B. T. Emmerson and B. R. Knowles. Triglyceride concentrations in primary gout and gout of chronic lead nephropathy, *Metabolism 20*:721 (1971).
19. V. Batuman, J. K. Maesaka, B. Haddad, E. Tepper, E. Landy, and R. P. Weeden. The role of lead in gout nephropathy, *N Engl J Med 26*:520 (1981).
20. H. Duncan and A. S. Dixon. Gout, familial hyperuricemia, and renal disease, *Q J Med 29*:127 (1960).
21. J. G. Evans, I. A. M. Prior, and H. P. B. Harvey. Relation of serum uric acid to body bulk, haemoglobin, and alcohol intake in two South Pacific populations, *Ann Rheum Dis 27*:239 (1968).
22. R. Jeremy and J. Towson. Serum uric acid levels and gout in Australian males, *Med J Aust 1*:116 (1971).
23. R. Klein, B. E. Klein, J. C. Cornoni, J. Mareaby, J. C. Cassel, and H. A. Tyrolier. Serum uric acid. Its relationship to coronary heart disease risk factors and cardiovascular disease, Evans County, Georgia, *Arch Intern Med 132*:401 (1973).
24. W. M. O'Brien, T. A. Burch, and J. J. Bunim. Genetics of hyperuricemia in Blackfeet and Pima Indians, *Ann Rheum Dis 25*:117 (1966).
25. K. Yano, G. G. Rhoads, and A. Kagan. Epidemiology of serum uric acid among 8000 Japanese-American men in Hawaii, *J Chronic Dis 30*:607 (1977).
26. U. Goldbourt, J. T. Medalie, J. B. Herman, and H. N. Neyfeld. Serum uric acid: Correlation with biochemical, anthropometric, clinical and behavioral parameters in 10,000 Israeli men, *J Chronic Dis 33*:435 (1980).
27. R. M. Acheson and Y. K. Chan. New Haven survey of joint diseases: the prediction of serum uric acid in a general population, *J Chronic Dis 21*:543 (1969).
28. L. E. Hollister, J. E. Overall, and H. L. Snow. Relationship of obesity to serum triglyceride, cholesterol, and uric acid, and to plasma glucose level, *Am J Clin Nutr 20*:777 (1967).
29. K. Brochner-Mortensen. Review of 21 diagnostic criteria and known etiological factors in gout, The Epidemiology of Chronic Rheumatism, Blackwell Scientific Publications, Oxford, F. A. Davis, Philadelphia, 1963, pp. 140–155.
30. N. Zollner. The treatment of gout, *Germ Med Mth 2*:253 (1957).
31. J. T. Scott. Obesity and hyperuricemia, *Clin Rheumat Dis 3*:25 (1977).
32. B. T. Emmerson. Alteration of urate metabolism by weight reduction, *Aus N Z J Med 3*:410 (1973).
33. J. B. Herman, J. H. Medalie, and U. Goldbourt. Diabetes, prediabetes and uricemia, *Diabetologia 12*:47 (1976).

34. F. N. Brand, D. L. McGee, W. B. Kannel, J. Stokes III, and W. P. Castelli. Hyperuricemia as a risk factor of coronary heart disease: the Framingham study. *Am J Epidemiol 121*:11 (1985).
35. J. Zalokar, J. Lellouch, J. R. Claude, and D. Kuntz. Epidemiology of serum uric acid and gout in Frenchmen, *J Chronic Dis 27*:59 (1974).
36. A. R. Myers, F. H. Epstein, H. J. Dodge, and W. M. Mikkelsen. The relationship of serum uric acid to risk factors in coronary heart disease, *Am J Med 45*:520 (1968).
37. L. G. Darlington, J. Slack, and J. T. Scott. Family study of lipid and purine levels in gout patients, *Ann Rheum Dis 41*:253 (1982).
38. J. H. Medalie, M. Snyder, J. J. Groen, H. N. Neufeld, U. Goldbourt, and E. Riss. Angina pectoris among 10,000 men. 5 year incidence and univariate analysis, *Am J Med 55*:583 (1973).
39. L. G. Darlington, J. Slack, and J. T. Scott. Vascular mortality in patients with gout and their families, *Ann Rheum Dis 42*:270 (1973).
40. D. S. Freedman, D. F. Williamson, E. W. Guntner, and T. Byers. Relation of serum uric acid to mortality and ischemic heart disease. The NHANES 1 epidemiologic follow-up study, *Am J Epidemiol 141*:637 (1995).
41. J. G. French, H. J. Dodge, M. O. Kjelberg, W. M. Mikkelsen, and W. J. Schull. A study of familial aggregation of serum uric acid levels in the population of Tecumseh, Michigan, 1959–1960, *Am J Epidemiol 86*:214 (1967).
42. S. M. Krane and E. D. Harris. Crystal-induced joint disease, SAM-CD, Scientific American Medicine, Inc., Enigma Retrieval Systems, Inc., New York, New York, 1997, chap. IX p. 13.

8

The Epidemiology of Filipino Hyperuricemia

LOUIS A. HEALEY
University of Washington, Seattle, Washington

In the 1960s, epidemiologic surveys of serum urate levels in different populations were popular. The mean urate value for adult males in North America and in Europe was remarkably constant at 5.0+ mg/100 ml. As discussed in detail by Mikkelsen in Chapter 7 surveys of South Pacific peoples revealed that some were hyperuricemic with serum urate levels of 6.1 to 7.3 mg/100 ml.

The story of one of these people, the Filipinos, is described in detail in this chapter. As this story gradually unfolded in a series of studies carried out over a period of 12 years, it was of inherent interest and also illustrated features of gout and hyperuricemia that have application to all patients regardless of race. These include the influence of heredity and environment on the urate level and the role of the kidney in development of hyperuricemia.

The story began in 1958 when John Decker came from Boston to start the Arthritis Service at the University of Washington School of Medicine in Seattle. He noted that among the patients with gout coming to the King County Hospital arthritis clinic there seemed to be a disproportionate number of Filipino men.

When this observation was tested statistically by review of hospital charts for a 5-year period, the impression proved correct. The incidence of clinical gout in Filipino men was 2.5% (7 cases out of 281 admissions) as compared to 0.13% for non-Filipinos (1). This paper presciently suggested that the environmental change these Filipinos had undergone might be playing an important role in explaining this phenomenon.

The next step was to determine the serum urate level in normal nongouty Filipino men. At that time, many of the Filipinos living in Seattle had migrated from the Philippine Islands to work in the salmon fishery. They worked in the canneries in Alaska during the summer salmon run and then returned to Seattle for the remainder of the year. In the summer of 1961, John Decker and James Lane traveled to Ketchikan to sample a group of healthy Filipino men working, eating, and living in three canneries there. They found that the mean serum urate level of 113 Filipino men was 6.3 mg/100 ml, contrasted with a mean level of 5.1 mg/100 ml for a group of Caucasian male inmates of the federal penitentiary at McNeil Island located in Puget Sound, Washington (2).

It was then desirable to refine conditions of the study and also to evaluate the effects of race, diet, environment, and body build. This opportunity was presented in the Hawaii State Psychiatric Hospital in Kaneohe, where the patient population, which roughly paralleled the ethnic distribution of the people of Hawaii, shared the same diet and environment. John Decker, John Caner, and I went to Hawaii to interview these patients, assess their body build, and draw serum samples for urate measurement.

The mean serum urate for the various racial groups of hospitalized patients is shown in Table 1. The Filipino value of 6.1 mg/100 ml was significantly higher than the mean for non-Filipinos of 5.3 mg/100 ml and for every other ethnic group except for the Hawaiians, whose sample was too small to give a reliable value. This difference could not be ascribed to diet, body build, or to other diagnoses such as hypertension, diabetes or hypercholesterolemia, either singly or in combination (3).

In light of these findings, it was puzzling that clinical gout was rarely observed by rheumatologists in the Philippines. This clinical impression was confirmed by the study of Manahan (4). She estimated the incidence of the diagnosis of gout in admissions to the Philippine General Hospital in Manila at only 0.01%. Only eight cases had been diagnosed over an 11-year span involving some 214,000 admissions to the same hospital (5). This experience was in marked contrast to the findings in Seattle (1) and also very different from a sur-

TABLE 1 Ethnic Group and Serum Urate Level

Ethnic group	Number	Serum urate (mg/100 ml)
Filipino	60	6.1
Japanese	73	5.4
Caucasian	43	5.2
Portuguese	38	4.7
Chinese	31	5.3
Hawaiian	11	6.4
Mixed Race	54	5.4

Source: Ref. 3.

vey in Hawaii that had determined an incidence of gout that was 0.68% for Filipinos admitted to the Queen's Hospital in Honolulu (6).

Although no anthropologic or genetic differences have been recognized among Filipinos, distinctions are drawn between the inhabitants of various regions based on language differences. Of the three largest language groups in the Philippines, lexicostatistical studies suggest that Iloko speakers have been separate from the Tagalog and Visayan people for 2000 years.

Historically, Filipinos—and other ethnic groups—immigrated to Hawaii to work in the sugar cane and pineapple plantations. The majority of these laborers came from a single area, the Ilocano speaking provinces of northwest Luzon island. About 85% of the Filipino cannery workers who had been studied in Alaska (2) were also of Ilocano origin, thus raising the possibility that hyperuricemia and gout were limited to that group of Filipinos. The next step was to survey urate levels of inhabitants of different linguistic areas, and this led us to the Philippine Islands themselves.

Maurice Skeith and I went to Manila and joined Pelagia Bayani-Sioson in this work (7). She was responsible for obtaining samples from 140 Tagalog-speaking male students and laboratory technicians at the University of the Philippines College of Medicine in Manila. Maurice Skeith and I sampled 115 cement workers and 82 farm laborers living in two small villages located in the Ilocano province of La Union. Through the kindness of Baruch Blumberg, we also received serum samples from 146 males attending a dermatology clinic on the island of Cebu where Visayan is the dialect spoken. The mean serum urate level for all four groups was 5.1 to 5.3 mg/100 ml, in good agreement with the value for control Caucasian populations in the previous studies (2,3).

Thus it was apparent that Filipinos who were born in the Philippines and migrated to Hawaii and the Pacific Northwest area of mainland United States had a high frequency of hyperuricemia. In contrast, linguistically identical Filipinos who remained in the Philippines did not. This difference must then have been due to some environmental change, and diet was the obvious difference. Filipinos in the United States ate more meat than those in the Philippines, where the staple diet was rice with little meat. However, the diet of the hyperuricemic Filipinos in the United States did not include more meat or purines than the usual Caucasian diet. This was clearly illustrated in the study in thc Hawaii State Hospital (3), where all the patients ate the same diet but only the Filipinos were hyperuricemic.

Since the obvious change was diet, we postulated that the Filipinos might become hyperuricemic because of an inability to increase renal excretion of urate to compensate for the increased load presented by a diet with more purine and protein. To test this hypothesis, Pelagia Bayani-Sioson and I studied the ability of normal Filipinos to increase the renal excretion of urate in response to a measured purine load and compared it to the response of normal Caucasians given the same purine load (8).

Nugent and Tyler (9) had suggested that in some patients with gout, hyperuricemia was due to an inability to increase urinary urate excretion in the face of a purine load. We followed the protocol outlined in their study. Serum urate level and 24-hour urinary urate excretion were measured both before and after a purine load consisting of 4 grams of yeast ribonucleic acid added to the usual diet for a period of 4 days. Subjects were 13 normal Filipino males in Manila and 10 normal Caucasian males in Seattle, where all the laboratory measurements were performed.

All 10 Caucasians increased their urinary urate excretion to the same degree as the control subjects in the study cited (9). Of the 13 Filipinos, 9 showed a similar increase in urate excretion, but 4 failed to show this increase. Their response, shown in Figure 1, is similar to the pattern of urate excretion seen in the Caucasian patients with gout (9).

We postulated that this renal defect in the Filipinos was not unique to them, but was the same as that present in the gouty Caucasian patients. It was possible for us to find it in normouricemic Filipinos because it was more common in that population. We assumed that many Filipinos inherit this less-effi-

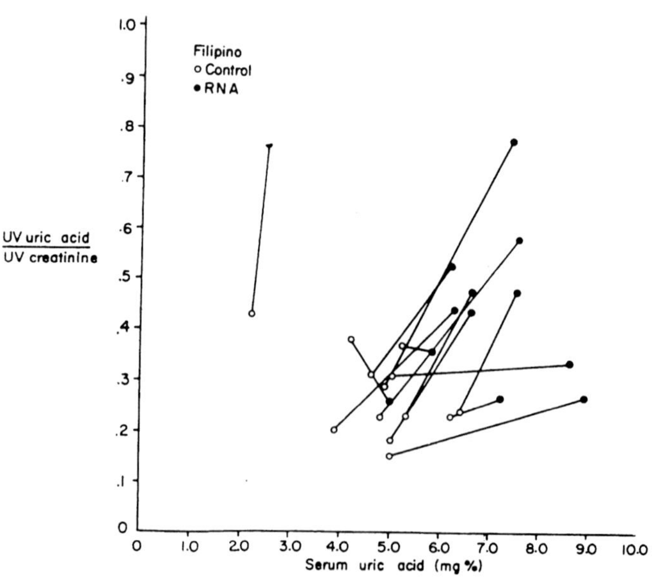

FIGURE 1 Urinary urate/urinary creatinine ratio for 13 normal Filipino subjects before and after purine load, shown in relation to serum urate levels. (From Ref. 8.)

cient system for urate excretion, but in the Philippines it did not lead to gout or hyperuricemia because the diet, mostly rice, was so low in purine. In the United States, the amount of purine presented by the amount of meat in the usual American diet was sufficient to exceed their renal capacity for excretion and led to hyperuricemia.

A similar mechanism has since been proposed for another Pacific people also noted to have an increased prevalence of gout and hyperuricemia, the Maori of New Zealand. Hyperuricemic men with gout as well as normouricemic Maori had reduced fractional urate clearance when compared to normal non-Maori males (10). A subsequent study demonstrated a similar defect in renal urate handling in Polynesian women as well (11). These Pacific peoples are not the same ethnically. The Maori are Polynesian and Filipinos are a mixture of Malay and Mongoloid. All might share a common origin from Indonesia some 30000 years ago. It should also be noted that Filipinos do not share the Polynesian tendency to obesity.

The nature of this renal defect is not known. It is assumed, but not proven, that it is the same defect which leads to hyperuricemia in the majority of Caucasian patients with gout as discussed in Chapter 10. It seems to be a genetic defect that occurs more commonly in Filipinos and in other Pacific peoples but does not manifest as hyperuricemia as long as they eat a diet low in purine.

REFERENCES

1. J. L. Decker, and J. J. Lane. Gouty arthritis in Filipinos, *New Engl J Med 261*:805 (1959)
2. J. L. Decker, J. J. Lane, and W. E. Reynolds. Hyperuricemia in a male Filipino population, *Arthritis Rheum 5*:144 (1962).
3. L. A. Healey, J. E. Z. Caner, and J. L. Decker. Ethnic variations in serum uric acid I. Filipino Hyperuricemia in a controlled environment, *Arthritis Rheum 9*:288 (1964).
4. L. A. Manahan. Rheumatic Diseases in the Philippines, Proceedings Australian Rheumatism Conference, 1963, pp. 20–22.
5. G. Castillo, P. C. Campos, and T. Maramba, Gouty nephropathy, *J Philippine Med Assn 34*:289 (1958).
6. G. Rosenblatt, J. L. Decker and L. A. Healey, Gout in hospitalized Filipinos in Hawaii, *Pacific. J. Med. Surg. 74*:312 (1966).
7. Healey, M. D. Skeith, J. L. Decker, and P. S. Bayani-Sioson. Hyperuricemia in Filipinos: Interaction of heredity and environment, *Am J Human Genetics 19*:81 (1967).
8. L. A. Healey and P. S. Bayani-Sioson. A defect in the renal excretion of uric acid in Filipinos, *Arthritis Rheum 14*:721 (1971).
9. C. A. Nugent and F. H. Tyler. The renal excretion of uric acid in patients with gout and in nongouty subjects, *J. Clin. Invest. 38*:1890 (1959).

10. T. Gibson, R. Waterworth, P. Hatfield, G. Robinson, and K. Bremner. Hyperuricemia, gout and kidney function in New Zealand Maori men, *Brit J Rheumatol 23*:276 (1984).
11. H. A. Simmonds, M. B. McBride, P. J. Hatfield, R. Graham, and J. Jackson. Polynesian women are also at risk for hyperuricemia and gout because of a genetic defect in renal urate handling, *Br J Rheumatol 33*:932 (1994).

9

Metabolism of Purines and Genetic Defects Leading to Hyperuricemia and Gout

J. EDWIN SEEGMILLER
University of California—San Diego, La Jolla, California

I. ROLE OF HYPERURICEMIA AND SUPERSATURATION OF URATE IN GOUT

The recognition of the functional equivalence of degree of hyperuricemia (above 7.0 mg/dl serum) and the degree of supersaturation (above 6.8 mg/dl) for monosodium urate in serum provides a unifying concept for considering the chemical origin of gouty arthritis. The higher the serum urate concentration above normal, the higher the degree of supersaturation and the greater the chance of precipitating the first needle-shaped crystal of monosodium urate monohydrate into the surrounding tissues as the first step. This supersaturation and deposition is further enhanced by the lower temperature observed in the cooler joints of the upper and lower extremities, thus creating a priority site for crystal deposition accounting for the highest prevalence of acute gouty attacks in these joints (1). The inflammatory reaction to subcutaneous injection of a suspension of urate crystals (2) suggesting a critical threshold of invading crystals must then be exceeded to trigger the second step—the initiation of the same type of inflammatory response used by the body to combat an invading micro-organism. The result is the exquisitely tender and painful, red, swollen, and warm joints characterizing the first acute attack of gouty arthritis, which must be distinguished from a septic infection by culture and by the demonstration of urate crystals in synovial fluids. The most rational approach to its permanent management in a preventive mode is to remove the cause by lowering the hyperuricemic

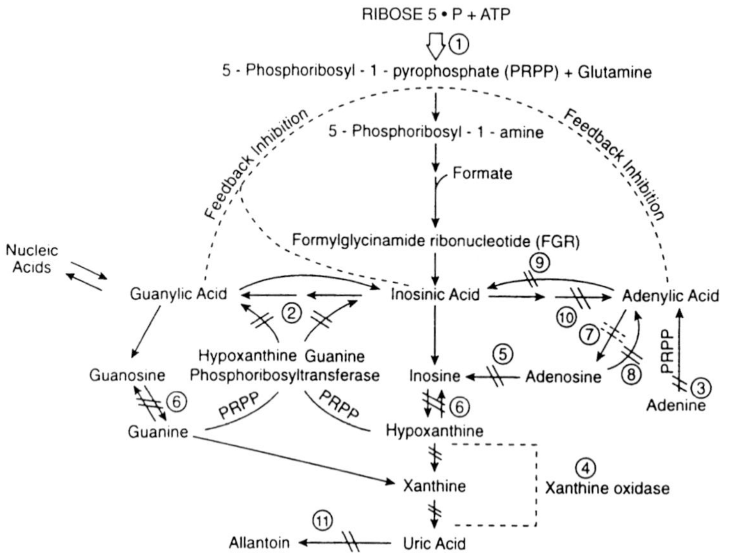

FIGURE 1 Known enzyme defects in human purine metabolism. 1, Increased phosphoribosylpyrophosphate synthetase activity in patients with overproduction of uric acid and gout. 2, Gross deficiency of hypoxanthine guanine phosphoribosyltransferase in children with Lesch-Nyhan disease and partial deficiency of the same enzyme in patients with overproduction of uric acid and gout. 3, Adenine phosphoribosyltransferase deficiency in patients with kidney stones composed of 2, 8-dioxyadenine that are often confused with uric acid stones. 4, Xanthine oxidase deficiency in patients with xanthinuria who are at increased risk for xanthine calculi of the urinary tract and, in occasional patients, myalgia from xanthine crystals in the muscle. 5, Adenosine deaminase deficiency associated with severe combine immunodeficiency disease. 6, Purine nucleoside phosphorylase deficiency associated with isolated defect in T cells. 7, Purine 5′-nucleotidase activity is low in lymphocytes of patients with agammaglobulinemia that may be secondary to loss of B cells. 8, Adenosine kinase deficiency has so far been developed only in human lymphoblast cell lines. Its counterpart in patients is yet to be identified. 9, Myoadenylate deaminase deficiency is associated in some patients with development of weakness and muscle cramps after vigorous exercise and failure to show a rise in venous blood ammonia in response to muscle exercise. 10, Adenylosuccinate lyase deficiency has been found in occasional patients with childhood autism and other neurologic disorders. 11, Evolutionary uricase deficiency makes uric acid the endproduct of purine metabolism in humans, thus setting the stage for their development of gout.

serum urate to the normal unsaturated range and thereby dissolve away all preformed crystals and maintain it there indefinitely to prevent their return.

The chance observation in 1948 that a new drug, caronamide, developed for retaining penicillin in the body would actually enhance the body's excretion of uric acid launched the successful development and clinical trial of a more potent drug, probenecid (Benamid), which effectively reduced the serum urate concentration of most patients studied to the normal range unless renal function was impaired by gouty nephropathy (3,4). In 1956, another new and more potent drug, allopurinol, tailor-made to inhibit the enzyme xanthine oxidase was developed primarily to enhance the effectiveness of a drug being used for chemotherapy of cancer (5). By partially blocking xanthine oxidase the final enzyme of uric acid synthesis (Figure 1), it also lowered the serum urate to normal in gout patients, including those with an excessive rate of purine synthesis and/or impaired renal function, thus providing a more potent agent for lowering the serum urate (6). This success provided concrete evidence of the primary role of hyperuricemia in the development of gouty arthritis. A number of reviews have been published (7–12b).

A. Role of an Evolutionary Defect of Purine Metabolism

The evolutionary loss of the enzyme uricase in the prosimian ancestor of man and the higher apes makes the whole human race unable to oxidize uric acid to the much more soluble product, allantoin, used by all other mammals for excretion. Remnants of this inactive gene have been identified in the human genome (13). This genetic loss forces the human species to excrete the very sparingly soluble uric acid as the end product of purine metabolism and sets the stage for developing of the crystal deposition diseases of gouty arthritis and its nephropathy.

B. Hyperuricemia: Definition, Mechanisms, and Consequences

Hyperuricemia is defined by a serum urate concentration above the upper limit of the normal range, 3.3 to 7.0 mg/dl, for adult males as determined in serum by a variety of highly specific enzymatic tests now in common use (14). The hyperuricemia can be asymptomatic for many years, even a lifetime. The presence of an urate binding protein (15), or similar colloidal agents, may enhance this stability. The deposition of the first crystal of monosodium urate monohydrate marks the turning point for eventual development of gouty arthritis. Since virtually all patients with gout are hyperuricemic, this chemical test is also useful clinically as an aid to the diagnosis of gout (7). Only rarely is it in the upper range of normal during the acute attack, presumably from the stress of the attack.

Serum content of uric acid can be increased to this hyperuricemic range by a heterogenous group of physiologic, genetic, and environmental factors and their interaction affecting its synthesis and excretion, as shown in Table 1 (7). Also included are a variety of changes in normal endocrine function with age and a wide group of "primary diseases" that are capable of producing a "secondary gout." In 10–15% of patients, the hyperuricemia results primarily from a genetically determined excessive synthesis of the purine precursors of uric acid.

TABLE 1 Contributors to Hyperuricemia and Gout

Physiological
Puberty in males
Menopause in females
Endocrine disorder
Hypothyroidism or hyperthyroidism
Hypoadrenal states
Pathological
Myeloproliferative disorders
Idiopathic hypercalciuria
Psoriasis
Environmental
Obesity
Alcohol consumption
High purine foods
Starvation
Ketogenic diet and high-fat diet
Lead poisoning
Pharmacologic
Salicilates, less than 3 g/day
Numerous diuretics
Radio-contrast agents
Genetic
Glycogen storage disease types 1, 3, 5, and 7
Disorders of fructose metabolism
Maple syrup urine disease

In others, the majority, purine synthesis is normal, and a diminished renal excretion of uric acid is responsible. In still others, both mechanisms contribute. The hyperuricemia may also be a risk factor for development of such disorders as cardiovascular disease and diabetes mellitus (16).

Patients with only a modest degree of hyperuricemia may remain asymptomatic throughout life, and thus do not warrant treatment until gout or its nephropathy develops. The mean serum urate of women is about 1.0 mg/dl below that of men until after menopause, thus providing substantial protection for women against the development of gout. Consequently, women account for only 5–10% of gout cases, with most being postmenopausal. Hippocrates noted in the fourth century B.C. that men do not take the gout until they reach sexual maturation and women do not take the gout until their menses cease (11). These observations are in keeping with the sharp rise of serum urate in young males by the end of puberty and the more modest rise of the serum urate in postmenopausal females (16). When hyperuricemia is identified, the patient should be informed of the possibility of development of gout so that the proper diagnosis might be made with the first acute attack.

C. Possible New Role for Hyperuricemia as a Free Radical Scavenger

For many generations, uric acid was regarded as merely a waste product to be eliminated from the body. However, this was at odds with the remarkably efficient renal mechanism eventually found in the human for the conserving of uric acid (see Chapter 10 by Klinenberg). This conservation results in the human male having the highest serum urate of any mammal (17). The mean serum urate is 5.1 ± S.D. 0.98 mg/dl in normal males and 4.0 ± S.D. 0.93 mg/dl in premenopausal females.

A previously unsuspected biological role for serum urate has been found. Ames and associates hypothesized (18) and later demonstrated a very effective action of urate as an antioxidant scavenger of free radicals generated during normal metabolism within the cell (19). Urate was not quite as effective as ascorbic acid, vitamin C, which is used up first and is regarded as the first line of defense against free radicals. However, it may well have an advantage over vitamin C which, itself, generates free radicals when it encounters atoms of iron, copper, or other trace metals as a ready source of free radicals (19). Since humans also lack the final enzyme for synthesizing vitamin C, this same substitute role for uric acid has been proposed as a reason for the human species having the longest lifespan of any mammal (17). If this is indeed so, then gouty arthritis in only the hyperuricemic segment of the population may well be the price paid by the human race for their longevity. Opposing this view is the generally good health of xanthinuria patients. Since they are incapable of synthesizing uric acid from their genetic loss of the enzyme xanthine oxidase (9), they should show an increase in pathology from oxidative damage by free radicals. Instead they show relatively normal health except for a high risk of xanthine stones forming in the urinary tract and of xanthine crystals in muscle causing myalgia in an occasional patient (9).

D. Inflammatory Action of Urate Crystals

The development of acute attacks of gouty arthritis in response to the intra-articular injection of a suspension of urate crystals demonstrated a causative role for the crystals (2,8,20). Evidently, the acute attack will be initiated by exceeding a critical threshold of crystals. The body interprets this invasion of crystals to be the equivalent of invading micro-organisms. The typical acute attack develops as it mobilizes its usual defenses by accumulating macrophages and appropriate cytokines in the joint space to battle the invaders by phagocytosis of the crystals. Indeed, microscopic examination with crossed polarizing filters of synovial fluid obtained during a spontaneous or an induced acute attack reveals over 90% of urate crystals now located within phagocytes (21). Furthermore, even though the enzyme uricase is absent, the strongly oxidizing action of other free-radical-generating enzymes released into the lysosomes during defensive phagocytosis can destroy urate crystals in studies in vivo and in vitro by a nonbacterial uricolysis (22) and an even smaller portion from the bacterial uricolysis observed in studies using ^{15}N-urate (23). The almost routine development of an acute attack of gout shortly after initiation of long-term treatment of their hyperuricemia revealed the same presence of numerous crystals undergoing phagocytosis despite several days or weeks of a normal serum urate. Since no new crystals can be formed, these crystals must arise from dense crystalline aggregates seen in tophi during their dissolution in sufficient number to exceed the critical threshold for initiating an acute attack.

E. Clinical Significance of Hyperuricemia

Since the upper range of normal serum urate is 7.0 mg/dl, the normal distribution places a 3–5% segment of the population in the hyperuricemia range, which is also above the limit of solubility, 6.8 mg/dl of monosodium urate in biological fluid. This supersaturated state may continue throughout life or for many decades without symptoms before precipitation of the first needle-shaped crystals of monosodium urate monohydrate. This crystal should then be able to serve as a seed crystal for the eventual deposition of a myriad of crystals of monosodium urate monohydrate in extracellular body fluids, leading eventually to the formation of solid nodules—the "tophi" characteristic of more advanced stages of gout. The moderately lower temperature in the ears and about the joints of upper and lower extremities should result in a slight decrease in solubility of monosodium urate and even greater supersaturation with a greater tendency for crystal deposition. It could well account for not only the high frequency of acute attacks in joints of the extremities but also the substantially greater prevalence of urate tophi in not only the outer border of the helix of the ears but also in peripheral joints of the extremities (7).

II. GOUT ASSOCIATED GENETIC DISORDERS

In Figure 1, an outline of the pathway of purine synthesis and metabolism in mammals is presented with the location of known enzyme defects of purine metabolism with a brief summary of their clinical features (7).

An excessive production of uric acid with marked hyperuricemia is associated with two types of genetic defects of purine metabolism. Both of them produce a substantial increase in the rate-limiting substrate phosphoribosyl pyrophosphate (PRPP) for the first reaction of purine synthesis. A virtually complete deficiency of the enzyme hypoxanthine guanine phosphoribosyltransferase (HGPRT) involved in the thrifty reutilization of these two purine bases (12,12a) results clinically in the severe neurological and behavioral disorder of Lesch-Nyhan disease (24). Other mutations producing an overactivity of PRPP synthetase can also produce a somewhat different set of neurological impairment along with a marked overproduction of uric acid (25,26). In both disorders the clinical presentation is substantially attenuated by mutations producing a less severe metabolic defect (discussed below).

III. ENZYME DEFECTS ASSOCIATED WITH GOUT

A. Heterozygote for Hereditary Fructose Intolerance

This most recently described gout-associated enzyme defect may account for a substantial portion of patients with a family history of gouty arthritis since it is a rather common recessively inherited abnormality of fructose metabolism. The dominantly inherited defect is found with a frequency of 1 in 80 individuals in Switzerland and 1 in 250 in England. This defect is the heterozygous state for phosphofructoaldolase (aldolase B) deficiency, which in the homozygote results in hereditary fructose intolerance (27). The defect has been identified by a noninvasive method using ^{31}P magnetic resonance spectroscopy over the liver. Homozygote children, when given as little as 1.5 g of fructose orally, show a gross decrease in inorganic phosphate and a marked increase in phosphomonoesters, presumably fructose phosphate. When family members were given 50 g of fructose, the heterozygotes showed a similar pattern. Of the nine heterozygotes detected, three were affected with gouty arthritis (27). In a subsequent study of 11 patients in the community with a family history of gout as well, two had this pattern in response to a fructose load. All of these patients were producing a normal amount of uric acid in the 24-hour urine collected before the study. Other affected members were found in one of the families studied, including the postmenopausal mother who had a normal serum urate but had close relatives with gout. Evidently, the hyperuricemia in this disorder may be modified by other factors (28). However, the affected members all showed a threefold greater rise in serum urate than was found in the nine nonaffected individuals. This defect might well account for the fructose-induced hyperuricemia (29).

B. Glycogen Storage Disease

A marked hyperuricemia and modest overproduction of uric acid leading to the development of gouty arthritis in early adult life has been found in over 40 patients with hepatic glucose-6-phosphate deficiency [glycogen storage disease type 1 (30) as well as in type 3, 5 and 7 (8,31)]. Clinical features include hepatomegaly, retarded rate of growth and sexual development, bleeding tendencies with frequent epistaxis, early development of severe cardiovascular disease, and an eating pattern in adult life of frequent small starchy meals rather than full meals. Blood shows a marked lactic acidemia, hyperuricemia, marked hyperlipidemia, and fasting hypoglycemia. A number of theories have been proposed to account for the hyperuricemia. The lactic acidemia and fasting hypoglycemia interferes with renal excretion of uric acid, but, in addition, it was found that patients show evidence of an increased rate of purine synthesis (9,30,31). Correction of hyperuricemia by continuous nocturnal drip indicates a major role for carbohydrate deprivation and resulting ketonemia in its genesis (33).

C. Lesch-Nyhan Disease

Lesch-Nyhan disease presents clinically as an incapacitating neurologic disorder, limited to males who present with choreoathetosis, spasticity, mild mental retardation "cerebral palsy," and compulsive self-mutilation (24). Affected children also produce the most excessive quantities of uric acid yet seen, which forms the basis for a relatively simple screening test (34,35), in which the ratio of uric acid to creatinine in the morning urine sample is measured. Lesch-Nyhan patients with the full syndrome show ratios between 2.0 and 5.3 compared to 0.2–0.6 for normal individuals. Some overlap with the normal may be found in the first few months of life as a result of high ratios observed at birth in normal infants followed by a marked age-related decline until puberty (34,35). Although most patients also show an elevation of serum urate, particularly in later stages of the disease, this test cannot be used to fully rule out this disorder as around 5–10% of affected infants may show a normal serum urate, particularly in early life.

A structural gene on the X chromosome coding for the synthesis of the enzyme hypoxanthine-guanine phosphoribosyltransferase (HPRT), is grossly deficient in this disorder (12). Less severe deficiencies of the same enzyme results in a clinical attenuation or even absence of the neurologic dysfunction, with a less marked but still excessive purine synthesis, giving rise to severe gouty arthritis with onset in early adult life and, in most cases, with the production of kidney stones composed of uric acid (36). Recurrence of the severe forms of the disease in families carrying the gene may now be prevented through monitoring of pregnancies and prenatal diagnosis on amniotic cells (37). Several reviews have been published (7–9,11).

1. Clinical Features

At birth, children with Lesch-Nyhan disease appear entirely normal and show normal development during the first months of life. A brownish to red-orange sand in the diapers, particularly noticeable when the infant becomes dehydrated, is the first indication of the disease to many mothers. Some of the infants are very irritable and have episodes of screaming, suggesting the possibility of renal colic. The first indication of impaired motor development is the inability to support the head at 4 to 6 months of age with hypotonicity during the next year of life. Voluntary movement of both athetoid and choreoform types are present by the latter part of the first year, with an increase in muscle tone as the first extrapyramidal sign. Pyramidal symptoms consisting of increased deep tendon reflexes, a sustained ankle clonus, scissoring of the lower extremities, and extensor plantar responses are usually present by 1 year of age. An increased incidence of dislocation of the hips and club feet may in some way be related to the early hypotonicity.

Motor and physical development of affected children are grossly impaired, with subnormal height and weight. Some show dysphagia and vomiting as prominent symptoms. An occasional patient is able to sit in a normal manner during the first year, but this ability is subsequently lost with the onset of the neurologic symptoms. They have a characteristic dysarthric speech, although they can usually make themselves understood to those caring for them. Severely affected children are never able to walk (37,38).

2. Behavioral Abnormalities

Compulsive aggressiveness and self-mutilation are the most unusual and variable features of Lesch-Nyhan disease (24,38) and are expressed in most of these children by biting away their lips, tongue, and ends of their fingers if given the opportunity. Biting can, in some cases, begin with the eruption of incisors. In other patients, it may be delayed until early adolescence. In any given patient it can be highly variable in expression, with patients going through periods of extensive self-mutilation and other periods when there is no problem. Self-mutilation tends to be correlated, at least in some cases, with emotional stress.

Lesch-Nyhan disease and its variants are the first well-documented example of a compulsive stereotyped form of behavior that is associated with a genetic and biochemical aberration. Since a harmless biting of lips and fingernails is a relatively common response to stress in members of the normal population, the genetic and biochemical changes could be merely producing an exaggerated response to an environmental stress.

Aggressive acts—kicking, biting, hitting, spitting—against others are also included in the bizarre behavior of these children. Eyeglasses are common targets for their aggression, so physicians soon learn to transfer them to a pocket before examining the child. Frequent projective vomiting is also used by older children as one of their weapons, especially when the child becomes upset emotionally.

Some, but not all, of the patients with less severe deficiencies of the HPRT enzyme with resulting minimal neurologic dysfunction have also shown a compulsive behavior (38). One such patient had a compelling urge to put his hand in the cog wheels of machines, which he had done on at least one occasion. He also recounted having an uncontrollable impulse to jump from a motorcycle or automobile while traveling at high speed, which had resulted in severe injuries to himself and the vehicles (39).

3. Pathology

At lease 11 patients have shown at autopsy no characteristic anatomic finding in histologic preparations that could be of value in characterizing the neurological disease. Kidneys are a target for extremely severe damage from deposits of urate, leading to cardiovascular disease and death in uremia. The most advanced gouty nephropathy seen at the National Institutes of Health was found in one of Dr. Nyhan's original patients, who died at age 12 after only one acute attack of gout in the knee (7).

4. Biochemical Features

Children with the full Lesch-Nyhan disease show the most extreme degree of excessive purine synthesis yet encountered in humans, some three to four times normal, and a full clinical expression of the disease (9,12,24,37). The urine also contains increased amounts of the uric acid precursors 4-amino-5-imidazole carboxamide and hypoxanthine. Hyperuricemia is the eventual outcome of this overproduction but may take a number of years to develop in some patients.

5. Primary Enzyme Defect

Normally, the HPRT enzyme is expressed in all cells of the body with the highest specific activity found in cells of the basal ganglia and testes. These values correlate with the brain area that, if damaged, can cause analogous disorders of movement and the later failure of sexual maturation and atrophic testes found in patients with the most severe enzyme deficit (40). A gross deficiency of the HPRT enzyme is found in all patients with full Lesch-Nyhan disease or its variants (12,12a,38). In patients with the most severe enzyme defect, HPRT activity is virtually absent from all cells of the body. In patients with less severe deficiencies, the HPRT activity in dialyzed erythrocyte lysates may range from less than .01% to 10% or 20% of the normal, using hypoxanthine as a substrate (36,38).

A concurrent increase in the activity of the analogous enzyme concerned with conversion of adenine to its nucleotide, adenine phosphoribosyltransferase (APRT), is a consistent finding in erythrocytes of all patients who show a severe virtually complete HPRT deficiency in erythrocytes (12,12a), but is not found in their fibroblasts nor is this increase found in erythrocytes of patients with a partial HPRT deficiency (12b). HPRT activity in erythrocytes of affected children is invariably substantially higher than is found in their fibroblasts with values of around 1% to 3% of the activity found in normal fibroblasts. The amount of residual activity in fibroblasts correlates inversely with the severity of clinical symptoms (41).

6. Heterozygote Detection

A consistent pattern of X-linked inheritance has been found in all pedigrees until very recently when two females with the disease were found. One study showed a new mutation in a heterozygote female. The other showed crossing over of chromosomes as a mechanism for loss of all activity. Definitive proof came with the demonstration by radioautography of both normal and mutant phenotypes in fibroblasts grown from skin biopsies of the mothers and this remains a very reliable method for heterozygote detection (7). Such a finding is entirely consistent with the single X-inactivation hypothesis proposed independently by Lyon (42). Demonstration of the presence of both normal and mutant cells can also be done by cloning or by selection for the mutant phenotype in the mother's fibroblasts with thioguanine or 6-azaguanine. Heterozygotes can also be detected by assaying hair roots (43).

Erythrocyte activity of mothers of severely HPRT-deficient children invariably show HPRT in the normal range. A selective advantage of the normal stem cell over the mutant phenotype at some stage of fetal or cellular development seems to be the most satisfactory explanation. Only in heterozygotes of partial HPRT deficiency have normal and mutant erythrocytes been demonstrated.

7. Properties of Normal and Mutant Enzymes

HPRT has been purified to homogeneity with complete amino acid sequence (45), which agrees with the cDNA sequence (44). The purified native enzyme is composed of four identical subunits, each containing 217 amino acids not counting the N-terminal methionine with a molecular mass of 24.47 KDa (45). Magnesium and sulfhydryl groups are required for its catalytic activity and its substrates are magnesium PRPP and either hypoxanthine or guanine. It reacts with xanthine at a rate of only 0.3% of that of hypoxanthine. It also reacts with 6-mercaptopurine, 8-azaguanine, allopurinol, and 6-thioguanine to form the respective ribonucleotides, but fails to react with adenine, uric acid, uracil, azathioprine, or oxypurinol (46). 8-Azaguanine is frequently used for selective media, since normal cells that incorporate this purine analog into nucleotides fail to survive, while HPRT-deficient cells are unaffected as they are unable to form the toxic nucleotide.

A large heterogeneous group of mutations have been found. A total of 89

HPRT-deficient patients or families showed 70 different mutations in the HPRT coding region (47). Of these, 32 different mutations predictably produced either a smaller or larger than normal size of the translated protein. Mutations in either the start or stop condons or from single base substitutions have caused splicing errors at an intron/exon boundary, which can cause an alteration of the rate of mRNA synthesis, stability, or translation into protein. Each of the remaining 38 mutations in the HPRT coding regions produced a single amino acid substitution resulting in 24 patients with the full Lesch-Nyhan syndrome and 14 with a partial enzyme deficiency. Of the above 89 patients, 54 had unique single base pair substitutions with the highest number occurring on exons 5 and 7 and the lowest occurrence on exon 2. In more than one unrelated patient, 12 of the mutations have been identified suggesting the presence of mutational "hot spots" in certain locations. Recent determinations of the crystal structure of human HPRT enzyme bound with GMP (48) should allow a greatly enhanced resolution of the functional centers of the HPRT molecule.

8. Mechanism of Purine Overproduction

The most reasonable explanation for the excessive purine synthesis is the increased amount of PRPP accumulating as a result of the HPRT mutation. Fibroblasts cultured from affected patients show a two- to threefold accumulation of PRPP and their erythrocytes a tenfold accumulation over normal values. PRPP is a rate-limiting substrate for the presumed rate-determining reaction of purine biosynthesis catalyzed by the enzyme PRPP glutamine amidotransferase.

The excessive rates of purine synthesis observed in Lesch-Nyhan patients are also found in their fibroblasts (12) and lymphoblasts. When hypoxanthine is omitted from the medium, normal cells increase their rate of purine synthesis to values quite comparable to that of the HPRT-deficient lymphoblasts presumably from formation in normals of feedback inhibitors (49).

Recent studies of mutant fibroblasts suggest a feedback regulation of both PRPP synthetase and amidophosphoribosyltransferase by end products with the latter reaction being more sensitive to small changes in the inhibitory activity of purine nucleotide concentrations (50). HPRT-deficient mice show a normal content of brain purines despite a four- to fivefold increase in ^{14}C formate incorporation, even though they show a complete loss of HPRT (50a).

9. Mechanism of Neurologic Dysfunction

HPRT deficiency substantially decreases dopamine neurotransmitter function and dopamine content of the mouse and the human brain. This is compared to 10–30% of normal in HPRT-deficient mice and Lesch-Nyhan patients (51,52). The dopamine-containing neurons in vivo showed a 50–63% reduction in dopamine neurotransmitter function in 12 Lesch-Nyhan patients in the caudate and a 64–75% reduction in putamen of Lesch-Nyhan disease patients compared to the normal control group. Volumetric magnetic resonance imaging detected a 30% reduction in the caudate volume of these patients. A rigorous correction of data for this volume difference resulted in an even greater decrease in the caudate cerebellar ratio (52a). Positron-emission tomography measuring presynaptic accumulation of fluorodopa ^{18}F showed a low ratio (30–50%) of control in Lesch-Nyhan brains of 12 patients indicative of decreased dopa decarboxylase activity and dopamine storage. They are pervasive and appear to be developmental in origin suggesting a possible role in neuropsychiatric manifestations of the disease (52b). In a mouse model of Lesch-Nyhan syndrome (53), the dopamine deficiency was also identified, despite the lack of the neurologic symptoms of Lesch-Nyhan disease (54). The decreased dopamine in the mouse was accompanied by a decrease in tyrosine hydroxylase activity as a rate-limiting step in dopamine synthesis (55). Dopamine deficits were 48–64% of normal. Thus, there seems to be a fairly specific deficit in the basal ganglia dopamine system in both the human and the mouse model. Although a wide range of experimental approaches to therapy have been attempted, none have been of lasting value for control of the neurologic problems, particularly those of behavior (52,56).

10. Molecular Genetics

The normal human cDNA coding for HPRT has been cloned (44) and inserted into a lymphoblast line cloned from a child with Lesch-Nyhan disease (57) using a defective retrovirus as a vector. The gene insertion produced clones with 2% to 21% of normal HPRT activity indicating a random insertion of the gene into various sites in the chromosome. Nevertheless, it produced a substantial correction of this aberration of purine metabolism, including the excessive rate of purine synthesis. This same vector efficiently transferred the genetic material into stem cells cultured from human bone marrow (58). The possibility of providing a therapeutic benefit to the neurologic dysfunction from a similar genetic correction of bone marrow stem cells of affected patients was suggested by reports of a thymic origin for glial cells of the brain (59). Furthermore, evidence of a partial correction of mutant cell activity by close proximity to a normal cell through the mechanism of metabolic cooperation (60) has been demonstrated with the use of glial cells (58). Although transplantation of normal bone marrow cells into a 21-year-old Lesch-Nyhan patient failed to modify the central nervous system abnormality (61), some promising results are being obtained in other centers.

The prospect of inserting genes for correction of defects in the central nervous system has been discussed with the possibility of using surrogate cells grafted to the brain or by direct delivery of the vector to brain cells in vivo (62). More recently, stable transfection has been reported for other genes into nondividing cells by using a lentiviral vector (63).

11. Treatment

General measures for treatment include avoidance of dehydration by assurance of high fluid intake of at least 50 ml/kg per day will diminish the chance of forming urinary concretions composed of xanthine that have been noted occasionally in children treated with allopurinol, and making certain that nutrition is adequate. Many of these children take a very long time to eat and in an understaffed institution may actually be malnourished. Sites of chronic irritation in the mouth from sharp edges of teeth can be eliminated by a dentist; hands can be kept away from the mouth and yet left free for use by constructing a loose-fitting wrap around fabric splints for the elbows, containing wooden or plastic ribs in a fabric pocket, and secured in place with the tightness desired by Velcro fasteners. These children seem to be incapable of learning from punishment, but they do respond to positive experiences, and some success in behavior modification has been achieved by simply turning away from the child when their aberrant behavior is in evidence (63). Partial improvement in the self-mutilating behavior has been reported from the use of both positive and negative conditioning programs (64).

Allopurinol is very effective in preventing damage to kidneys produced by the excessive amounts of uric acid excreted in the urine. Allopurinol at doses up to 20 mg/kg of body weight per 24 hours produces a striking decrease in uric-acid content of both urine and serum, but fails to decrease the total purine synthesis as is observed in other types of purine overproduction (9). Hypoxanthine and xanthine merely replace the deficit in uric acid in the 24-hour urine. Established renal calculi composed of uric acid can thereby be substantially reduced in size. Unfortunately, no rational therapy has yet been found satisfactory for treating the neurologic dysfunction. Orotic acid decreased purine synthesis but failed to prevent the neurological deficit (32). Children treated with diazepam (Valium) are more tractable and less spastic. Hydroxytryptophan has been reported to reduce self-mutilation in children in Japan (65–66), but was not effective in reducing self-mutilating behavior in numerous other studies (67–69). Despite clinical trials with a large number of agents, no successful treatment of the neurologic problem has been found (54,70).

12. Prenatal Diagnosis

Until a more effective therapy for the neurologic aspects of this disease is developed, prevention of the disease by monitoring pregnancies is indicated. This is best done by identifying heterozygous females among the relatives of an index case (71). The identification of 7 affected fetuses in 25 heterozygote females monitored is very close to the expected 25%, suggesting that HPRT deficiency does not trigger spontaneous abortions.

D. Increased Phosphoribosylpyrophosphate Synthetase

The excessive production of uric acid found in over 20 families with gouty arthritis has now been traced to an increased activity of the enzyme phosphoribosylpyrophosphate synthetase. The increased intracellular concentration of PRPP found in fibroblasts or lymphoblasts cultured from patients with this disorder provides another example, with a different mutation, of the correlation of PRPP concentration and excessive production of uric acid (38,50,72). This correlation provides additional evidence in support of the concept outlined above of the central role of PRPP concentrations as one important factor governing the rate of purine synthesis de novo in vivo. All families showed gouty arthritis and an excessive rate of purine synthesis, ranging from 1.0 to 2.4 g of uric acid excreted/24 hours while maintained on a purine-free diet. In addition, a high incidence of renal calculi composed of uric acid was also present in these families (50). Other clinical features in two other families included deafness (73,74). A wide range of different mutations in this same gene have been identified (75). Both the HPRT enzyme and PRPP synthetase enzyme are located in close proximity on the long arm of the X chromosome (73).

REFERENCES

1. J. N. Loeb. The influence of temperature on the solubility of monosodium urate. *Arth Rheum 15*:189 (1972).
2. J. E. Seegmiller, R. R. Howell, and S. E. Malawista. The inflammatory reaction to sodium urate: Its possible relationship to the genesis of gouty arthritis, *J Amer Med Assn 180*:469 (1962).
3. T.-F. Yu and A. B. Gutman. Mobilization of gouty tophi by protracted use of uricosuric agents. *Am J Med 11*:765 (1951).
4. J. H. Talbot, C. Bishop, B. M. Norcoss and L. M. Lockie. The clinical and metabolic effects of Benemid on patients with gout. *Trans Assoc Am Phys 64*:372 (1951).
5. R. K. Robbins. Potential purine antagonists. I: Synthesis of some 4,6-substituted pyrazole-3,4-pyrimidines. *J Am Chem Soc 78*:784 (1956).
6. R. W. Rundles, J. B. Wyngaarden, and G. H. Hitchings. Effects of a xanthine oxidase inhibitor on thiopurine metabolism, hyperuricemia and gout. *Trans Assoc Am Phys 76*:126 (1963).
7. J. E. Seegmiller. Diseases of purine and pyrimidine metabolism. In: Metabolic Control and Disease, 8th Ed. (P. K. Bondy and L. E. Rosenberg, eds.), W. B. Saunders Co., Philadelphia, PA, 1980, pp. 777–937.
8. J. B. Wyngaarden and W. N. Kelley. Gout and Hyperuricemia, Grune and Stratton, New York, NY, 1976, pp. 360–375.
9. J. E. Seegmiller, Disorders of purine and pyrimidine metabolism. A. Emery and D.L. Rimoin Principles and Practice of Medical Genetics, 3rd Ed. (D. Rimoin, J.M. Connor, and R.E. Pyeritz, eds.), Churchill Livingstone, Inc., New York, NY, 1997, pp. 1921–1943.

10. P. A. Simkin. Gout and hyperuricemia, *Curr Opin in Rheumatol 9*:268 (1997).
11. J. E. Seegmiller. Conquest of gouty arthritis, Landmark Advances in Rheumatology (Daniel J. McCarty, ed.), American Rheumatology Association, Atlanta, GA, 1985, pp. 89–101.
12. J. E. Seegmiller, F. Rosenbloom, and W. N. Kelley. Enzyme defect associated with a sex-linked human neurological disorder and excessive purine synthesis. *Science 155*:1682 (1967).
12a. J. E. Seegmiller. Inherited deficiency of hypoxanthineguanine phosphoribosyltransferase in X-linked uric aciduria (the Lesch-Nyhan syndrome and its variants). *Adv Hum Genet 6*:75 (1976).
12b. B. T. Emmerson. The management of gout. *New Engl J Med 334*:445 (1996).
13. X. Y. Wu, C. C. Lee, D. M. Muzny, and C. T. Caskey. Urate oxidase primary structure and evolutionary implications, *Proc Natl Acad Sci USA 23*:9412 (1989).
14. L. Liddle, J. E. Seegmiller and L. Laster. The enzymatic spectrophotometric method for determination of uric acid. *J Lab Clin Med 54*:903 (1959).
15. J. O. Alvsaker. Uric acid in human plasma. Isolation and identification of plasma proteins interacting with urate. *Scand J Clin Lab Invest 18*:227 (1966).
16. W. J. Fessel, A. B. Siegelaub, and E. S. Johnson. Correlates and consequences of asymptomatic hyperuricemia. *Arch Intern Med 132*:44 (1973).
17. R. G. Cutler, Antioxidants, aging and longevity. Free Radicals in Biology, Vol. I (W. A. Pryor, ed.), Plenum Press, New York, NY, 1984, pp. 371–405.
18. B. N. Ames, R. Cathcart, E. Schiviers, and P. Hochstein. Uric acid provides an antioxidant defense in humans against oxidant and radical caused aging and cancer: a hypothesis, *Proc Natl Sci USA 78*:6858 (1981).
19. B. Frei, L. England, and B. N. Ames. Ascorbate is an outstanding antioxidant in human blood plasma, *Proc Natl Acad Sci USA 76*:5366 (1989).
20. D. J. McCarty. Phagocytosis of urate crystals in gouty synovial fluid, *Arth Rheum 4*:425 (1961).
21. J. S. Faires and D. J. McCarty. Acute arthritis in man and dog produced by intrasynovial injection of sodium urate crystals, *Clin Res 9*:329 (1961).
22. J. B. Wyngaarden and D. Stetten, Jr. Uricolysis in normal man. *J Biol Chem 209*:9 (1953)
23. J. D. Benedict, M. Roche, T-F. Yu, E. J. Bien, A. B. Gutman, and D. W. Stetten, Jr. Incorporation of glycine nitrogen into uric acid in normal and gouty man, *Metabolism 1*:3 (1952).
24. M. Lesch, and W. L. Nyhan. A familial disorder of uric acid metabolism and central nervous system function. *Am J Med 36*:561 (1964).
25. O. Sperling, P. Boer, and S. Persky-Brosh. Altered kinetic property of erythrocyte phosphoribosylpyrophosphate synthetase in excessive purine production. *Rev Eur Etud Clin Biol 17*:703 (1972).
26. M. A. Becker, L. J. Meyer, A. W. Wood, and J. E. Seegmiller. Purine overproduction in man associated with increased phosphoribosylpyrophosphate synthetase activity, *Science 179*:1123 (1973).
27. R. D. Oberhaensli, B. Rajagopalan, and D. J. Taylor. Study of hereditary fructose intolerance by use of 31-P magnetic resonance spectroscopy, *Lancet 2*:931 (1987).

28. J. E. Seegmiller, R. M. Dixon, G. J. Kemp, P. W. Angus, T. E. McAlindon, P. Dieppe, B. Rajagopalan, and G. K. Radda. Fructose-induced aberration of metabolism in familial gout identified by 31-P magnetic resonance spectroscopy, *Proc Natl Acad Sci USA 87*:8326 (1990).
29. F. Stirpe, E. Della Corte, E. Bonnetti, and A. Abbondanza. Fructose-induced hyperuricemia, *Lancet 2*:1310 (1970).
30. F. P. Alepa, R. R. Howell, J. R. Klinenberg, and J. E. Seegmiller. Relationships between glycogen storage disease and tophaceous gout. *Am J Med 47*:58 (1967).
31. S. Jakovcic and L. B. Sorensen. Studies of uric acid metabolism in glycogen storage disease associated with gouty arthritis, *Arth Rheum 10*:129 (1967).
32. W. N. Kelley, M. L. Greene, I. H. Fox, F. M. Rosenbloom, R. I. Levy, and J. E. Seegmiller. Effects of orotic acid on purine and lipoprotein metabolism in man. *Metabolism 19*:1025 (1970).
33. P. J. Benke and S. Gold. Purine metabolism in therapy of Von Gierke's disease, *Pediatr Res 1*:837 (1977).
34. J. M. Kaufman, M. L. Greene, and J. E. Seegmiller. Urine uric acid to creatinine ratio: a screening test for inherited disorders of purine metabolism. *J Pediatr 73*:583 (1968).
35. R. McInnes, P. Lamm, C. L. Clow, and C. R. Scriver. A filter paper sampling method for the uric acid:creatinine ratio in urine: normal values in the newborn. *Pediatrics 49*:80 (1972).
36. W. N. Kelley, F. M. Rosenbloom, J. F. Henderson, and J. E. Seegmiller. A specific enzyme defect in gout associated with overproduction of uric acid. *Proc Natl Acad Sci USA 57*:1735 (1967).
37. W. Nyhan. Behavior in the Lesch-Nyhan syndrome. *Ann Progr in Child Psych and Child Devel*:175 (1977).
38. T. Page, and W. L. Nyhan, The spectrum of HPRT deficiency: an update, Purine and Pyrimidine Metabolism in Man, Vol. 6, Part A (K. Mikanagi, K. Nishioka, and W. N. Kelley, eds.), Plenum Press, New York, NY, 1989, pp. 129–133.
39. A. Geerdink, W. H. M. DeVries, and J. Willemse. An atypical case of hypoxanthineguanine phosphoribosyltransferase deficiency (Lesch-Nyhan syndrome). *Clin Genet 4*:348 (1973)
40. R. W. E. Watts, R. Harkness, E. Spellacy, and N. F. Taylor. Lesch-Nyhan syndrome: growth delay, testicular atrophy and a partial failure of the 11b-hydroxylation of steroids. *J Inherited Metabol Disor 10*:210 (1987).
41. T. Page and W. L. Nyhan. Abnormalities of purine and pyrimidine metabolism. *Neurol Aspects of Pediatrics*:177 (1992).
42. M. F. Lyon. Gene action in the X-chromosome of the mouse. *Nature 190*:372 (1961).
43. B. Bakay, C. Tucker-Pian, and J. E. Seegmiller. Detection of Lesch-Nyhan Syndrome carriers: analysis of hair roots for HPRT by agarose gel electrophoresis and autoradiography. *Clin Genet 17*:1 (1980).
44. D. J. Jolly, H. Okayama, P. Berg, A. C. Esty, D. Filpula, P. Bohlen, G. G. Johnson, J. E. Shively, T. Hunkapillar, and T. Friedmann. Isolation and characterization of a full length, expressible cDNA for human hypoxanthine guanine phosphoribosyltransferase. *Proc Natl Acad Sci USA 80*:477 (1983).

45. J. Wilson, G. Tarr, W. Mahoney, and W. Kelley. Human hypoxanthine-guanine phosphoribosyltransferase: complete amino acid sequence of the erythrocyte enzyme. *J Biol Chem 257*:10978 (1982).
46. T. A. Krenitsky, R. Papainnou, and G. B. Elion. Human hypoxanthine phoribosyltransferase. I. Purification, properties, and specificity. *J Biol Chem 244*:1263 (1969).
47. D. A. Sculley, P. A. Dawson, B. T. Emmerson, and R. B. Gordon. A review of the molecular basis of hypoxanthine-guanine phosphoribosyltransferase (HPRT) deficiency. *Hum Genet 90*:195 (1992).
48. J. C. Eads, G. Scapain, and Y. Xu. The crystal structure of human hypoxanthine-guanine phosphoribosyltransferase with bound GMP. *Cell 78*:325 (1994).
49. M. S. Hershfield and J. E. Seegmiller. Regulation of de novo purine synthesis in human lymphoblasts: similarities of de novo synthesis during growth by normal cells and mutants deficient in hypoxanthine-guanine phosphoribosyltransferase activity. *J Biol Chem 252*:6002 (1977).
50. M. A. Becker and M. Kim. Regulation of purine synthesis de novo in human fibroblasts by purine nucleotides and phosphoribosylpyrophosphate, *J Biol Chem 262*:14531 (1987).
50a. H. A. Jinnah, T. Page and T. Friedmann. Brain purines in a genetic mouse model of Lesch-Nyhan disease, *J Neurochem* 2036 (1993).
51. K. G. Lloyd, O. Hornykiewicz, and L. Davidson. Biochemical evidence of dysfunction of brain neurotransmitters in the Lesch-Nyhan syndrome. *New Engl J Med 305*:1106 (1981).
52. W. L. Nyhan, H. G. Johnson, I. A. Kaufman, and K. L. Jones. Serotonergic approaches to the modification of behavior in the Lesch-Nyhan syndrome, *ppl. Res Ment Retardation 1*:25 (1980).
52a. D. F. Wong, J. C. Harris, N. Sakkubai, F. Yokoi, S. Marenco, R. F. Dannals, H. T. Ravert, M. Yaster, A. Evans, O. Rousset, R. N. Bryan, A. Giedde, M. J. Kuhar, and G. R. Breese. Dopamine transporters are markedly reduced in Lesch-Nyhan disease in vivo, *Proc Natl Acad Sci USA 93*:5539 (1996).
52b. M. Ernst, A. J. Zametkin, J. A. Matochik, D. Pascualvaca, P. H. Jons, K. Hardy, J. G. Hankerson, D. J. Doudet, and R. M. Cohen. Presynaptic dopaminergic deficits in Lesch-Nyhan disease, *New Engl J Med 334*:1568 (1996).
53. M. Hooper, K. Hardy, and A. Handyside. HPRT-deficient (Lesch-Nyhan) mouse embryos derived from germline colonization by cultured cells. *Nature 326*:292 (1987).
54. H. A. Jinnah, B. E. Wojcik, and M. Hunt. Dopamine deficiency in a genetic mouse model of Lesch-Nyhan disease, *J Neurosci 14*:1164 (1994).
55. H. A. Jinnah, P. J. Langlais, and T. Friedmann. Functional analysis of brain dopamine systems in a genetic mouse model of Lesch-Nyhan syndrome. *J Pharmacol Exp Ther 263*:596 (1992).
56. T. Page and W. L. Nyhan. Biochemical correlates of auto-aggressive behavior, Application of Basic Neuroscience to Child Psychiatry (S. I. Deutsch, W. Weizman, and R. Weizman, eds.), Plenum, New York, NY, 1990, pp. 297–311.
57. R. C. Willis, D. J. Jolly, A. D. Miller, M. M. Plent, A. C. Esty, P. J. Anderson, H-C

Chang, O. W. Jones, J. E. Seegmiller, and T. Friedmann. Partial phenotypic correction of human Lesch-Nyhan (hypoxanthine-guanine phosphoribosyltransferse-deficient) lymphoblasts with a transmissible retroviral vector. *Proc Nat Acad Sci USA 259*:7842 (1984).

58. H. E. Gruber, K. D. Finley, and R. M. Hershberg, Retroviral vector-mediated gene transfer into human hematopoietic progenitor cells. *Science 230*:1057 (1985).
59. S. Frujita, and T. Kitamura, Origin of brain macrophages and the nature of the microglis, *Pro Neuropathol 111*:1 (1976).
60. T. Friedmann, J. E. Seegmiller, and J. H. Subak-Sharpe. Metabolic cooperation between genetically marked human fibroblasts in tissue culture, *Nature 220*:272 (1968).
61. W. L. Nyhan, T. Page, H. E. Gruber and R. Parkman. Bone marrow transplantation in Lesch-Nyhan disease, *Birth Defects 22*:113 (1986).
62. T. Friedmann and H. A. Jinnah. Gene therapy for disorders of the nervous system, *Trends in Biotechnol 11*:192 (1993).
63. L. Naldini, U. Blomer, and P. Gallay. In vivo gene delivery and stable transduction of nondividing cells by a lentiviral vector, *Science 272*:263 (1996).
64. P. McGreevy and M. Arthur. Effective behavior treatment of self-biting by a child with Lesch-Nyhan Syndrome, *Dev Med Child Neurol 29*:529 (1987).
65. T. I. Mizuno and Y. Yugari. Self-mutilation in the Lesch-Nyhan syndrome, *Lancet 1*:761 (1974).
66. T. Mizuno and Y. Yugari. Prophylactic effect of 1-5-hydroxytryptophan on self-mutilation in the Lesch-Nyhan syndrome, *Neuropaediatrie 6*:13 (1975).
67. L. T. Anderson, L. Hermann, and J. Dancis. The effect of 1-5-hydroxytryptophan on self-mutilation in Lesch-Nyhan disease: negative report, *Neuropaediatrie 7*:439 (1976).
68. R. D. Ciaranello, T. F. Anders, and J. D. Barchas. The use of 5-hydroxytryptophan in a child with Lesch-Nyhan syndrome, *Child Psychiatry Hum Dev 7*:127 (1976).
69. C. D. Frith, E. C. Johnstone, and M. H. Joseph, Double-blind clinical trial of 5-hydroxytryptophan in a case of Lesch-Nyhan syndrome, *J Neurol Neurosurg Psychiatry 39*:656 (1976).
70. K. Sege-Peterson, J. Chambers, T. Page, O. W. Jones, and W. L. Nyhan. Characteristics of mutations in phenotypic variants of hypoxanthine phosphoribosyltransferase deficiency. *Hum Mol Genet 1*:427 (1992)
71. J. E. Seegmiller. Amniotic fluid and cells in the diagnosis of genetic disorders. Amniotic Fluid: Physiology, Biochemistry, and Clinical Chemistry, Vol. 1 (S. Natael-son, A. Scommegna, and M. B. Epstein, eds), I. Wiley, New York, NY, 1974, pp. 291–316.
72. F. M. Rosenbloom, J. F. Henderson, and I. C. Caldwell. Biochemical bases of accelerated purine biosynthesis de novo in human fibroblasts lacking hypoxanthine-guanine phosphoribosyltransferase. *J Biol Chem 243*:1116 (1968).
73. M. A. Becker, R. C. K. Yen, and P. Itkin. Regional localization of the gene for human phosphoribosylpyrophosphate synthetase on the x-chromosome, *Science 203*:1016 (1980).

74. M. A. Becker, K. O. Raivio, and B. Bakay. Superactive phosphoribosylpyrophosphate synthetase with altered regulatory and catalytic properties, *Adv Exp Med Biol 122A*:387 (1980).
75. M. A. Becker, J. M. Nosal, and R. I. Switzer. Point mutations in PRP1, the gene encoding the PRPP synthetase (PRS) 1 isoform underlie X-linked PRS superactivity associated with purine nucleotide inhibitor resistance, *Adv Exp Med Biol 370*:707 (1994).

10
Renal Handling of Urate

James R. Klinenberg
Cedars Sinai Medical Center and University of California at Los Angeles School of Medicine, Los Angeles, California

In a chapter entitled, "Renal Exchange of Urate," Talbot (1) states that "since the renal exchange of urate is intimately involved in the etiology of the dyscrasia considerable attention has been given to the role of urate excretion." It is noted that the concentration of urate in glomerular filtrate is presumed to be similar to that of a protein-free filtrate of plasma, while the concentration of urate in bladder urine may be from 3 to 15 times greater. The mechanism whereby the kidney removes the great quantity of water and urate from glomerular filtrate and excretes a urine of higher urate content than serum is of considerable significance. The determination of the rate of formation of glomerular filtrate—the initial essential function—may be measured by the clearance of inulin or mannitol. It was suggested at that time that the mechanism whereby the bladder urine is more concentrated with respect to urate than the glomerular filtrate could be one by which water is selectively removed from the glomerular filtrate, thus concentrating urate in the urine.

I. RENAL URATE EXCRETION IN NORMAL MAN

In the past 30 years, much has been learned about the handling of uric acid by the kidney in normal humans. Evidence has been gathered to allow the present concept of renal tubular urate handling, which proposes a four component model. This includes (1) glomerular filtration, (2) tubular reabsorption, (3) active tubular secretion, and (4) postsecretory reabsorption. It has also been demonstrated that many patients with gout have decreased renal excretion of urate resulting in urate retention.

II. REGULATION OF URIC ACID EXCRETION IN PATIENTS WITH GOUT

In normal humans, about two-thirds of the uric acid formed in the body is excreted by the kidneys and one-third is eliminated via the intestinal tract, where uric acid is decreted by intestinal bacteria. Uric acid excretion by the kidneys involves glomerular filtration, tubular reabsorption, tubular secretion, and postsecretory reabsorption. Under ordinary circumstances, 99% of the filtered urate is reabsorbed by the renal tubules. That which escapes reabsorption amounts to less than 20% of the uric acid excretion in urine and the major portion is derived from tubular secretion.

III. RENAL URIC ACID EXCRETION IN PATIENTS WITH GOUT

Theoretically, the decreased excretion of uric acid could be due to: (1) reduced filtration of urate, (2) enhanced reabsorption, or (3) decreased tubular secretion. Attempts to localize the site of the defect of urate transport in the nephron have been hindered by limitations of the techniques used to definitively answer this question. Surely, there are some examples of hyperuricemia related to decreased glomerular filtration of urate, but this occurs primarily in patients with evidence of decreased ability to clear other waste products, mainly patients with some degree of azotemia, and this has surely not been the case in the average gouty patient. Therefore, decreased glomerular filtration does not appear to be a viable explanation for the decreased renal excretion of uric acid in most gouty patients. There is no evidence to support increased tubular reabsorption either in the initial reabsorptive phase or in the postsecretory reabsorption. Therefore, most of the emphasis in studies of the decreased renal clearance of urate in the gouty patient have emphasized decreased tubular secretion.

A. Glomerular Filtration of Uric Acid

Glomerular filtration of uric acid was first demonstrated with micropuncture studies in the frog, demonstrating that the concentration of urate in the glomerular fluid were the same as that in plasma. Similarly, micropuncture studies have been done in the rat. No such studies in humans have ever been performed. However, it is generally believed that urate in plasma is freely filterable at the glomerus, although some studies have suggested that there might be a small amount of urate that is bound to plasma proteins. It is currently thought that the amount of urate bound to plasma proteins is less than 5% and, therefore, it is appropriate to suggest that urate filtration at the glomerular is almost complete.

B. Reabsorption of Uric Acid

Comparison of the renal clearances of uric acid with those of inulin or creatinine in human subjects disclose a mean ratio of about 0.07–0.10. If we suggest that there is complete glomerular ultrafiltration in human subjects, then there is 90–93% reabsorption of the filtered urate. Most studies of uric acid reabsorption indicate that the process takes place in the proximal tubules. Available evidence also suggests that urate absorption also occurs by a mechanism of active transport. There seems to be a close link between the reabsorption of sodium and the reabsorption of a number of other components in the glomerular filtrate, such as phosphate, calcium, glucose, bicarbonate, and uric acid. Thus, in conditions associated with an increase in proximal reabsorption sodium, the clearance of uric acid is also reduced; in conditions leading to decreased proximal reabsorption of sodium, the clearance of uric is increased. Since highly acidified distal tubular fluid uric acid is likely to be minimally ionized, one might assume that uric acid would then undergo reabsorption by nonionic diffusion. However, if so, the contribution to urate reabsorption is so small that it is not readily detected and therefore does not seem to play a major role in uric acid reabsorption.

C. Tubular Secretion of Uric Acid

The first evidence for uric acid secretion in man was published by Praetorius and Kirk in 1952, when they reported the case of a young man with plasma urate concentration of less than 0.6 mg in the urate inulin clearance ratio of 1.46 mg. Subsequently, Gutman and coworkers achieved urate/inulin clearance ratios as high as 1.23 in normal subjects following urate loading, mannitol diuresis, and larger doses of probenecid. Each of these studies indicated net tubular secretion of urate in humans under these very special circumstances. The biphasic effects of salicylate upon uric acid excretion were interpreted as representing inhibition of urate secretion with urate retention at low salicylate doses plus inhibition of urate reabsorption with urate diuresis at higher salicylate doses. Diamond and his colleagues have suggested that the apparent paradoxical effect of salicylate on uric acid excretion is due to inhibition of reabsorption by salicylate itself with inhibition of excretion due to a metabolite, salicylurate. Irrespective of the mechanism, bidirectional transport of uric acid is apparent. The site within the nephron where uric acid secretion occurs has not definitely been established.

D. Postsecretory Absorption

A number of observations have proved difficult to accommodate within the model of filtration, early proximal reabsorption, and later proximal secretion. In patients with Wilson's disease and some people with Hodgkin's disease there is hyperuricemia associated with increased renal urate clearance ratios, and in these patients, pyrazinamide suppresses the hyperuricosuria.

The effects of pyrazinamide are explained in terms of reduced secretory delivery to the late reabsorptive sites. The location of the postsecretory reabsorptive process could be coextensive with the secretory mechanism and are separate and distal to it. Additional, in two kindreds with familial hyperuricemia due to diminished renal clearance of urate it was proposed that the defect was due to decreased postsecretory reabsorption. Thus, the postsecretory reabsorption may be more important than previously recognized.

ADDITIONAL READING

1. J. H. Talbot, Gout, Grune & Stratton, New York, N. Y., 1964, p. 53.
2. T. D. Palella and W. N. Kelley, Purine and deoxypurine metabolism, & Textbook of Rheumatology, 2nd Ed., In: Kelley, Harris, eds., W. B. Saunders, Philadelphia, Pa., 1981, pp. 343–346.
3. I. M. Weiner, the renal handling of urate, In: The Kidney in Gout and Hyperuricemia, Futura Publishing Co., Inc., 1982, pp. 17–60.
4. T.-F. Yu, Chapter 46, In: W. A. Katz, ed., Diagnosis and Management of Rheumatic Diseases, J. B. Lippincott Company, 1988, pp. 544–545.

11

Trends in the Treatment of Gout

HARRY SPIERA and TSAI-FAN YÜ
Mount Sinai School of Medicine, New York, New York

I. INTRODUCTION

Gout has been a scourge for mankind for many years. It was well-recognized before the Common Era (1). References to the disease can be found in ancient manuscripts, including the Yeroshalmi Talmud (2). A discussion of the trends in the treatment of gout must be viewed in historical perspective, to understand the modalities that came to be available.

Since gout is such a severely painful disease, and its manifestations are obviously striking, it quickly came to demand medical attention over the years. Moreover, with the perception that gout was related to a gluttonous, intemperate lifestyle, and often affected the rich, wealthy, and intelligent, there developed a long history of descriptions of the disease in both written texts and illustrations. A magnificent review of the art of gout was presented by the late Dr. Rodnan (3). As an extremely painful and visible illness in which attacks would occur and then subside, it became the subject of speculation as to its cause or causes, and an incredible variety of treatments were used. These speculations and treatments were naturally reflective of the medical theories, dogmas, and modalities extant at any given time. Precisely because each acute attack would usually get better spontaneously, it was easy to ascribe improvement to whichever modality was used. An unending series of salves, poultices, physical treatments, religious incantations, and invasive procedures were attempted (4). It was believed that the patient's lifestyle and venery were not only contributory, but actually causative of the disease, which led to the concept that the disease was in some way a divine punishment, and that the victim could be blamed for his or her predicament.

Over the years, a number of clinical and pathological observations were made that helped develop a better understanding of gout, and prepared the way for the important observations that led to a fuller understanding and successful treatment. These observations included the fact that it was primarily a male disease, and that patients with gout would develop joint and/or soft tissue deposits called tophi, and that gout patients were more likely to be subject to kidney stone formation.

The modern era of the study of gout dates back to Dr. Thomas Sydenham's description of gout (a disease from which he personally suffered) (5). He, as many before him, recognized the presence of "chalk stones" deposited about the joints and ligaments, which we now recognize as deposits of uric acid.

It was Karl Wilhelm Scheele, in 1776, who began the serious scientific study of gout (6). He demonstrated that the kidney stones passed by patients with gout were not calcium in nature, but rather made of a heretofore unidentified organic acid, which he called "lithic acid." It was subsequently renamed uric acid. He also demonstrated the presence of uric acid in normal urine. In 1797, William Hyde Wollaston discovered that tophi were formed from a "neutral compound consisting of lithic acid and mineral alkali" (7). Thus, it was established that the vector of tophaceous gout was sodium urate.

In 1848, Garrod described the presence of uric acid in the serum of patients with gout (8). He introduced the "thread test," in which a thread was soaked in the acidified serum of gout patients and then evaporated. The test was positive when uric acid crystals grew on the thread. He also described the presence of extensive tophaceous deposits about joints, bones, and ligaments in the autopsies of gouty patients. He identified the presence of urate crystals in articular cartilage and in the pyramidal portions of the kidney.

Garrod postulated a series of 10 propositions as to the "true nature of gout," which were remarkably accurate in light of subsequent scientific study. His work stating that tophaceous gout was the result of urate deposition was irrefutable. However, the nature of the acute gouty attack remained unexplained. As late as 1959, Hensch wrote "it would appear that urates have little or nothing to do with acute gouty arthritis" (9).

It was not until the early 1960s, after a series of brilliant experiments by McCarty and associates (10), that it was clearly demonstrated that the acute gouty attack resulted from the precipitation of crystalline urate leading to the acute inflammatory reaction in the joint, which we now recognize as the acute gouty attack. Not only was he able to demonstrate that, in virtually every attack of gout, intracellular urate crystals could be demonstrated in the affected joint, but that the injection of urate crystals could produce an acute gout-like attack, not only in gouty men, but in those who had never previously had gout. He also demonstrated in dogs that the presence of white cells capable of phagocytosing the urate crystals are necessary for the development of acute gout. The observation that it was not necessarily the chemical composition of the crystal that was important, but rather its physical properties, led to an understanding of a totally new biological phenomenon. He demonstrated that amorphous urate would not induce an attack of gout when injected into the joints of dogs or people, but microcrystalline urate would. Other crystals, such as sodium orotate, a crystal which is similar in shape to the urate crystals, were found to cause the same physiological response. Thus arose the concept of crystalline arthropathy, which led soon to the description of calcium pyrophosphate deposition disease (CPDD) (11).

Studies of renal physiology and purine and protein biochemistry established that urate was the end product of purine and protein metabolism (12). It was also established that most gout patients did not show overexcretion of uric acid in the urine, and that a fair number of gout patients did produce uric acid calculi (13).

Specific treatment for acute gout began in 1764 when Baron Anton Von Steuch introduced the use of colchicine, which was often remarkably effective for the treatment of the acute attack (14). The introduction of phenylbutazone in the late 1940s, and eventually the whole group of nonsteroidal anti-inflammatory agents, particularly Indomethacin, made treatment of acute gout simpler (15,16). adrenocorticotropic hormone (ACTH) and synthetic steroids provided another powerful way to treat acute attacks (17,18).

In the late 1940s, penicillin was found to be an effective drug for controlling infections, but the drug was rather expensive (19). By using probenecid together with penicillin, the penicillin dosage could be reduced (20). It was also found that serum uric acid became lower on such a regimen (21). By prolonged use of probenecid in tophaceous gout, the size of the subcutaneous or osseous tophi became smaller or even disappeared (22). The increased urinary excretion of uric acid, however, sometimes increased the formation of uric acid calculi in the kidney, particularly if urine pH was low (23). The subsequent discovery of allopurinol, a xanthine oxidase inhibitor that reduced uric acid production, introduced another phase in the treatment of gout (24).

In 1948, an article entitled "A Perverse, Ungrateful, Maleficent Malady" in *The New Yorker* magazine describes what a terrible illness gout was, and how it adversely affected the lives of many men (25). It is remarkable to contemplate that by 1963, most of the major clinical problems of gout had been solved, and the basis for modern treatment of gout developed. Thus gout quickly became a disease easy to treat effectively in all of its manifestations, and complications were prevented. It probably remains the prototype of medical conquest of a disease through modern medical science.

II. TREATMENT

The treatment of gout is best considered by looking at the disease as a series of stages, which often represent a continuum. They are asymptomatic hyperuricemia, acute gout, interval gout, and chronic tophaceous gout. To some extent, uric acid stones must also be considered as part of the spectrum.

A. Asymptomatic Hyperuricemia

An elevated serum uric acid is found far more commonly in nongouty than gouty persons (26). This observation was clearly made when multichannel chemical analysis came into broad use. It was found at that time that between 2.3% and 17.6% of men were hyperuricemic (27). Before that time, routine uric acid determinations were made only as indicated by a particular clinical condition. Tests were expensive, and medical insurance for such tests was not generally available. Thus before the 1960s, the clinical decision as to whether to treat asymptomatic hyperuricemia was rarely an issue. It came up primarily when family members of gout sufferers were studied. At that time, treatment recommendations for patients with asymptotic uricemia would include strict dietary modification, avoidance of alcohol, and weight reduction (28).

With the introduction of probenecid as a uricosuric agent in the 1950s, it became the drug of choice.

With the introduction of allopurinol in the 1960s, in combination with the widespread chemical screening with the use of multipanel chemistries, there was a tendency on the part of many physicians to treat asymptomatic hyperuricemia. Evidence of the efficacy of this approach has not been conclusively determined, and this question still remains controversial. Most authorities do not advocate treating asymptomatic hyperuricemia with drugs, though they still recommend weight reduction and avoidance of alcohol and purine-rich foods. Patients with very high uric acid (greater than 10.0 mg/dl) were found to have a 90% chance of eventually developing gout. Whether this in itself would justify treating all such patients with a uric-acid-lowering drug is still an individual clinical decision. An exception to the above is the hyperuricemia associated with blood dyscrasias, and their treatment, in which allopurinol is an accepted indication (29). The avoidance of allopurinol in routine treatment of asymptomatic hyperuricemia is advocated not only because of the expense of such treatment, but because of the rare but potentially serious complications of the use of allopurinol and uricosuric agents. In a study from a university medical center, Wallace reported that patients who died of allopurinol toxicity usually did not have a good indication for its use (30).

B. Acute Gout

Perhaps the most dramatic manifestation of gout is the acute gouty attack, which has historically received the most attention. It is the excruciatingly painful gouty attack, usually involving the first metatarsophalangeal (MTP) joint, that has been the subject of such attention over the years. Before the introduction of colchicine in 1783 as a specific treatment for acute gout, all manners of treatment were employed, with varying degrees of success. Dr. Rodnan, in his review of ancient therapeutic arts in the gout, lists baptism, amulets, salves of varying composition, application of blistering ointments, putting nails and hair into a tree, counterirritants, cautery, leeching, cupping, moxibustion, acupuncture, and myriad others. Indeed, any agent that was available to treat anything was used. Again, because of the often self-limited nature of gout, any improvement was often attributed to the treatment used.

After the introduction of colchicine as an effective method of interrupting the course of the acute gouty attack, it gradually became the mainstay for the treatment of acute gout. It was found to be effective in about 90% of patients, particularly when used early in the gouty attack (31). Aspirin, of course, and other analgesics were used. In the early 1950s, phenylbutazone and oxyphenylbultazone became available. They were extremely effective in treating gout in the vast majority of patients. Almost simultaneously, ACTH was introduced, which was also virtually always successful in the treatment of acute gout. Synthetic corticosteroids were also somewhat effective, but there remained the impression that they were less effective than ACTH, for reasons that are still unclear. It was observed that flares of gout would occur when ACTH was discontinued, but the use of colchicine prophylaxis in conjunction with ACTH effectively solved that problem. Thus by the early 1950s, with the use of colchicine, phenylbutazone, and ACTH, the treatment of acute gout was virtually always effective, with some rare exceptions. Phenylbutazone, however, had significant toxicity, particularly agranulocytosis, which could be fatal. Its use was superseded by the development of indomethacin in the early 1960s, and indeed phenylbutazone is no longer marketed in the United States. Other nonsteroidal anti-inflammatory agents (NSAIDs), such as naproxen and fenoprofen have also been found to be useful. At present, most clinicians use indomethacin for the treatment of acute gout. Colchicine is still used, both intravenously and orally, by many clinicians. It is used particularly when the diagnosis of gout is doubtful and when fluid cannot be obtained for crystal analysis.

In patients with chronic renal disease and other medical problems where the use of NSAIDs may be contraindicated, ACTH has been found to be remarkably effective and safe when used for a short duration (32).

A vexing exception to this virtually always-successful treatment of acute gout is a patient with organ transplants, particularly those treated with cyclosporine (33). NSAIDs are considered to be contraindicated, and attacks are often refractory to colchicine and ACTH. The lack of response to ACTH may reflect on the lack of responsiveness of the adrenal gland, possibly relating to long-term corticosteroid use. In such transplantation patients, colchicine and synthetic corticosteroids are the treatments of choice.

C. Interval Gout

Interval gout refers to the asymptomatic phase of gout, which occurs once the acute attack has been successfully treated or has spontaneously subsided. There are some patients who have one attack only, and even without treatment do not develop another one for years. More commonly, in patients who are untreated, attacks occur often with increasing frequency and severity, and lead to chronic gout (10).

Initially, treatment of the interval phase consisted of lifestyle changes, such as abstinence from alcohol, weight loss, restriction of diet, and exercise. This approach was subsequently modified when powerful uricosuric drugs became available in the 1950s. It then became practice by many physicians to treat gout and hyperuricemia with the use of probenecid. It was remarkably effective in lowering uric acid levels, but seemed paradoxically to initiate more frequent gouty attacks. Eventually, as uric acid levels were decreased, the attacks decreased in frequency, and eventually ceased in most cases.

The next important observation was made in the 1950s by Drs. Yu and Gutman, who found that colchicine in daily doses of 0.6 to 1.2 mg q.d. would effectively prevent acute gouty attacks in the vast majority of patients (30). Thus was born the concept of treating interval gout with a combination of a uric-acid-lowering agent and prophylactic colchicine. This is the basis of the modern treatment of gout. With such a combination, acute attacks in most patients can be prevented and tophi diminished or prevented from forming.

With the use of allopurinol as a uric-acid-lowering agent in patients with no medical complications, dietary reduction of purines and proteins was less strict. However, weight loss in obese patients and avoidance of alcohol was still deemed advisable.

D. Chronic Tophaceous Gout

Chronic tophaceous gout refers to the phase of gout in which deposition of urate appears over the joints, tendons, and other soft tissues. Probably included in this would be urate deposition in the kidney, as well as kidney stones. Though colchicine was available for the treatment of acute gout by the end of the 18th century, treatment of tophaceous gout was not available until the 1950s, when uricosuric drugs became available. Yü and Gutman clearly demonstrated that Probenecid could often cause dissolution of urate deposits. Tophi were also prevented. Though other uricosuric agents such as sulfinpyrazone, zoxazolamine, and high doses of salicylates were often used, Probenecid remained the favorite drug. It was effective and relatively safe. High fluid intake and alkalinization of urine was used to prevent urate stone formation in the kidney and the collecting system.

Allopurinol was introduced in the early 1960s. It was initially studied as an anticancer drug, but was found to inhibit the enzyme xanthine oxidase, the enzyme responsible for the biosynthesis of urate acid and the conversion of xanthine to hypoxanthine and hypoxanthine to uric acid. It has come to replace probenecid for lowering uric acid, particularly in patients whose uric acid results from urate overproduction. In most patients, hyperuricemia is related to decreased excretion of uric acid. Similarly to probenecid, allopurinol might precipitate and prolong gouty attacks. Thus allopurinol is used in conjunction with colchicine in the prevention of gouty attacks and the treatment of tophaceous gout.

In chronic gouty arthritis with persistent joint pain, the NSAIDs have been found to be effective.

In rare circumstance, surgery may still be used to remove deeply-seated tophaceous deposits.

E. Uric Acid Stones

Uric-acid-stone formation can obviously occur in patients with gout and patients who do not have gout. Before the use of allopurinol, the treatment of urate-stone formation involved high fluid intake and alkalinization of the urine. Probenecid increased the urate excretion, and thus was felt to be problematic in patients who were urate overexcretors. However, with the use of allopurinol, urate stones could be successfully prevented in a large percentage of patients.

III. CONCLUSION

In summary, gout is a disease that goes back to ancient days. In the 15 years between 1948 to 1963, the painful, crippling, and at times life-threatening disease was virtually conquered as a clinical problem. The beneficiaries, of course, were the large number of patients with gout and its complications. For the clinician treating gout, the advances afforded by a modern scientifically oriented approach to the etiology and treatment of gout has been a great gift.

There are, of course, remaining problems, such as the exact biochemical and genetic defects that underline gout, the treatment of gout in transplant recipients, and other patients who are either intolerant of or who do not have a positive response to the current treatment modalities available. However, for the overwhelming majority of patients, if a proper diagnosis is made, successful treatment is virtually assured.

REFERENCES

1. G. R. Rodnan. *Arth Rheum 8*:599–609 (1965).
2. Talmud Yerushalmi, Shabat VI: 8.
3. G. R. Rodnan. *Arth Rheum 4* (1961) (1st part Feb., 2nd part April).
4. G. R. Rodnan. *Arth Rheum 6*:317–339 (1963).
5. T. Sydenham. A treatise of gout and dropsy. In: The Works of Thomas Sydenham, M.D. Vol. 2 (R. G. Latham, translator), The Sydenham Society, London, England, 1850, pp. 119–162.
6. K. W. Scheele. Analysis of the calculus vesicae (1776). In: The Chemical Essays of Charles William Scheele Translated from Transactions of the Academy of Sciences at Stockholm, J. Murray, London, England, 1786, p. 199.
7. W. H. Wollaston. On gouty and urinary concretions. *Phil Trans* (*Royal Soc Lond*) *87*:386 (1797).
8. A. B. Garrod. Observations on certain pathological conditions of the blood and urine in gout, rheumatism, and Bright's disease, *Med-Chir Trans 31*:83 (1848).
9. P. S. Hench. In: *Textbook of Medicine* (Cecil and Loeb, eds.), W.B. Saunders, Philadelphia, PA, 1959, p. 602.
10. D. J. McCarty. The inflammatory reaction to microcrystalline sodium urate. *Arth Rheum 8*:726–734 (1965).
11. D. J. McCarty, N. Rohn, J. S. Farris. The significance of calcium pyrophosphate crystals in the synovial fluid of arthritis patients: The pseudogout syndrome. I: Clinical aspects. *Ann Int Med 56*:711 (1962).
12. A. B. Gutman and T. F. Yü. Gout, a derangement of purine metabolism. *Adv Int Med 5*:227 (1952).
13. A. B. Gutman and T. F. Yü. Renal function in gout, with a commentary on the renal regulation of urate excretion, and the role of the kidney is the pathogenesis of gout. *Am J Med 23*:600 (1957).
14. A. Storck. An essay on the use and effects of the root of the colchicum autumnale, or meadow saffron. Translated from Latin by T. Becket and P. A. De Honot, 1764.
15. W. C. Kuzell, R. W. Schafarzick, B. Brown, and E. A. Mankle. Phenylbutazone (Butazocidin) in rheumatoid arthritis and gout. *JAMA 149*: 729 (1952).
16. C. J. Smyth, E. E. Velayos, and C. Amoroso. Influence of new anti-inflammatory drug: indomethacin in acute gout. *Acta Rheum Scand 9*:306 (1963).
17. W. Q. Wolfson, H. D. Hunt, C. Cohn, W. D. Robinson, and I. F. Duff. ACTH and colchicine in the clinical treatment of acute gouty arthritis. *J Mich State Med Soc 49*:1058 (1950).
18. A. B. Gutman, and T. F. Yü. Effect of adrenocorticotropic hormone (ACTH) in gout. *Am J Med 9*:24 (1950).
19. H. W. Florey. The use of microorganisms for therapeutic purposes. *Yale J Biol Med 19*:101–118 (1946).
20. R. H. Beyer, H. F. Russo, E. K. Tillson, A. K. Miller, W. F. Verney, and S. R. Bass. Benamid (P-(D1-N propylsulfamyl)-benzoic acid): its renal affinity and its elimination. *Am J Physiol 166*:625–640 (1951).

21. A. B. Gutman and T. F. Yü. Benemid (P-(D1-N-propylsulfamyl)-benzoic acid) as uricosuric agent is chronic gouty arthritis. *Trans Am Assoc Phys 64*:279 (1951).
22. T. F. Yü and A. B. Gutman. Mobilization of gouty tophi by protracted use of uricosuric agents. *Am J Med 11*:765 (1961).
23. A. B. Gutman. The search for uricosuric agents suited to the management of tophaceous gout. *New York State J Med 63*:576 (1963).
24. R. W. Rundles, J. B. Wynngarden, G. H. Hitchings, G. B. Elion and H. R. Silberman. Effects of a xanthine oxidase inhibitor on thiopurine metabolism, hyperuricemia, and gout. *Trans Am Assoc Phys 76*:126 (1963).
25. B. Roueche. "A perverse, ungrateful, maleficent malady." *The New Yorker*, 13 March, 1948.
26. H. E. Paulus, A. Coutts, J. J. Calabro, et al. Clinical significance of hyperuricemia in routinely screened hospitalized men. *JAMA 211*:277 (1970).
27. W. N. Kelly. Gout and related disorders of purine metabolism. In: Textbook of Rheumatology (Kelley, Harris, Ruddy, Sledge, eds.), W.B. Saunders, Philadelphia, PA, 1981.
28. C. S. Smyth. In: Arthritis and Allied Conditions: A Textbook of Rheumatology (J. L. Hollander, ed.), Lea & Febiger, Philadelphia, PA, 1960, p. 884.
29. T. F. Yü. Gout, In: Current Therapy in Endocrinology and Metabolism (C.W. Bardin, ed.), Mosby, Philadelphia, PA, 1991, pp. 176–182.
30. J. Z. Singer and S. L. Wallace. The allopurinol hypersensitivity syndrome: unnecessary morbidity and mortality. *Arth Rheum 29*:82–87 (1986).
31. S. L. Wallace, D. Bernstein, and H. Diamond. Diagnostic value of the colchicine therapeutic trial. *JAMA 199*:525 (1967).
32. J. M. Ritter, L. D. Kerr, J. Valeriano-Marcet, and H. Spiera. ACTH revisited: effective treatment for acute crystal-induced synovitis in patients with multiple medical problems. *J Rheum 21*:21–24 (1994).
33. B. A. Baethge, J. Work, M. D. Landreneao, and S. C. McDonald. Tophaceous gout is patients with renal transplants treated with cyclosporin A. *J Rheum 20*:718–720 (1993).
34. T. F. Yü and A. B. Gutman. Efficacy of colchicine in prophylaxis of gout: prevention of gouty arthritis over a mean period of five years in 208 gouty subjects. *Ann Int Med 55*:179–192 (1961).
35. A. B. Gutman and T. F. Yü. Uric acid urolithiasis. *Am J Med 45*:756 (1968).

12

Diagnosis and Differential Diagnosis of Gout and Hyperuricemia

JOHN H. BLAND
University of Vermont College of Medicine, Burlington, Vermont

I. INTRODUCTION

Gout has been identified since great antiquity and descriptions of the disease date back to Babylonian times (c2100–698 BC). Babylon, an ancient city on the lower Euphrates River in what is now central Iraq, was the capital of Babylonia, noted for wealth, luxury, and wickedness. Gout was certainly well known and extensively described by Hippocrates (460–c377 BC), the Father of Medicine. Evidence of the disease has been found in early skeletal remains, and lead concentrations detected in some of those remains suggest the possibility that some gout may have been saturnine (sluggish, gloomy, morose, grey, taciturn—the alchemist's term for lead, which they considered to be very cold, like the planet Saturn), having lead poisoning being one of the etiologies of gout.

Though true that many of the advances in the comprehension and optimum therapy of gout have emerged in the 20th century, it still is worth noting that some of the fundamental discoveries, e.g., the identification of crystals of urate and the demonstration of urate in tophi, date back to the 17th and 18th centuries.

II. MONOSODIUM URATE

Monosodium urate (MSU) crystals result from hyperuricemia. The other MSU constituents, water and sodium, are abundant and are not limiting factors. Commonly renal urate retention causes the hyperuricemia. However, a host of reasons for urate overproduction are well known. Overproducers and undersecreters are conveniently separated by determination of the urate secretion in a 24-hour urine specimen. A value greater than 800 mg/day on a standard diet (or 600 mg for 24 hours in a reliable and compliant patient on a low purine diet) indicates overproduction. This differentiation also assists in diagnosis and in determining which hypouricemic agent is most suitable for a given patient. Cautious interpretation is required by a host of influences on the urinary determination, including diet, many medications, methodology and, not least, the completeness of the collection of a 24-hour specimen.

Whatever the cause of hyperuricemia, at 37°C MSU crystals form in physiologic solutions when the urate concentration exceeds 6.5 mg/ml. Local factors may increase urate concentrations beyond systemic (plasma) levels. For example, Simkin and coworkers describe a more rapid clearance of water from joints compared with urate (1). Thus, dependent joints such as the great toe (first metatarsal phalangeal) may accumulate water and urate while the person is upright and while the joint is traumatized, walking about or running, during waking hours. At night preferential resorption of water could result in local hyperuricemia, favoring crystal formation or growth of pre-existing small crystals. This scheme fits well with the observation that attacks of Podagra occur frequently at night. The solubility product of MSU is temperature dependent and precipitates form at concentrations as low as 4.5 mg/ml at 4°C. This may explain characteristic deposition in the cooler peripheral acral joints. Finally matrix abnormalities may influence MSU precipitation. A number of older women with chronic hyperuricemia due to hypertension or thiazide treatment have developed gout in their Heberden's nodes! Loss of proteoglycans, which normally inhibit crystal deposition, may potentiate the deposition at this site.

III. CLINICAL MANIFESTATIONS AND DIAGNOSIS

Gout is a relatively common irritable disorder generally found in middle-aged men and to a lesser extent postmenopausal women. This disease is a disorder defined by the metabolic consequences of hyperuricemia and tissue deposition of urate (Table 1).

The presence of either criterion A or criterion B is enough to make the diagnosis. Both A and B involve microscopic identification of MSU crystals using polarized light microscopy (Figures 1A–C) Since the treatment of gout often involves lifelong medication, making a precise definitive and permanent diagnosis is of great importance. Therefore, crystal identification is highly urged whenever possible. Clinical diagnosis may be made and the therapy started, but the more ultimate secure diagnosis by crystal identification is mandatory.

Attacks of gout occur most commonly in the lower extremities, particularly at the first metatarsal-phalangeal (MTP) joint. But great caution should be

TABLE 1 Diagnostic Criteria for Gout

A. Characteristic urate crystals documented in joint fluid (Figures 1A–C) or
B. Tophus documented to have urate crystals (Figures 3A and B) or
C. In some cases, the presence of 6 out of the following 12 clinical, laboratory, and X-ray criteria (note that criterion on A or B are preferable):
    1. More than one acute arthritis attack
    2. Maximal inflammation within 24 hours
    3. Episode of monarticular arthritis
    4. Joint redness
    5. First metatarsal-phalangeal joint swelling or pain (big toe) (Figure 2)
    6. Unilateral MTP joint inflammation
    7. Unilateral tarsal joint inflammation
    8. Possible tophus
    9. Hyperuricemia
    10. Asymmetric swelling in a joint on x-ray study
    11. X-ray study showing subcortical cysts without erosion
    12. Negative bacterial culture of joint fluid during attack

observed in assuming that an arthritic episode at the first MTP joint is always due to gout. Conditions such as pseudogout (discussed later), hydroxyapatite deposition disease, rheumatoid arthritis, osteoarthritis, and Reiter's syndrome are among other conditions that can involve this joint (2).

Sometimes the diagnosis of gout needs to be made in a patient who is not having an acute attack. In such cases it has been shown that urate crystals can be identified even in asymptomatic MTP and knee joints. It is important to examine joint fluid within hours of aspiration, since crystals may become more difficult to recognize and artifactual, confusing crystals may form (3–5).

If six of the 12 clinical, laboratory, and X-ray criteria are present, a diagnosis of gout may be safely made. However, crystal identification is always preferable and should be pursued. The important aspects of gouty arthritis are brought out by these criteria. Note that response to colchicine was not listed as a diagnostic factor, since the response is not thought nowadays to be sufficiently specific. Gout attacks tend to reach their peak of clinically evident inflammation quickly, a distinctive clinical criterion, certainly within 24 hours and may even present with extensive enlarging areas of erythema that may be suggestive of cellulitis. The skin may even desquamate afterward. Early in the gouty process there is often only one joint involved, particularly the first MTP or a tarsal joint. Commonly enough a contiguous joint becomes involved shortly (Figure 2).

Over time, tophi may form, representing large local deposits of urates. They occur particularly at the helix of the ear, around the olecranon bursa, along the Achilles tendon, and on the ulnar forearm. Those patients with tophi are

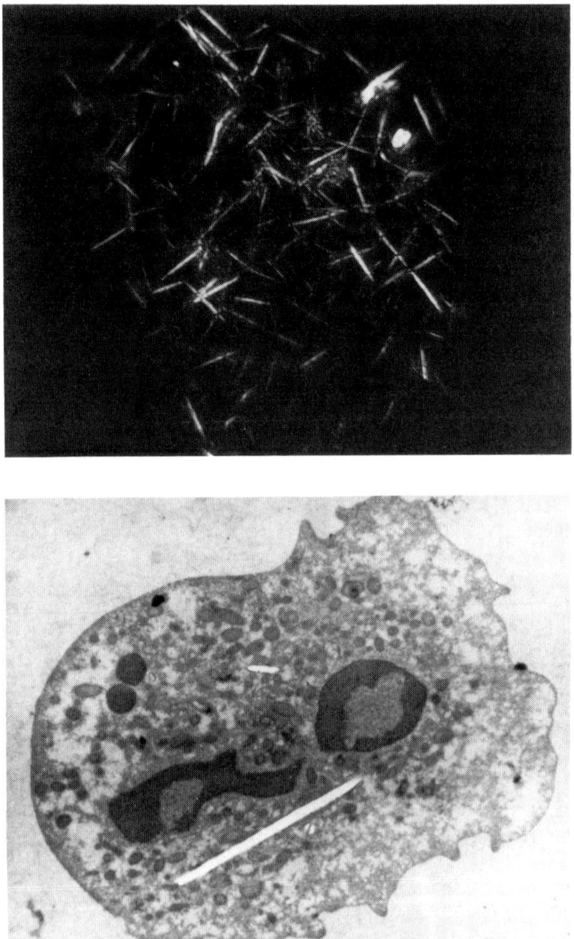

(A)

(B)

FIGURE 1 (A) Monosodium urate crystals observed by polarizing microscopy. (B) Monosodium urate crystal in a polymorphonuclear leukocyte. (C) Urate crystals viewed in a gouty tophus.

much more likely to have associated joint abnormalities, such as subcortical cysts and subsequent joint damage. (Figures 3A and B) Tophi tend to be firmer in consistency than the subcutaneous nodules of rheumatoid arthritis and/or lupus erythematosus.

Kidney stones are an important complication of gout and hyperuricemia. The presence of urate kidney stones suggest that the patient is an overproducer of uric acid with high levels of urinary urate. Late in the course of gout, some pa-

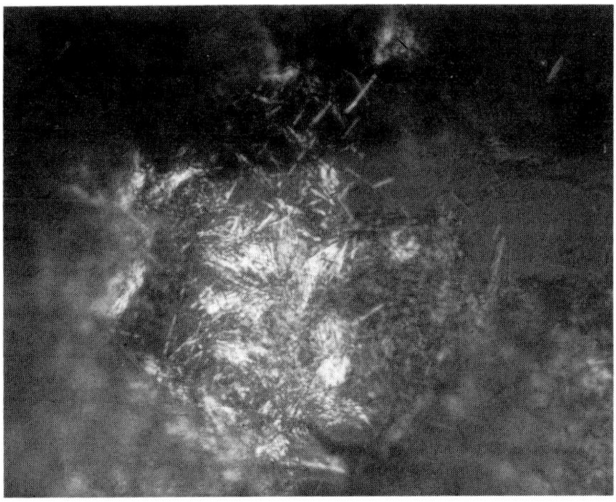

(C)

FIGURE 1 Continued

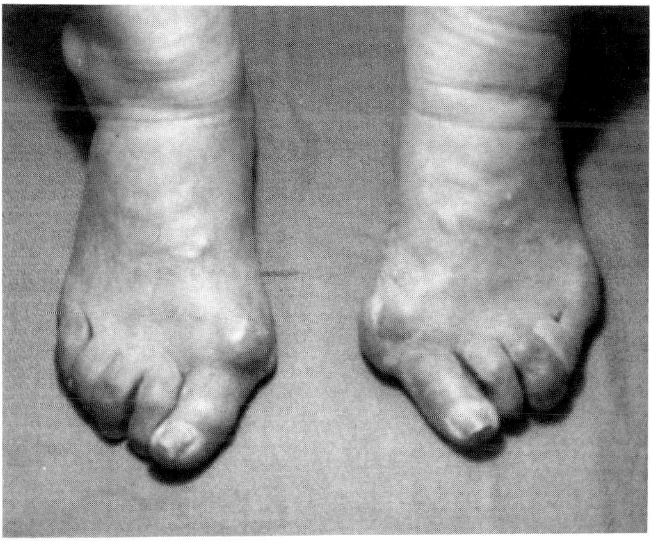

FIGURE 2 Large tophi right ankle and both MTP joints.

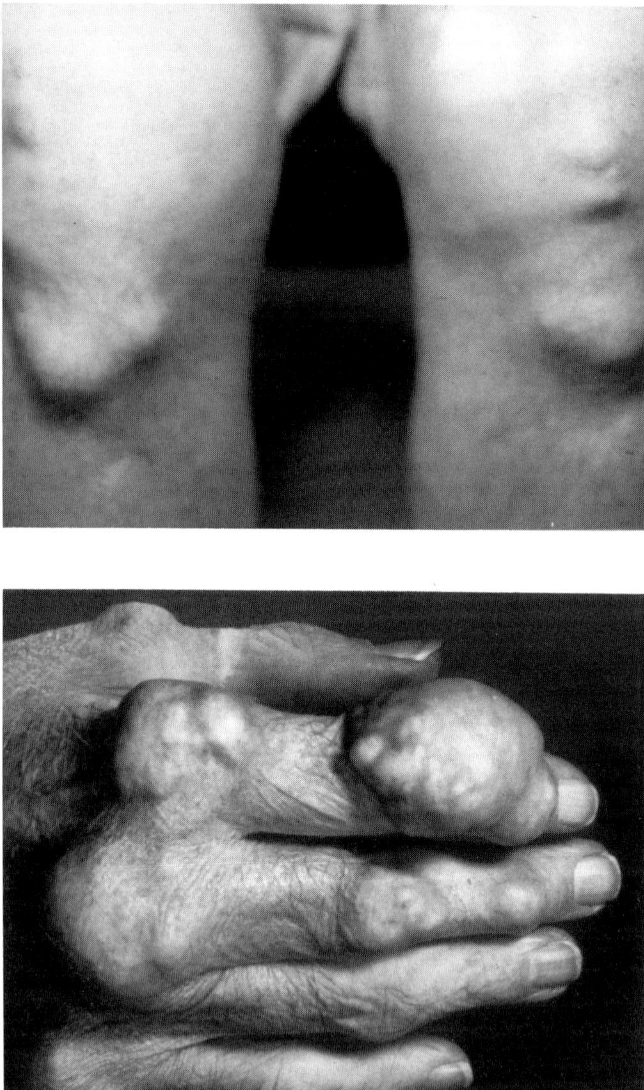

(A)

(B)

FIGURE 3 (A) Large tophi about both knees. (B) Enormous tophi index and middle fingers.

tients develop a chronic polyarticular arthritis. Absence of symmetrical typical X-ray changes and crystal identification are aids in separating this condition from other chronic arthropathies.

Only a very small percentage of patients with gout have identifiable enzyme defects leading to hyperuricemia. Most patients with idiopathic gout have hyperuricemia on the basis of decreased excretion of uric acid. A large number of factors may either cause gout or worsen already manifest gout by virtue of increasing serum uric acid concentrations. These factors, for example, obesity and excessive alcohol consumption, may work by increasing uric acid production (6).

Some other factors decrease the excretion of uric acid, including renal vascular disease, the use of diuretics, lead nephropathy, and cyclosporin (7).

IV. CLINICAL GOUT

Problems in determining the exact incidence rate and prevalence of gout is a consequence of the remitting and relapsing nature of the disease as well as the propensity to misdiagnosis by patients and, to a lesser extent, by clinicians. This problem is highlighted by the higher prevalence noted with patient-reported gout compared with physician-diagnosed gout, a disparity that is even greater in females than in males. The epidemiology of gout is undergoing change (e.g., the ratio of males to females afflicted with gout was formerly 20:1 but is now 2–7:1). This is surely due to changes in lifestyle, drugs, and increasing longevity. Nevertheless, gout is still recognized as the most common inflammatory arthropathy in males over 40 years of age.

Gout is rare in children and premenopausal females and is uncommon in males under 30 years of age. The peak age of onset in men is between 40 and 50 years; it is somewhat later in females, often associated with identifiable causes of hyperuricemia such as associated thiazide diuretic therapy.

The single most important determinant of the risk of developing gout is the plasma urate concentration. It seems the risk of developing gouty arthritis is the same in men and women for a particular urate concentration. This suggests that the lower prevalence of gout in females is likely a reflection of their normal lower urate concentrations. Table 2 is a summary of the epidemiology of gout.

Regarding epidemiology, many studies including children will give lower incidence rates and prevalence figures than those examining only adults. Although studies do show racial differences in prevalence of hyperuricemia and gout, the relative importance of genetic and environmental factors (especially with respect to diet) is difficult to determine. Gout was previously uncommon in ethnic Chinese as well as several groups of Polynesians, but the prevalence has increased in recent years in these races. Moreover, ethnic Chinese, Polyne-

TABLE 2 Epidemiology of Gout

Peak age in years	Males 40–50, Females over 60
Sex distribution (M:F)	Males 2–7: Females 1
Prevalence rate (per 1000)	Males 5–28; Females 1–6
Annual incidence (per 1000)	Males 1–3; Females 0.2
Geography	Worldwide regional differences may reflect environmental factors as well as racial predisposition.
Genetic associations	Inherited enzyme abnormalities and inherited urate underexcretion.
Environmental associations	Diet, drugs, toxins (e.g., lead)

The serum or plasma urate concentration is the major determinant of risk for the development of gout.

sians, and Filipinos in different countries exhibit prevalences of hyperuricemia and gout that vary from those in their native countries. These studies suggest that the increased prevalence of hyperuricemia and gout in these races is due to environmental factors (predominantly diet) superimposed upon a basic underexcretion of urate. On the other hand, a study of New Guinea people demonstrated hyperuricemia in two population groups in absence of obesity or a westernized diet.

The prevalence of tophi has decreased over the period 1948–1973, surely related to improved therapy. Yu et al. reported that 53% of the patients in the period 1948–1953 had tophi in comparison with 17% in the period 1969–1973 (9). Even now, however, tophaceous gout remains common in patients with untreated or inadequately treated gout.

V. ASYMPTOMATIC HYPERURICEMIA

One must recognize the clear distinction between hyperuricemia and gout. Hyperuricemia is certainly a risk factor for the development of gout, the risk increasing with higher urate concentrations. Still, many years of hyperuricemia have usually elapsed before the development of acute gouty arthritis, and in some hyperuricemic people gout may never develop. Nonetheless acute, severe overproduction of urate as may occur with cytotoxic chemotherapy is associated with a high risk of acute renal failure from uric acid crystal deposition in the renal tubules.

The risk of damage beyond the musculoskeletal system from protracted hyperuricemia or recurrent attacks of gout is small. Calculi are uncommon, with the annual incidence being approximately 1% in gout and 0.3% in otherwise asymptomatic hyperuricemia (10). These may consist of either uric acid or calcium oxalate. Such calculi may cause an obstructive nephropathy and renal impairment. However, the calculi are usually passed or surgically removed with resolution of any transient renal impairment. In addition, microtophi may be deposited in the renal parenchyma and interstitial renal damage is likely to be found after 10 years of inadequately treated gout.

VI. ACUTE GOUT

Sydenham's classical description of gout still demonstrates the important clinical characteristics used to diagnose a typical attack of acute gout (11):

> The victim goes to bed and sleeps in good health. About two o'clock in the morning he is awakened by pain in the great toe; more rarely in the heel, ankle or instep. This pain is like that of a dislocation, and yet the parts feel as if cold water were poured over them. Then follows chills and shivers and a little fever. The pain, which was at first moderate, rapidly becomes more intense. With its intensity the chills and shivers increase. After a time this comes to its full height, accommodating itself to the bones and ligaments of the tarsus and metatarsus. Now it is a violent stretching and tearing of the ligaments. Now it is a gnawing pain and now a pressure and tightness. So exquisite and lively meanwhile is the feeling of the part affected that it cannot bear the weight of bedclothes nor the jar of a person walking in the room. The night is passed in torture, sleeplessness, turning of the part affected and perpetual change of posture; the tossing about of the body being as incessant as the pain of the tortured joint, and being worse as the fit comes on. Hence the vain effort by change of posture both in the body and the limb affected to obtain an abatement of the pain.

Acute gout is characterized by the rapidity of onset and buildup of pain, the exquisite nature of the pain, and the swelling with associated redness of the affected joint. In more than half of the initial attacks this occurs in the first metatarsal-phalangeal joint (great toe) and in time this joint is affected in some 90% of patients with gout. Almost any joint can be affected, however the lower limbs are involved much more often than the upper limbs. Symptomatic involvement of the axial joints is rare. After the first metatarsal-phalangeal joints the order of frequency of involvement is the instep, heel, ankle, and knee. Gout does not always need to be articular, with involvement of several sites including the olecranon bursa and the Achilles tendon being well recognized. Redness overlying the affected part is a feature that sets gout apart from most other noninfective arthropathies. Swelling can be marked and involve an entire region. The natural history of the acute attack is variable and dependent in part on its severity. Mild attacks may resolve within 1–2 days. More severe attacks exhibit rapidly increasing pain reaching its peak usually within a few hours, remaining at this level for 1–3 days, then slowly remitting such that the attack has often subsided within 7–10 days. It may take several weeks before very severe attacks settle completely.

About 90% of initial attacks are monarticular (12). Associated systemic features are mild or absent. Even so, occasional patients with just a single joint affected may have severe systemic features with high fever and leukocytosis, even suggestive of sepsis. Subsequent attacks may affect the same joint or progress to involve other joints. Later in the disease process the incidence of polyarticular attacks increases, sometimes with an associated increase in the severity of systemic features. Nevertheless, these attacks will resolve completely with symptom-free intervals until finally chronic gout, in which symptoms resolve incompletely between exacerbations, becomes established. Occasionally gout may present early in its course with polyarticular involvement, and is then easily confused with other arthropathies.

In the elderly, gouty arthritis is usually more indolent than that arising in younger patients, and may be mistaken for osteoarthritis with a resultant delay in accurate diagnosis. This is further complicated by the coexistence of gout and osteoarthritis at times in the same joint (especially Heberden's nodes), (13). More than one joint is involved in the initial attack in about 50% of patients. Antecedent or intercurrent medical disorders are common in this group.

Pauci or polyarticular onset of gouty arthritis is more common in women than men. This may largely reflect the age of onset since gout is predominantly found in women over the age of 60. In addition tophi and concurrent diuretic use are all more common in women than in men (14).

Several factors have been noted to precipitate acute attacks of gout, e.g., acute illness, trauma, surgery, alcohol (especially beer and wines), and drugs that either increase or decrease the plasma urate concentration.

The periods between attacks when the patient is asymptomatic has sometimes been termed intercritical gout. Since many patients with a single attack of gout are either not diagnosed or are overlooked in epidemiologic studies, it is not possible to determine the proportion of patients who have subsequent attacks. Nevertheless it would appear that a significant majority of patients will have more than one attack, with a second attack usually occurring with one or two years. In a small minority, many years may elapse between attacks.

VII. CHRONIC GOUT

Failure of resolution of attacks early in the course of gout usually indicates a concurrent arthropathy, usually osteoarthritis. Symptom-free periods, characteristic of the early phase of gout, rarely may not be seen and the disease may become chronic from an early stage. The proportion of patients who develop chronic gout is uncertain and depends upon the number whose hyperuricemia is not controlled.

Tophi appearing within the first two years of gout are extremely rare and patients have usually suffered from gout for at least 10 years before tophi develop. Exceptions exist, particularly in juvenile forms with severe hyperuricemia, when tophi occasionally appear concurrent with an early or even the first attack of gout and secondary gout associated with myeloproliferative disorders.

Tophi appear as firm nodular or fusiform swellings (Figures 3A and B). If there is associated significant local inflammation, the overlying skin may be erythematous. When they are indolent and the tophi are close to the skin surface, they may appear yellowish in color. In ulcerated tophi, white chalky material may easily exude. Tophi may appear at virtually any site with the most common locations being the digits of the hands and feet. The olecranon bursa is frequently involved and tophi of the helix or antihelix of the ear are classical, albeit less common locations for gouty tophi.

The inflammatory process in chronic gout is often mild except when acute attacks supervene. Much of the disability in chronic gout is due to the presence of tophi. These may be associated with destructive deforming arthritis and may ulcerate in which case secondary infection may be a problem.

Tophi may give rise to diagnostic difficulties when they arise in an unusual site, especially when there is no accurate history of recurrent attacks of acute gout. Some reported locations for gouty tophi are different parts of the eye, other structures within the head and neck, the heart (particularly cardiac valves), and the carpal tunnel and spine, causing back pain and rarely quadriparesis (15).

VIII. DIFFERENTIAL DISORDERS

The concurrence of the clinical features of gout and a wide variety of rheumatic and nonrheumatic disorders with hyperuricemia are common. For effective management, it is necessary that such associations be recognized and that therapy be patterned accordingly. In Table 3 is a list of the most frequently obtained conditions where this differential diagnosis needs to be made.

1. Strong association of obesity with hyperuricemia and gout, usually reflecting dietary excesses.
2. Hypertension associated with hyperuricemia three ways apart from that due to diuretic therapy.
   a. Hypertension reduces renal excretion of urate
   b. Renal damage from interstitial microtophi may lead to secondary renal hypertension
   c. Excessive alcohol consumption

TABLE 3 Differential Diagnosis

1. Infection: differentiation by observance of streaks, lymph node hypertrophy.
2. Response to treatment: Often acute attacks have subsided before laboratory confirms presence of synovial fluid monosodium urate crystals.
3. Typical gouty deformities from previous attacks (tophaceous deposits with residual deformities).
4. 90% of patients have involvement of the first metatarsophalangeal joint, great toe, sometime during their history.
5. Asymptomatic hyperuricemia reported in the history prior to onset of the first episode of gout, usually postpubertal.
6. History of previous episodes similar to the present attack.
7. History or presence of renal calculi.
8. 85–90% percent of first attacks of gout are in a single joint.
9. First attack is commonly at night.
10. Hypertriglyceridemia: 75–80% of patients with gout.[a]
11. Obesity commonly associated with gout.
12. 8.3% of all joints involved in gout are in the lower extremity.
13. Radiologic findings typical of tophaceous deposits and gout.
14. Tophi in unusual locations, notably the ears.

[a]Ref. 16.

3. Hyperlipidemia frequently occurs in gouty patients, the common associated disorder being hypertriglyceridemia type IV lipoproteinemia.
4. Association between gout and vascular disease, probably dependent upon several factors other than hyperuricemia, i.e., hypertension, obesity, platelet adhesiveness, and possible hyperlipidemia.
5. Some studies, not all, have suggested an association between gout and diabetes mellitus or abnormal glucose tolerance. However, plasma urate concentrations are lower in diabetic subjects than normal subjects in the absence of renal impairment.

A summary of conditions to be considered in the differential diagnoses of gout and with the findings of an elevation of serum urate are listed in Table 3.

REFERENCES

1. P. A. Simkin. The pathogenesis of Podagra. *Annals Intern Med 86*:230 (1977).
2. A. G. Fam and J. Rubenstein. Hydroxyappetite Pseudopodagra: a syndrome of young women. *Arth Rheum 32*:741 (1989).
3. A. Weinberger, H. R. Schumacher Jr., and C. A. Agudelo. Urate crystals in asymptomatic metatarsal-phalangeal joints. *Ann Int Med 91*:56 (1979).

4. J. S. Bomalski, G. Lluberas, and H. R. Schumacher Jr. Monosodium urate crystals in the knee joints of patients with asymptomatic non-tophacious gout. *Arth Rheum 29*:1480 (1986).
5. G. Kerolus, G. Clayburne, and H. R. Schumacher Jr. Is it mandatory to examine synovial fluids promptly after arthrocentesis? *Arth Rheum 32*:271 (1989).
6. J. Faller and I. H. Fox. Ethanol induced hyperuricemia: evidence for increased urate production by activation of adenine nucliotide turnover. *New Eng J Med 307*:1598 (1982).
7. V. B. Batuman, et al. The role of lead in gout nephropathy. *New Eng J Med 304*:520 (1981).
8. H. Y. Linh, et al. Cyclosporin induced hyperuricemia and gout. *New Eng J Med 321*:287 (1989).
9. T. F. Yu, et al. Milestones in the treatment of gout. *Am J Med 56*:676–685 (1974).
10. W. J. Fessel. Renal outcomes of gout and hyperuricemia. *Am J Med 67*:74–82 (1979).
11. J. B. Wyngaarden and W. N. Kelley. Gout and Hyperuricemia, Grune and Stratton, New York, NY, 1976, pp. 152–153.
12. G. V. Lawry, P. T. Fan, and R. Bluestone. Polyarticular versus monoarticular gout, a prospective comparative analysis of clinical features. *Medicine (Baltimore) 67*:335–343 (1988).
13. E. V. Lally, B. Zimmerman, and G. Kaplan Ho Sr. Urate mediated inflammation in nodal osteoarthritis. Clinical and roentgenographic correlations. *Arth Rheum J 32*:86–90 (1989).
14. D. G. MacFarlane and P. A. Dieppe. Diuretic induced gout in elderly women. *Brit J Rheumatol 24*:155–157 (1985).
15. T. W. Stark, and R. H. Hirokawa. Gout and its manifestations in the head and neck. *Otolaryngolog Clin North Am 15*:659–664 (1982).
16. T. G. Bendek. Correlations of increased serum acid and lipid concentration in normal, gouty and atherosclerotic men. *Ann Int Med 66*:851 (1967).

13

Acute Gout

Diagnosis and Management

A. LEÓN RIVELIS*
Hospital for Special Surgery, New York, New York and Instituto de Reumatología, Buenos Aires, Argentina

ANA CARINA RIVELIS
Hospital Ramos Mejía, Buenos Aires, Argentina

I. DIAGNOSTIC APPROACH

Acute gout is suspected by evidence of its characteristic clinical pattern, and a diagnosis is definitively established by the presence of urate sodium monourate crystals in the synovial fluid.

The clinical picture is often typical and was described since the time of Hippocrates (5th Century BC), who included some of its aspects in his six famous aphorisms. The best clinical description of an acute attack was written by Dr. Thomas Sydenham, published in London in 1683, and reproduced in most rheumatology texts (1), and partially says:

> The victim goes to bed and sleeps in good health. About two o'clock in the morning he is awakened by pain in the great toe; more rarely in the heel, ankle or instep. This pain is like that of a dislocation, and yet the parts feel as if cold water were poured over them.
>
> Then follows chills and shivers and a little fever. The pain, which is at first moderate, becomes more intense. With its intensity the chills and shivers increase. After a time this comes to its full height, accommodating itself to the bones and ligaments of the tarsus and metatarsus. Now it is a violent

*Retired.

> stretching and tearing of the ligaments, now it is a gnawing pain and now a pressure and tightness. So exquisite and lively meanwhile is the feeling of the parts affected, that it cannot bear the weight of bedclothes nor the jar of a person walking in the room. The night is passed in torture, sleeplessness, turning of the part affected, and perpetual change of posture; the tossing about of the body being as incessant as the pain of the tortured joint, and being worse as the fit comes on. Hence the vain effort by change of posture, both in the body and the limb affected, to obtain an abatement of pain.

This is a typical attack of gout in the most frequent location of metatarsophalangeal joint of the great toe (Podagra), but any diathrodial joint could be affected.

The diagnosis and differential diagnosis of gouty arthritis made a great step forward with the work of Drs. McCarty and Hollander in 1961, when they reported the finding of urate crystals in synovial fluid of most patients suffering of acute attack (2).

Both in monoarticular and polyarticular acute onset, the only way to establish a definite diagnosis is to aspirate synovial fluid and examine it by a polarized light microscope. The fluid contains large numbers of needle-shaped crystals within the polymorphonuclear leukocytes that are strongly negatively birefringent. Hyperuricemia and a negative synovial fluid culture are also important. The preliminary diagnostic criteria proposed by Wallace et al. in 1977 are generally accepted today and endorsed by the American Rheumatism Association (ARA) and American College of Rheumatology (ACR) (3). They are based on the presence of urate crystals in the joint fluid and/or tophus of six or more of 12 clinical, radiology, and laboratory findings (Table 1).

TABLE 1 Preliminary Criteria for Classification of Acute Arthritis of Primary Gout

Major Criteria

1. Monosodium urate monohydrate microcrystals in joint fluid during attack.
2. Tophus (proved).

Minor Criteria

1. Maximum inflammation developed within one day.
2. More than one attack of acute arthritis.
3. Monoarthitis attacks.
4. Redness observed over joints.
5. First metatarsophalangeal joint attack.
6. Unilateral first metatarsophalangeal joint attack.
7. Unilateral tarsal joint attack.
8. Tophus (suspected).
9. Hyperuricemia.
10. Asymmetric swelling within a joint on x-ray examination.
11. Subcortical cysts without erosions on x-ray examination.
12. Joint fluid culture negative for organisms during attack.

Requires: one mayor criterion or any six of the 12 minor criteria.
Source: Ref. 3. Accepted by the ARA and ACR.

Until some years ago, diagnosis was also supported by a dramatic good response to colchicine, but improvement was also observed in patients with arthritis in pseudogout, familial mediterranean fever, rheumatoid arthritis, sarcoidosis, erythema nodosum, and hydroxyapatite calcific tendinitis. Still there are rheumatologists in the world that consider a rapid response to colchicine of diagnostic value in acute gout when used in the first hours of the attack, especially when arthrocentesis and/or identification of urate crystals cannot be carried out (4).

A. Clinical Aspects

The first attack of acute gouty arthritis has clinical aspects that should enable one to suspect a probable or definite diagnosis. One important hallmark is the predilection of the first metatarsophalangeal joint (MTP) of the great toe (Podagra) in 50% of the patients and in 90% sometime during the course of the disease. Other frequent locations are the insteps, ankles, heels, knees, wrists, fingers, elbows, and rarely in the shoulders, hips, and sacroiliac, acromioclavicular, sternoclavicular, temporomandibular, and vertebral joints. Any synovial joint can be affected. Acute inflammation may be located in nonarticular areas such as bursae (patellar or olecranon), tendon sheets (Achilles), or a Baker's cyst. In 85–90% of the patients, the first attack is monoarticular and in only 10–15% is it polyarticular. Most have a sudden onset, usually during the night, with dramatic pain and explosive inflammation. Within hours, the affected joint becomes progressively swollen, red, hot, tender, and, in severe cases, may resemble a septic arthritis or cellulitis. Systemic manifestations like fever (up to 40%) and chills may be present (4). The duration of the first untreated attack is variable from 3 to 10 days and subsides spontaneously. A light attack may last 24 hours and a severe one more than a week. Desquamation and pruritus on the skin over the affected joint occur at the resolution of a severe flare.

Afterward, the patient recovers and feels completely well and then enters the so-called intercritical period. Attacks become recurrent; the second one should be expected in 75% of the patients during the following two years. Subsequent flares in untreated patients occur more frequently and with shorter asymptomatic intervals. The flares become polyarticular and severe with more systemic manifestations, slowly reaching the chronic stage.

Polyarticular onset in primary gout is seen in 10–15% of the patients, predominantly in postmenopausal women. The first attack of primary gout occurs in the middle decades of life (40–60 years of age), predominantly in males (95%).

The number of patients with secondary gout has increased in the last 10 years due to the frequent use of diuretics and cyclosporine A in organ transplants. The sex distribution and age of onset of acute gout in these patients depends on the underlying disease. In young patients (under 30 years), acute attacks are usually severe; they are monoarticular in 90% of the cases with strong family history of gout. In elderly patients (more than 65 years), the onset is polyarticular, predominantly subacute in upper extremities, and generally in women. Also in the elderly, after a relatively short period, tophi deposition in

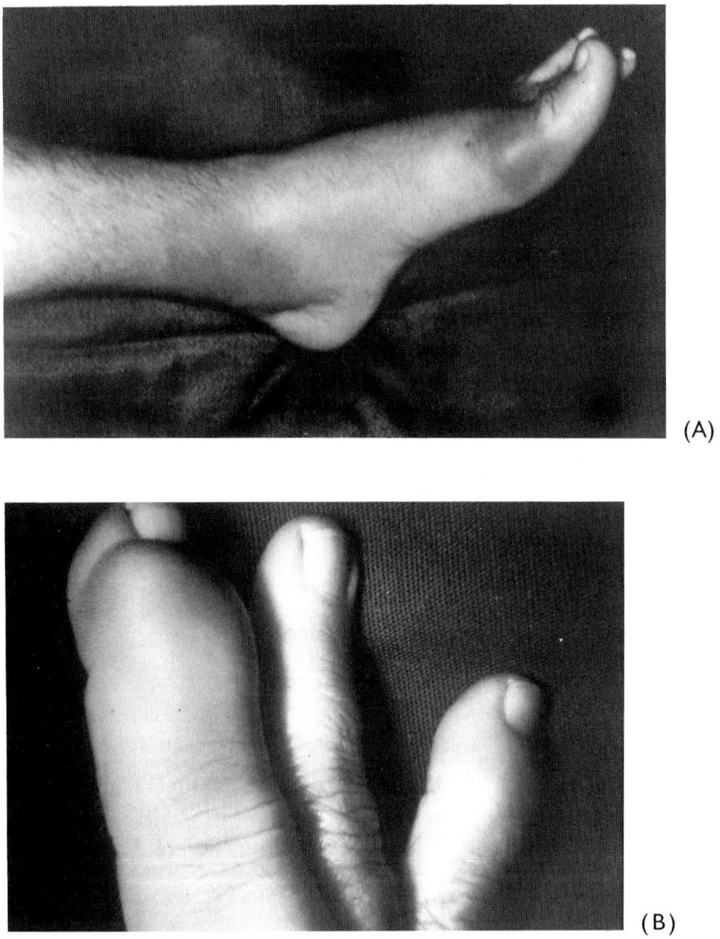

FIGURE 1 (A) Acute gout of the MTP joint of the toe and ankle (redness and swelling). (B) Swelling of the distal interphalangeal joint (Heberden's node) in acute gout. (C) Desquamation of the skin over MTP joint of the toe. (D) Desquamation of the skin over a meta carpophalangeal joint of a finger. Reprinted from the Clinical Slide Collection on the Rheumatic Diseases, Copyright © 1991, 1995, 1997. Used by permission of the American College of Rheumatology.

Heberden's nodes may occur. This combination is noted to be increased by the use of diuretics. At this age, associated diseases are frequently seen, such as hypertension, congestive heart failure, and chronic renal or hepatic failure.

It is known that the coexistence with osteoarthritis modifies the clinical presentation and course of gouty arthritis. Premonitory mild symptoms are referred by some patients. The most frequent are light pain and paresthesia on

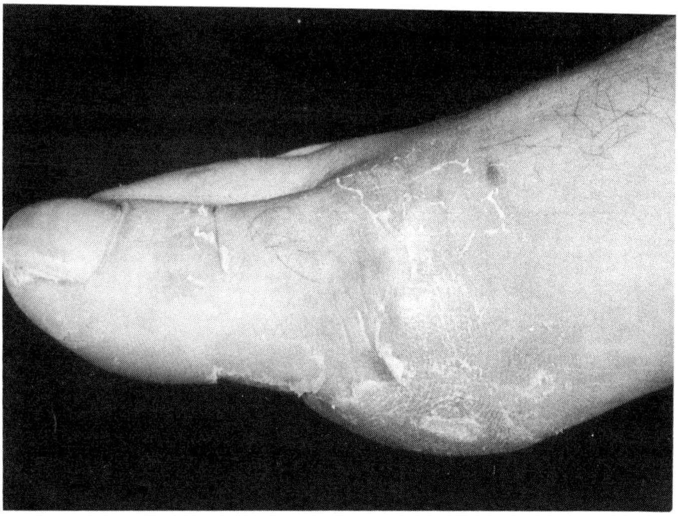

(C)

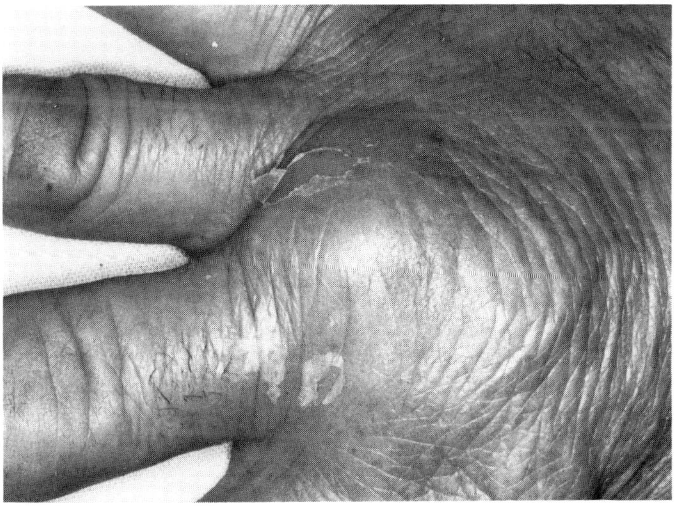

(D)

FIGURE 1 Continued

the great toe or other joints, dyspepsia, insomnia, anorexia, and headache. (If recognized, preventive treatment with a moderate dose of nonsteroidal anti-inflammatory drugs (NSAIDs) could abort the attack.)

1. Ocular Abnormalities

The most frequent finding are the "red eyes" (75%), characterized by bilateral ocular redness caused by hyperemia of the episcleral and conjunctival vessels. This is a chronic sign not related to crystal deposit and may be seen in all stages of gout (7).

B. Precipitating Factors

In the first acute attack most patients do not recognize an inciting cause. During the following episodes of recurrent arthritis, a number of possible precipitating factors are recalled by patients and/or their physicians (4, 5). They may include one or more of the following:

1. Initiation of antihyperuricemic therapy (uricosurics or allopurinol) without colchicine prophylaxis due to the mobilization of serum uric acid.
2. Dietary excess, rich foods in purine or fats.
3. Starvation diets (rapid loss of weight).
4. Alcohol overindulgence and/or sexual debauchery.
5. Emotional stress (of different types).
6. Physical injury (direct blow or strain).
7. Changes in weather conditions.
8. Acute infection (mild or severe).
9. Surgery procedures, minor or major, usually in the first 3 days.
10. After arthroscopy, cytoscopy, and gastroscopy studies.
11. Acute myocardial infarction.
12. Hemorrhages or blood transfusions.
13. After hemodialysis (in chronic renal failure).
14. Use of drugs such as vitamin B12, insulin, folic acid, cytotoxins, sulfadrugs, liver extracts, thiamine chloride, penicillin, foreign protein therapy, intravenous nitroglycerin, omeprazole (recent report).

A special consideration among drugs is the current frequent use of diuretics (fursemide, chlorathiazide); cyclosporine (in organ transplant recipients), and intravenous heparin. All of these increase urate serum level and may induce an acute attack (6). Several of the above factors, if recognized, can be corrected or avoided during the management of the disease.

1. Postsurgical Gout

In 1933, Dr. Hench emphasized the concept of postsurgical gout (6). In recent decades, with the development of new surgical procedures such as carpal tunnel release and arthroplasties (hips, knees, hands, elbows), the number of such reported cases has increased. The acute attack usually occurs 1–10 days after surgery. It affects the lower extremities, is febrile, and with leucocytosis. If the surgeon is not aware, it could get confused with a possible septic complication. To rule out an infection, it is necessary to do laboratory studies, especially of the synovial fluid of the affected joint (crystals, culture). The basic treatment of acute gout resolves the attack. If any surgical procedure is planned on a gouty patient, the use of prophylaxis with colchicine, 1 mg daily for a few days before and after surgery, is very important because it reduces the possibility of an attack in the proportion of 9 to 1 (4).

2. Changes in Weather Conditions

The observation that acute gout is seasonal belongs to Hippocrates, who, in one of his famous aphorisms, stated that the incidence of acute gout is more frequent in autumn and spring. In recent years, several studies done in the United States, Sweden, and Israel mentioned that heat stress and low barometric pressure are important factors and that acute flares are also more frequent in spring and autumn.

C. Differential Diagnosis

During the first attack and in the intercritical period, acute gout may affect one or several joints. For that reason, it is necessary to include some of the possible causes of acute monoarthritis and polyarthritis in the differential diagnosis. The most important causes among the acute monoarthropathies are as follows.

1. Septic Arthritis

Septic arthritis is seen in both sexes at all ages, but more in elderly people. The most commonly affected areas are the knee and ankle. Factors of risk are chronic alcoholism, diabetes, rheumatoid arthritis, joint replacements, tumors, blood dyscrasias, and antitumoral and/or corticosteroid treatments. It is mandatory to perform arthrocentesis, and a complete synovial fluid study: Gram stain, culture, white blood cells (WBC) (with differential), and search of crystals. The usual findings are a turbid synovial fluid with low viscosity and WBC count of 50,000–100,000 cells/mm^3. The rapid demonstration of micro-organism on Gram stain smear is evidence of an infection. The culture of the joint fluid is positive. Bacterial findings in decreasing order are: *Staphylococcus aureus, Streptococcus, Entamoeba coli, Gonococcus.* Urate crystals are not present. Early diagnosis and treatment are mandatory. Septic arthritis should be considered a life-threatening emergency, but is curable. In case of doubt, if the clinical findings suggest infection while waiting for laboratory results, the proper course of action is to initiate antibiotic therapy and monitor the response. Acute gout and septic arthritis may rarely coexist in the same joint. Synovial fluid studies will confirm the diagnosis.

2. Pseudogout (CPPD)

Differential diagnosis is made by identification of the synovial fluid of CPPD crystals of rod or rhomboid shape with weak positive birefringence. The knees and wrists are the joints most affected and radiographs frequently show chondrocalcinosis. In acute gout, crystals are rod- or needle-shaped with negative birefringence. Joints of the feet are more frequently involved. Radiographs show only soft tissue swelling. Coexistence of gout and pseudogout were reported in elderly patients.

3. Traumatic Hemarthrosis

The diagnosis of traumatic hemarthrosis is easy to make from the history. As acute gout may be precipitated by trauma; arthrocentesis and study of the synovial fluid is indicated. Fluid is bloody and otherwise normal. Radiographs may show may show a bone fracture.

In polyarticular presentations of gout, the differential diagnosis should be made to rule out rheumatoid arthritis, seronegative spondylarthropathies (e.g., ankylosing spondylitis, psoriatic arthritis, Reyter's syndrome), and some flares of osteoarthritis. The characteristic clinical, radiological, and specific laboratory findings will help in the differentiation. In doubtful cases, study of the joint fluid and identification of urate crystals will make the definitive diagnosis of gout. Coexistence of gout and other rheumatic diseases has been rarely reported.

D. Laboratory Findings

During an acute attack, mild leukocytosis (from 2,000 to 75,000 cells/mm_3) and a moderately elevated erythrocyte sedimentation rate are usually noted. Serum uric acid is increased in only 50% of the cases and it is of little value for diagnosis.

In the first attack, arthrocentesis and study of the synovial fluid is highly recommended for a definite diagnosis and to rule out other treatable diseases like septic arthritis. It should include viscosity, color, white cell count (with differential), crystal content, Gram stain, and culture. The identification of urate crystals is specific for acute gout, but they are not present in 5–15% of patients. There were reports of synovial effusions containing massive quantities of urate crystals, deeming the aspect of "urate milk" (7).

E. Radiological Findings (See Chapter 19)

X-rays of the affected joints in acute gout shows only soft tissue swelling with preserved joint spaces. They could be useful for differential diagnosis with pseudogout (chondrocalcinosis), septic arthritis (juxta-articular osteopenia, cartilage loss, bone erosion), and traumatic hemarthrosis (bone fracture).

F. Histopathology Studies: Synovial Biopsy

In only a few doubtful cases, a synovial biopsy is indicated when it is impossible to get synovial fluid for studies, as well as for differential diagnosis with other possible diseases (infections or tumors). The findings in acute gout are a diffuse and perivascular neutrophil infiltration in the synovium, with fibrin exudate and proliferation of the lining cells (5).

G. Pathogenesis of Acute Gout

Acute gout results from the deposition of urate crystals in oversaturated joint fluid of hyperuricemic patients. The reason why only a minority of the patients develop acute episodes is not understood. The frequent incidence of the attacks in the feet (podagra) is explained by the lower temperature of those joints, which decreases urate solubility, and by the microtrauma to which they are exposed. It is a well-known fact that in an acute attack, urate crystals are found in the synovial fluid, along with an increased number of polymorphonuclear leukocytes. Both have an important role in gouty inflammation.

The first step in acute gout is the precipitation of urate crystals into the synovial fluid (formed in vivo or by shedding from synovial deposits). The crystals are coated by Immunoglobulin G (IgG) that activates the neutrophils and monocytes after which the phagocyte crystals and phagolysosomes are formed. It follows a chemical digestion and rupture of the phagolysosome membrane with release of enzymes and oxygen radicals into cytoplasm. The cells are destroyed producing a great number of inflammatory mediators and further deposition of crystals into the synovial fluid. This further reinitiates the cycle and new neutrophils ingress the area. It seems that other crystals are coated by an Apo-lipoprotein that produces an inhibition of the phagocytosis of the neutrophils and monocytes. This balance between pro- and anti-inflammatory factors and the observed changes in the size of the crystals may explain the clinical observation of the self-limited duration of the acute gouty arthritis (switch-off mechanism). (see Chapter 1) (5–8).

II. TREATMENT

After a probable or definite diagnosis, which is not difficult to make, it is mandatory to start treatment promptly. The aim is to stop the acute attack and bring rapid relief to the patient. Standard modern management preferred by most rheumatologists includes one of the NSAIDs, and, when contraindicated or in refractory cases, glucocorticosteroids and colchicine. In the first hours, rest of the affected joints, cold packs, and analgesic are helpful.

A. General Measures

In an acute attack, immobilization should be recommended the first two days, followed by use of splints or crutches to rest the affected joints and avoid trauma. Local ice therapy (cold packs) have proven helpful. It is analgesic and reduces swelling; 30 minutes 4 times a day, until the attack subsides, is the recommended schedule.

B. Analgesics

Analgesics are indicated in patients resistant to standard treatments or in the first 12 hours of an acute attack until the NSAIDs start to relieve the inflammation. The following analgesics could be prescribed: acetaminophen alone or with codeine, propoxyphene hydrochloride, tramadol, and meperidine, if necessary in dramatic painful episodes.

C. Nonsteroidal Anti-Inflammatory Drugs

NSAIDs are effective analgesic and anti-inflammatory agents. One of the known mechanisms of action is by inhibition of the enzyme prostaglandin H synthase and modulation of the function of a variety of cell like neutrophils, lymphocytes, chondrocytes. The inhibition of the COX_2 enzyme at the synovial level, is responsible for the analgesic and anti-inflammatory action and of the COX_1 side effects at the gastrointestinal, renal, and hepatic levels.

Therapeutic research now is trying to develop an NSAID that inhibits only COX_2, and already some products that have partial action have appeared on the market. There are many NSAIDs that are useful in acute gouty arthritis (AGA). The first NSAID, used since 1952, is phenylbutazone. It was discontinued a few years ago due to the development of serious hematological side effects, noted mostly in chronic rheumatic diseases like rheumatoid arthritis (cases with agranulocytosis and aplastic anemia). Since 1962, indomethacin has been the most frequently prescribed NSAID for AGA and is still included in most comparative studies with new drugs (4–9).

Reports were published, given here in chronological order, on the efficacy of indomethacin, naproxen, piroxicam, ibuprofen, diclofenac, flubiprofen, tenoxicam, ketoprofen, sulindac, etodolac, aceclofenac, fenoprofen, and nabumetone. More frequently used in the United States are indomethacin, ibuprofen, naproxen, diclofenac, ketoprofen, and oxaprozin (Table 2). Pain relief is noted in 1–3 days, faster if used in the first few hours of the attack, but also when started later. Complete clinical resolution takes place in 5–7 days in 90% of cases. The selection of an NSAID depends on the patient's age and general health and the physician's experience. In gout, NSAIDs recommended have a short half-life, rapid absorption and distribution, and a reasonable high blood concentration, but all are useful. In general, there are infrequent side effects in middle-aged patients, without risk factors. These occur mostly in the gouty patients who only need treatment during a short period of 5–10 days. The strategy is to use the largest dose initially, in the first 24–48 hours, and to taper it gradually over 7 days.

Serious side effects are rare in acute gout, but are frequently reported in long-term treatment (more than 6 months) and in other chronic rheumatic diseases such as rheumatoid arthritis or osteoarthritis.

All NSAIDs are contraindicated in patients with an active peptic ulcer, a history of allergy or hypersensitivity to aspirin and to other NSAIDs, and during pregnancy and breast feeding. Caution should be taken with elderly patients and with those who are taking anticoagulants or who have a history of peptic ulcer, inflammatory bowel diseases, renal, hepatic or heart failure.

A summary of the major possible, but infrequent, side effects in acute gout are:

TABLE 2 Treatment of Acute Gout with Nonsteroidal Anti-inflammatory drugs

Drug	Commercial name	Dose (mg)/day	Divided in
Indomethacin	Indocin	50–200	2–4 doses
Ibuprofen	Motrin	1200–3200	3–4 doses
Naproxen	Naprosyn	500–1500	2–3 doses
Diclofenac sodium	Voltaren	100–150	2 doses
Diclofenac potassium	Cataflam	75–100	2 doses
Ketoprofen	Orudis	150–300	3–4 doses
Oxaprozin	Daypro	1200–1800	a single dose
Etodolac	Lodine	400–1200	1–4 doses
Piroxicam	Feldene	20–40	a single dose
Sulindac	Clinoril	300–400	2 doses
Flubiprofen	Ansaid	200–300	2–3 doses
Fenoprofen	Nalfon	900–2400	3–4 doses
Ketorolac	Toradol	up to 40 Inj*:up to 120	4–6 doses
Mefenamic acid	Ponstel	1000	4 doses
Nabumetone	Relafen	500–1000	1–2 doses
Tolmetin	Tolectin	1200–1800	3 doses
Meloxicam	Mobic	7, 5–15	a single dose

Start with full doses for 1 or 2 days, then taper to 0 within 7 days according to clinical response. Ketorolac : no more than 5 days.
*Inj = parenteral.

1. Allergy or hypersensitivity: rare (from minor rush to bronchial asthma). These cannot be prevented and are probably caused by inhibition of prostaglandin E).
2. Gastrointestinal: 50% are dyspeptic symptoms and ulcers diagnosed by gastroscopy and clinically asymptomatic.

The main risk factors in elderly patients (more than 65 years) are past history of gastric ulcer and/or gastrointestinal bleeding, concurrent use of other NSAIDs, corticosteroids, or warfarin. If diagnosed, the peptic ulcer could be treated (omeprazole 20–40 mg daily, or other drugs). In persons with high risk, misoprostol offers the best protection during treatment. In the small bowel and colon, side effects are rare colitis, bloody diarrhea, and dehydration.

3. Nephrotoxicity: of low incidence, but could be high in patients at risk (with congestive heart failure and liver cirrhosis). Reversible elevation of blood urea may be noted in some patients.
4. Hepatic: lesions are rare. Transient elevations of transaminase have been reported (1–4%).
5. Central nervous system: headaches (more often with indomethacin) and sometimes dizziness, depression, and insomnia, which resolves discontinuing the drug. In summary, severe side effects are seen more often in long-term treatments. In acute gouty arthritis, most NSAIDs have a good effect and safety ratio.

D. Glucocorticoid Therapy

It is now well established that systemic steroids are useful in the treatment of acute gout and prescribed by an increasing number of rheumatologists as a second alternative, in refractory cases to NSAIDs, and preferred to colchicine for the lower incidence of side effects. Relapses of acute attacks, which were a concern decades ago, are not more frequent than those observed with other forms of treatment (NSAIDs).

E. Intra-Articular Corticosteroids

Intra-articular corticosteroids are indicated in monoarticular or polyarticular acute gout when one or two joints are refractory or have contraindications to standard treatments. If possible, synovial fluid should be aspirated and studied to rule out a septic arthritis and in the first attack to confirm the diagnosis by a finding of urate crystals. Knees, feet, ankles, and olecranon bursa are the most frequent sites aspirated and injected.

The drugs more often employed are triamcinolone hexacetonide (Aristopan, 10–40 mg), triamcinolone acetonide (Aristocort), dexamethasone acetate (Decadron), and methylprednisolone acetate (Depomedrol, 30–40 mg), but several others are also effective. The selection is made by the preference and experience of the physician, and the dose (Triamcinolone or equivalent steroid) depends on the size of the joint (10 mg for a finger and 40 mg for a knee). Improvement is noted rapidly and complete resolution of the symptoms in 12 to 24 hours; relapses are rare.

In general, with a proper sterile technique, iatrogenic infection is exceptional (1 in 50,000 injections). Also, atrophy and hypopigmentation of the skin due to drug leakage, and synovitis due to injection of corticoid crystals, are rare (1%). Contraindications are for patients with infectious arthritis, with joint prosthesis, with bacteremia, on anticoagulant therapy, and with periarticular cellulitis (10).

F. Systemic Adrenocortical Steroids

P. Hench was the first rheumatologist that encouraged the use of cortisone in acute gout 45 years ago. The dose was 200 mg/day for 4 days, and tapered in 7 to 14 days. He also stated that combination with colchicine is not necessary because rebounds are not seen when the dose and duration of the treatment is sufficient (6). In present times, the drug more prescribed is oral prednisone 30 to 50 mg/day as the initial dose, and tapered over 7–10 days monitoring clinical response. Relief of pain is usually noted within 12 to 48 hours, and complete resolution is within 4 to 10 days (11). Side effects are infrequent because of the short period of treatment and the progressive reduction of the dose (less than 20 mg/day at the end a week). It is necessary to take caution with elderly patients and diabetics, and to remember the contraindications: those with systemic fungal or bacterial infections, ocular herpes simplex, and severe osteoporosis.

1. Parenteral Corticosteroids

Parenteral corticosteroids are also effective, safe, and a good alternative therapy to NSAIDs in acute gout in refractory patients. In 1995, Werlen et al. (12) used a single intramuscular injection of 7 mg of betamethasone in a group of 10 patients. Also, they treated another group of 7 patients that were receiving anticoagulant therapy intravenously with a single dose of 125 mg of methylprednisolone. All patients improved in 7 days. Intramuscular triamcinolone (14) acetonide 60 mg in a single dose was used in acute gout patients (13). All the patients had a resolution of their attacks in one week, without side effects. Another study compared intramuscular ACTH (40 mg) and triamcinolone acetonide (60 mg) in a single dose. Both were effective, but the last group of patients had fewer side effects (9).

In summary, during the last decade several reports were published on the treatment of AGA with long-acting parenteral corticosteroids in a single dose. Triamcinolone acetonide, 60 mg (IM); betamethasone, 7 mg (IM); and methylprednisolone, 125 mg (IV), had effective results. Relief of pain was noted in hours, resolution of the attack in was 8 days, and side effects were infrequent. Some patients needed a second injection (10% of cases).

G. Adrenocorticotropin Hormone or Corticotropin

The first report of the use of adrenocorticotropin hormone or corticotropin (ACTH) in acute gout is from the years 1949–1950, but a few years later, coincident with the development of NSAIDs in 1952, they were almost left at the wayside and rarely prescribed. In 1988, ACTH was rediscovered by Axelrod and Preston, who used a single intramuscular injection of 40 IU of ACTH in 36 patients with good results and relief of pain in 3 hours, without side effects (14). They compared these results with a group of 40 patients treated with oral indomethacin (40 mg, 4 times daily) until pain abated. The relief of pain in this last group was in more than 24 hours, and half of the patients had dyspepsia or abdominal discomfort, headaches, and difficulty in mentation. In their comparative study, ACTH was more effective than indomethacin, with fewer side effects. Relapses of acute attacks were similar in both groups (5.6% and 7.5%). It is now recognized that corticotrophin is useful in the treatment of acute gout, producing a rapid relief of pain (in 4 hours) and resolution of the attack (in 5 to 6 days). It is another good alternative to NSAIDs and colchicine in severe refractory and polyarticular gouty patients. ACTH is available in aqueous and gel injectable solutions. It could be administered intravenously (IV) in variable doses and times adapted to the medical problems of the individual patients and intramuscularly 40–80 IU in a single dose or every 12 hours, for 1 to 3 days.

In 1994, Ritter et al. (15) treated patients with multiple coexisting medical problems (congestive heart failure, chronic renal insufficiency, and gastrointestinal bleedings) with ACTH (IM-IV and subcutaneously). In 97% of the cases, the attacks were resolved in 5.5 days, with good tolerance. Like most steroids, ACTH is contraindicated for use in those with systemic fungal infections, ocular herpes simplex, severe osteoporosis, and diabetes mellitus.

In summary, ACTH was used only intermittently from 1949 until 1988, when a new dosage schedule was established and proved effective in acute gouty attacks in patients refractory to standard treatments (NSAIDs and colchicine).

H. Colchicine

Colchicine (see Chapter 14) has been used in the treatment of acute gout for many centuries. It is an alkaloid obtained from the plant colchicum autumnale and was crystallized in France by Houdee in 1884 (see Chapter 10).

The mechanism of action of colchicine is at the level of the microtubular proteins of neutrophils, altering its capacity of phagocytosis of crystals and interrupting the well-known cycle that permits the continuation of the acute attack (4–7). The dose of oral colchicine varies from 0.5 to 1 mg every 2 hours (with a maximum of 7 mg) until the attack improves, or one of the following gastrointestinal symptoms are noted: nausea, vomiting, diarrhea, or abdominal pains. These toxic side effects occur in 80% of the cases.

The rapid response to oral colchicine within 12 to 48 hours in 90% of patients was for decades considered diagnostic of gout, until it was also established that it improves the acute arthritis of other diseases such as pseudogout, sarcoidosis, erythema nodosum, rheumatoid arthritis, and familial mediterranean fever. Colchicine was the only effective remedy for acute gout until 1950, when NSAIDs and glucocorticoids were found to be equally useful with fewer side effects.

In the last 10 years, the use of oral colchicine has been in the middle of a controversy. In France it is prescribed as the first-line drug in the management of gout by nearly 65% of rheumatologists, in Brazil by 40%, and in Canada by only 11%. There is a tendency in the world today to use oral colchicine as an alternative to NSAIDs because of the inevitable gastrointestinal side effects. Intravenous colchicine (IV) is indicated in cases of active peptic ulcer or during surgical procedures. Benefits occur rapidly, in 6–12 hrs, with infrequent gastrointestinal side effects.

It is necessary to strictly follow the recommendations of Moreland and Ball (16) to avoid possible serious side effects such as local tissue necrosis or multiorgan failure, which may be fatal. When administering colchicine, 2mg should be diluted in 20 ml of normal saline and given in a freely running IV line over 20 minutes. If necessary, the doses could be repeated, but the patient should not receive more colchicine by any other route. The above dose should be reduced in older patients and in the presence of renal or hepatic disease. Absolute contraindications are combined hepatic and renal disease, creatinine clearance rates less than 10 ml/min, extrahepatic biliary obstruction, coexistent severe infections, preexistent bone marrow depression, or immediate prior use of oral colchicine (16).

One of the established and very effective indications of oral colchicine is to prevent recurrent attacks of acute gout during the intercritical period and before starting treatment with allopurinol or uricosuric drugs. The dose is 0.5 mg twice a day during months or years according to results and tolerance.

IV colchicine is available in the United States and a few other countries, and has been discontinued in others, such as Great Britain.

I. New Drug

In 1994, Dr. Schworer reported an interesting experience in a gouty patient with renal dysfunction, arterial hypertension, and hematemesis who suffered an acute attack of podagra (17). Having contraindications to all conventional treatments, he was treated with 5-hydroxytryptamine antagonist ondansetron (Zopran) at a dose of 8 mg intravenously. Pain was drastically reduced within 30 minutes, redness in 2 hours. This is a new drug that was effective in the treatment of a very difficult case (17).

J. Acute Gout in Organ Transplant

In the last decades, heart, kidney, lung, and liver transplantations were carried out in many patients in several countries (18). To prevent rejection, it is necessary to treat patients with high doses of immunosuppressive drugs such as corticosteroids and azathioprine. Progress was made with the addition of cyclosporine A, which allows a reduction of corticosteroids and diminished its severe side effects (osteoporosis, fractures, and osteonecrosis). Also, cyclosporine A produces hyperuricemia in 45–80% of the patients and, in a short period of months, recurrent episodes of acute gout occur in one or several joints (secondary gout). Tophi usually develop later in 5–17%. It is very difficult to treat these patients who always have some degree of renal insufficiency (19). NSAIDs and colchicine are contraindicated. Systemic corticosteroids and ACTH are ineffective for long-term steroid use. The best management in this circumstance is intra articular steroids, and to perform Gram stain and culture studies periodically for the high risk of infection.

In most organ transplants, it is necessary to use diuretics, which are an additional cause of hyperuricemia. Transplanted patients with renal insufficiency cannot take uricosurics. Allopurinol in low dose is the only choice, but because it potentiates azathioprine, this drug must be reduced 50–75% to avoid serious side effects.

K. Preventive Treatment

During the intercritical period, it is necessary to prevent recurrent attacks. This is achieved by the use of some drugs and general clinical measures. Since 1926, colchicine has been used as the first-choice drug in the prophylaxis of acute gouty arthritis in doses of 1 mg/day (taken as 0.5 mg twice daily). It is indicated in patients with frequent attacks, in some with coexisting medical complications, and when starting allopurinol or uricosuric therapy. The duration of the treatment is variable and tailored to each patient according to results, tolerance, age, level of serum urate, and frequency of attacks. The results were excellent in 82% of patients, satisfactory in 12%, and unsatisfactory in 5% of a large series of 208 patients treated during a period of several years by Drs. Gutman and Yu (20). Only six patients had episodes of diarrhea. Colchicine prophylaxis prevents or diminishes the rate of attacks independent of the presence of tophi and hyperuricemia. Side effects are minimal with the low dose employed in prophylaxis, but caution should be taken when the patient has renal and/or hepatic failure.

Compliance is important and patients should be educated and advised to avoid risk factors such as obesity, high purine diet, alcohol consumption, and diuretic therapy, which are controllable.

It is possible that a small dose of colchicine modulates immune responses in the synovial lining cells, resulting in cumulative suppression of chemotactic activity and reducing subclinical joint inflammation. The duration of the prophylaxis with colchicine should be continued for at least one year after the control of the serum urate level. One isolated case of myoneuropathy has been reported in a patient that had a creatinine clearance below 50 ml/min. If colchicine is not tolerated in small doses, an anti-inflammatory drug could be used as an alternative (indomethacin 25 mg/daily or equivalent of another NSAID).

Prophylaxis therapy also includes urate-lowering drugs such a uricosurics (e.g., probenecid, sulfinpirazone, or benzabromarone) or an xanthine oxidase inhibitor (allopurinol) with the aim of keeping serum urate levels below 6.0 mg/dl. The selection of the best drug, dose, and duration of treatment should be done on an individualized basis according to the clinical and laboratory findings of each patient. The combined prophylactic treatment of colchicine and one hypouricemic drug should be continued until serum uric level is normal and patient is asymptomatic for 6 months to 1 year.

In summary, preventive therapy during the intercritical period should include low dose of colchicine 1 mg/day and control of symptomatic hyperuricemia (in patients with frequent and severe recurrent attacks, presence of tophi or renal stones), and avoid factors that favor hyperuricemia such as obesity, alcohol intake, high purine diet, iatrogenic drugs, diuretics, and the recognized precipitating factors.

REFERENCES

1. T. Sydenham. A treatise of the gout and dropsy (G. Kettilby, ed.), London, 1683.
2. D. J. McCarty and J. L. Hollander. Identification of urate crystals in gouty synovial fluid, *Ann Intern Med 54*:452 (1961).
3. S. L. Wallace, H. Robinson, A. T. Masi, J. L. Decker, D. J. McCarty, and T.-F. Yu. Preliminary criteria for the classification of acute arthritis of primary gout. *Arth Rheum 20*:895 (1977).
4. J. H. Talbott and T.-F. Yu. Gout and Uric Acid Metabolism, Stratton Intercontinental Medical Book Corporation, New York, New York, 1976.
5. M. G. Cohen and B. T. Emmerson. Textbook of Rheumatology, (J. H. Klippel, P. A. Kieppe, eds.), Gout. Mosby Year Book, Europe, Philadelphia, 1994, p. 12.1–12.15.
6. P. S. Hench. Gout and gouty arthritis, Textbook of Medicine, 9th Edition, (Cecil-Loeb, eds.) Saunders, Philadelphia, 1953, p. 643–647.

7. W. N. Kelley and H. R. Schumacher, Jr. Crystal associated synovitis. In: Textbook of Rheumatology, 4th Edition, (Kelley, Havis, Ruddy, Sledge, eds.), Saunders, Philadelphia, PA, 1993, pp. 1292–1395.
8. R. A. Terkeltaub. What stops a gouty attack? *J Rheum 19*:1 (1992).
9. L. B. Siegel, J. A. Alloway, and D. J. Nashel. Comparison of Adrenocorticotropic hormone and Triamcinolone acetonamide in the treatment of acute gouty arthritis, *J Rheum 21*:1325–1327 (1994).
10. R. G. Gray, J. Tenenbaum, and N. L. Gottlieb. Local corticosteroid injection treatment in rheumatic disorders, *Sem Arth Rheumat 10*:231–254 (1981).
11. G. D. Gross, W. A. Franck, and D. A. Raddatz. Systemic steroid therapy for acute gout: A clinical trial and review of the literature, *Sem Arth Rheum 19*:329–336 (1990).
12. D. Werlen, C. Gabay, and Th. L. Vischer, Les glucocorticoides dans le traitment des acces microcristallins: une alterantive efficace aux anti-inflammatories non steroidienes, *Rev Rhum 63*:271–277 (1996).
13. S. A. Alloway, M. Moriarity, Y. T. Hoagland, and D. J. Nashel. Comparison of Triamcinolone Acetonide with Indomethacin in the treatment of acute gouty arthritis, *J Rheumat 20*:1383–1384 (1993).
14. D. Axelrod and S. Preston. Comparison of parenteral adrenocorticotropic hormone with oral indomethacin in the treatment of acute gout, *Arth Rheum 31*:803–805 (1988).
15. J. Ritter, L. Kerr, T. Valeriano-Marcet, and H. Spiera. ACTH revisited: effective treatment of acute crystal induced synovitis in patients with multiple medical problems, *J Rheumat 21*:696–699 (1994).
16. L. W. Moreland and G. V. Ball, Colchicine and gout, *Arth Rheum 34*:782–786 (1994).
17. H. Schworer and H. Ramadory. Treatment of acute gouty arthritis with 5-Hydroxytryptamine antagonist ondansetron, *Clin. Investig. 72*:801–814 (1994).
18. C. West, B. J. Carpenter, and T. R. Hakala. The incidence of gout in renal transplant recipient, *Am J Kidney Dis 10*:369–372 (1987).
19. S. Rozenberg, L. Frith, T. Lang, et al. Manifestations Rheumatologiques chez le transplantes cardiaques. Etudy transversale de 365 patients, *Rev Rheum 60*:10–15 (1993).
20. T.-F. Yu. The efficacy of colchicine prophylaxis in articular gout: A reappraisal after 20 years, *Sem Arth Rheumat 12*:2 (1982).

14
Colchicine

Yair Molad
Tel Aviv University
Tel Aviv, Israel

Bruce N. Cronstein
New York University School of Medicine
New York, New York

Stephen E. Malawista
Yale University School of Medicine
New Haven, Connecticut

I. INTRODUCTION

Today, when "natural" drugs have achieved a newfound popularity in the treatment of many ailments, colchicine, an anti-inflammatory drug in continuous use for as long as 3000 years, stands out as a long-tested agent whose roots are buried deep in the soil of natural remedies. Although the preparations of colchicine most commonly used today are synthetic, the drug was first isolated from *colchicum autumnale* (autumn crocus, meadow saffron). Colchicine is unique in its spectrum of action; it is a weak, general anti-inflammatory agent that is singularly active in the treatment and prevention of such neutrophil-mediated conditions as acute gouty arthritis and familial Mediterranean fever (1–4).

In ancient times, colchicum was considered to be a poison because of its pronounced gastrointestinal toxicity, which is rapid in onset, and the slower lethal effects of the agent (5). Although colchicum was first mentioned as a remedy (named hermadactyl or finger of Hermes) for acute gouty arthritis in the "Therapeutica" of Alexander of Tralles (550 AD), a drug that was probably identical to colchicine was described in the Ebers papyrus (1500 BC). Colchicine was later reintroduced as a drug for gout in 1764 by Baron Anton Von Storch, physician to Empress Maria Theresa (5). In 1820, Pelletier and Caventou were the first to extract colchicine as the active alkaloid of colchicum. Colchicine is still a potent drug in the management of acute attacks of gout although it is much more commonly used to prevent gouty attacks (6).

In this chapter we discuss the pharmacological and clinical aspects of colchicine as it is used in the management of gout.

II. PHARMACOKINETICS

Among the unique features of colchicine is its low therapeutic index: effective steady-state plasma concentrations after acute treatment range from 0.5 to 3 ng/ml, with toxic effects occurring at a level of approximately 3 ng/ml (7,8). Colchicine is a neutral and highly lipid soluble compound at physiologic pH (pKa = 12.8, MW = 398), which enables its rapid passage into body tissues. After an intravenous dose of 2 mg of colchicine, the plasma half-life is 19.3 ± 7.5 min (7,8). After oral administration, colchicine is absorbed in the jejunum and ileum with a single zero-order rate process, with 44% bioavailability (9). It binds with low affinity to albumin (32% bound) (10) and possesses a large steady-state volume of distribution (11). Serum colchicine concentration declines in a biexponential mode, reflecting its rapid clearance from the plasma and its rapid redistribution to leukocytes (12) and red blood cells (10). Most of the administered dose of the drug is metabolized; only 10–25% of an oral dose is recovered unchanged in the urine. Its peak plasma concentration following oral administration is achieved after about 2 hr and colchicine has a plasma half-life of about 4 hr, although it can be detected in leukocytes for up to 10 days after administration. Colchicine is excreted mainly in the urine hence its plasma half-life is prolonged in patients with renal dysfunction, especially in those with combined renal and liver diseases (13). Thus, patients with renal or liver diseases who take colchicine should be carefully monitored for possible toxic effects of the drug.

III. MECHANISM OF ACTION

Colochicine mediates its therapeutic effects in the treatment of acute gout by virtue of its capacity to inhibit inflammatory reactions, not by any effect on the formation or dissolution of the causative agent in the pathogenesis of acute gouty arthritis, monosodium urate crystals. Colchicine does not affect crystal formation, serum urate concentration, or the urinary excretion of uric acid (14). The fact that colchicine is a better prophylactic than therapeutic agent, and that in treatment it is most effective when used early, suggests that there is a critical, early, colchicine-sensitive, proinflammatory event(s) in acute gouty arthritis and in other colchicine-responsive disorders, which later on is less important for the propagation and amplification of the inflammatory response (1,15).

Investigations into the molecular mechanism by which colchicine modulates cellular behavior began nearly four decades ago and the findings of these early studies remain relevant to our understanding of the mechanism of action of colchicine. Colchicine was long known to inhibit cell division and proliferation, and early studies demonstrated that colchicine disrupts the mitotic spindle; dissolution of microtubules was subsequently shown to be responsible for the effect of colchicine on the mitotic spindle as well as cellular proliferation (reviewed in 1). Although colchicine was previously known to affect a variety of neutrophil functions, Malawista and Bensch (16) first demonstrated that, like other cells, neutrophils possess microtubules and colchicine disrupts them in a dose-dependent fashion, a discovery made independently by Bessis and Breton-Gorius (17). They further suggested that the effect of colchicine on neutrophil microtubules might underlie the capacity of colchicine to diminish inflammation (1,16,18–21). Microtubules are labile structures that lengthen or shrink by elongation at one end and dissolution at the other. Colchicine does not enhance the rate of microtubule dissolution but inhibits the process of microtubule self-assembly in a substoichiometric fashion by binding to β-tubulin with the formation of tubulin-colchicine complexes (19,22,23). Most of the pharmacological effects of colchicine on the cells involved in gouty inflammation appear to be related to the capacity of colchicine to disrupt microtubules.

Neutrophils constitute the vast majority of the cells present in the synovial fluid in acute gouty arthritis and their disappearance is associated with the end of the acute attack. Thus, it is logical to assume that colchicine modulates either the function or recruitment of neutrophils into the joints during acute gouty attacks. Inhibition of neutrophil motile function by colchicine would be expected to diminish neutrophil recruitment to the inflamed joints and thereby mediate the anti-inflammatory effects of colchicine in the treatment of gout (1). Colchicine inhibits neutrophil phagocytosis and, perhaps more importantly, release of lysosomal contents during phagocytosis (24,25). Since the effects of colchicine on neutrophil function were mimicked by other agents that disrupt microtubules (20,21) it was concluded from these experiments that microbutule disruption directly modulated neutrophil function (24,25). Subsequent studies have broadened our understanding of the relationship between colchicine's effects on microtubules and neutrophil function. Colchicine, via its disruption of microtubules, appears to activate an adenylate cyclase in neutrophils leading to the intracellular accumulation of cAMP (26–28). Increased intracellular cAMP markedly inhibits stimulated neutrophil function and could also explain the observed suppressive effect of colchicine on neutrophil function (26–28). Colchicine also selectively modulates monosodium urate crystal-induced tyrosine phosphorylation of proteins via an effect on microtubules (29,30). Colchicine exerts several other potentially anti-inflammatory effects including suppression of phospholipase A2 activation (31), selective inhibition of the crystal-induced increase in cytoplasmic calcium, and superoxide production by activated neutrophils (32), all of which are pivotal steps in the inflammatory response of neutrophils to crystals. Thus, these in vitro studies suggested that colchicine disrupts neutrophil microtubules that, either directly or indirectly, modulate neutrophil function in a fashion that would diminish both the recruitment of neutrophils to the acute gouty joint and the function of those neutrophils already present in the joint.

During inflammation a large number of soluble mediators are generated that may recruit and stimulate neutrophils; many of these mediators are thought to play a major role in the pathogenesis of acute gouty arthritis (33,34). Thus, over the years a number of investigators have questioned whether colchicine regulates the production of or response to the soluble mediators of inflammation by inflammatory cells. The monokine tumor necrosis factor α (TNFα) is produced by monocytes and synovial cells upon contact with monosodium urate crystals (33); colchicine inhibits the production of TNFα by macrophages and downregulates the surface expression of TNFα-receptor on macrophages and endothelial cells (35,36). Diminished TNFα secretion may, therefore, interfere with the "priming" effect of TNFα on neutrophils prior to their activation by monosodium-urate crystals (37). Colchicine may also diminish recruitment of neutrophils to the affected joint by inhibiting the urate crystal-induced (38) and ionophore-induced formation of leukotriene B_4 (LTB_4) (39), as well as suppressing the locomotion of neutrophils in in vivo studies (40,41). Monosodium urate–stimulated neutrophils secrete a high molecular weight chemotactic factor that has not been characterized and colchicine inhibits secretion of this chemoattractant (42). It should be noted that colchicine mediates the effects described above at concentrations that are generally not achieved in patients. That colchicine is rapidly partitioned to the leukocyte compartment in patients may explain how these lower, pharmacologically relevant concentrations of colchicine are magnified in the leukocytes of patients and thereby regulate inflammation. Even in vitro, colchicine effects are a function of both concentration and time of incubation (43,44).

Neutrophils are recruited into the gouty joint from the circulation and it has recently been appreciated that the endothelium plays an active role in neutrophil recruitment. When studied in an in vivo model of acute inflammation, colchicine reduces the adhesion of neutrophils to the vascular endothelium (45,46). The interaction of neutrophils and other circulating leukocytes with the vascular endothelium is mediated by a number of specific cell adhesion molecules on both the neutrophil and the endothelial cell; the molecules responsible for leukocyte-endothelial interaction include members of the integrin family (β_2 integrins on the neutrophil), immunoglobulin superfamily (ICAM-1 and ICAM-2 on endothelial cells), and selectin family (L-selectin on neutrophils, P-selectin, and E-selectin on endothelial cells) (reviewed in 47,48). When studied in vitro, colchicine abrogates the E-selectin–mediated adhesiveness of cytokine-stimulated vascular endothelium for neutrophils (49). The effect of colchicine on E-selectin–mediated endothelial adhesiveness is microtubule-dependent and occurs at concentrations of colchicine that are over a thousand-fold lower than those required to affect neutrophil function. Relatively low doses of colchicine are administered to patients in order to prevent acute gouty attacks and the capacity of very low doses of colchicine to modulate endothelial-mediated recruitment of neutrophils to gouty joints may account for the prophylactic effects of the drug. At higher concentrations (tenfold lower than those required to modulate neutrophil lysosomal enzyme release or LTB_4 secretion in vitro) colchicine reduces the surface expression of L-selectin on leukocytes and may, therefore, interfere with the interaction of neutrophils with the vascular endothelium. Administration of therapeutic doses (but not prophylactic doses) of colchicine markedly reduced L-selectin expression on the neutrophils of normal volunteers suggesting that this phenomenon also plays a role in diminishing the inflammation of acute gouty attacks (49).

Other effects of colchicine include inhibition of arachidonate release and 5-lipoxygenase action in alveolar macrophages (50), suppression of delayed hypersensitivity reactions (51), histamine (43,52), insulin (53) and parathormone release (54), and induction of apoptosis in mice cerebellar cells (55).

IV. INDICATIONS AND CLINICAL USE

Colchicine is currently indicated for the treatment of acute attacks of gout, for prophylaxis during the intercritical phase, and in the late chronic tophaceous phase of the disease. In the treatment of acute gouty attacks, colchicine works best if given early in the course of the episode.

Colchicine may be administered orally or intravenously for the treatment of acute attacks. Although nonsteroidal anti-inflammatory drugs (NSAIDs) are currently considered to be the drugs of choice for the treatment of acute gouty attacks (56), intravenous colchicine may be particularly useful when NSAIDs are contraindicated. Most patients who receive colchicine respond within 18 hr; joint inflammation subsides in 75–80% of the patients within 48 hr, (57). Only one double-blind placebo-controlled trial has been performed on the effectiveness of oral colchicine in the treatment of acute gout, and this study demonstrated clinical improvement in two-thirds of the colchicine-treated patients within 48 hr although the therapeutic effects were most often preceded by gastrointestinal side effects (58). The drug is usually administered orally in an initial dose of 1 mg, followed by 0.5 mg every 2 hr until gastrointestinal side effects occur or a total dose of 8 mg has been given. This procedure is usually safe unless the patient has renal or liver disease or is elderly (59). Although intravenous administration of colchicine is sometimes extremely useful, the drug must be employed properly to avoid serious and even fatal toxic effects. Should intravenous colchicine be administered, the following guidelines and restrictions are firmly recommended:

1. Nonsteroidal anti-inflammatory drugs, steroids, or corticotropins are preferred whenever oral colchicine is contraindicated or intolerable for the therapy of acute gouty arthritis.
2. Intravenous and oral colchicine therapy should not be given concomitantly. If the patient has not responded to therapeutic doses of oral colchicine, an alternative drug should be used in place of further colchicine.
3. The doses must be reduced by at least 50% in patients with renal or hepatic disease and in elderly patients. The drug should not be used at all if the patient has a creatinine clearance below 10 ml/min. It must be emphasized that colchicine is not removable by dialysis or exchange transfusion (60).
4. Colchicine should not be given to patients with combined liver and kidney disease.
5. The intravenous dose should be given cautiously and slowly to minimize the risk of extravasation.
6. Single intravenous doses should be no greater than 2–3 mg with a cumulative dose of no more than 4 mg.

Following the guidelines outlined above colchicine may be given intravenously as follows: an initial dose of 2 mg should be administered through an established intravenous line. Two more doses of 1 mg each may be administered at 6-hr intervals thereafter, but the total dose should rarely, if ever, exceed 4 mg (56).

Colchicine can be used to prevent acute gouty attacks, as has been shown in a placebo-controlled study (61). An oral dose of 0.5–1 mg/day diminished the frequency of acute attacks, whether or not the serum urate level was normal (57,62,63). In one study, 1 mg daily of oral colchicine reduced the number of white blood cells in the synovial fluid of asymptomatic knees of gouty patients during the intercritical phase (64). This clinical observation is consistent with the capacity of colchicine to diminish endothelial recruitment of neutrophils, as demonstrated in vitro (49). Therapy designed to diminish serum urate levels is often indicated in the prevention of acute gouty attacks and development of chronic tophaceous gout (See Chapter 11) and acute gouty attacks are often observed at the outset of urate-lowering therapy. It is therefore appropriate to administer prophylactic doses of colchicine to patients before the initiation of drugs to correct the hyperuricemia, and prophylaxis should be continued for at least a year after the serum urate concentration has returned to a normal level (56). Although prophylactic doses of colchicine are generally very well tolerated, in those patients with impaired renal function (creatinine clearance of 50 ml/min or less) a myoneuropathy has been reported during prophylaxis with colchicine (65–68).

V. ADVERSE AND TOXIC REACTIONS

When therapeutic or prophylactic colchicine is administered orally to patients with normal renal and hepatic function the drug is usually safe, although gastrointestinal discomfort occurs in most of the patients given the higher doses of the drug within 24 hr (56,57). Diarrhea, vomiting, and abdominal cramps are the most frequent side effects of high-dose colchicine, are often the first sign of toxicity, and are an indication that the drug should be stopped. In contrast, intravenous colchicine rarely produces gastrointestinal toxicity, provided that oral colchicine is not being given concomitantly. Prolonged high-dose oral colchicine therapy can lead to malabsorption. Bone marrow suppression is rarely seen in patients given either low-dose or high-dose colchicine. Long-term colchicine administration can result in ovarian and testicular dysfunction (69,70). Neuromuscular toxicity was reported in patients with renal failure, usually resolving after the drug is stopped (65,71). Poisoning from colchicine overdose, usually with suicidal intent, when the dose of 0.8 mg/kg is exceeded, has been uniformly fatal (69). Hill et al. concluded that a dose of 40 mg in adults with normal renal function is lethal (72). Colchicine intoxication is characterized by multiorgan failure, starting with gastrointestinal symptoms, dehydration and leukocytosis, followed by bone marrow suppression, renal failure, adult respiratory distress syndrome, arrhythmias and heart failure, fever, coagulopathy, acid-base disturbances, and neuromuscular involvement (69). Recently, colchicine-specific Fab fragments of immunoglobulin were reported as effective therapy for colchicine intoxication (73).

VI. CONCLUSION

There are very few drugs that have been in use as long as colchicine and the outlook for its continued use in the treatment and prevention of acute gouty attacks is excellent. Moreover, the lessons learned from studies of the mechanism of action of colchicine have broadened our understanding of both cell biology and of the pathogenesis and control of acute inflammation.

REFERENCES

1. S. E. Malawista. The actin of colchicine in acute gouty arthritis. *Arthritis Rheum 18*:835–846 (1975).
2. S. E. Malawista and J. E. Seegmiller. The effect of pretreatment with colchicine on the inflammatory response to injected urate. A model for gouty inflammation. *Ann Int Med 62*:648–657 (1965).
3. S. E. Malawista and V. T. Andriole. Colchicine: Anti-inflammatory effect of low doses in a sensitive bacterial system. *J Lab Clin Med 72*:933–942 (1968).
4. S. E. Goldfinger. Colchicine for familial Mediterranean fever. *New Engl J Med 287*:1302 (1972).
5. E. F. Hartung. History of the use of colchicum and related medicaments in gout. *Ann Rheum Dis 13*:190–200 (1954).
6 P. J. Pelletier and J. B. Caventou. Examen clinique de plusiers vegetaux de la famille des colchicees et du principe actif qu'ils enferment. *Ann Chim Phys 14*:69 (1820).
7. S. L. Wallace, B. Omokoku, and N. H. Ertel. Colchicine plasma levels. Implications as to pharmacology and mechanism of action. *Am J Med 48*:443–448 (1970).
8. S. L. Wallace and N. H. Ertel. Plasma levels of colchicine after oral administration of a single dose. *Metabolism 22*:749–753 (1973).
9. M. Rochdi, A. Sabouraud, C. Girre, R. Venet, and J. M. Scherrmann. Pharmacokinetics and absolute bioavailability of colchicine after intravenous and oral administration in healthy human volunteers and elderly subjects. *Eur J Clin Pharmacol 46*:351–354 (1994).
10. A. Sabouraud, O. Chappey, T. Dupin, and J. M. Scherrmann. Binding of colchicine and thiocolchicoside to human serum proteins and blood cells. *Int J Clin Pharmacol Ther 32*:429–432 (1994).
11. G. M. Ferron, M. Rochdi, W. J. Jusko, and J. M. Scherrmann. Oral absorption characteristics and pharmacokinetics of colchicine in healthy volunteers after single and multiple doses. *J Clin Pharmacol 36*:874–883 (1996).
12. O. N. Chappey, E. Niel, J. L. Wautier, P. P. Hung, M. Dervichian, D. Cattan, and J. M. Scherrmann. Colchicine deposition in human leukocytes after single and multiple oral administration. *Clin Pharmacol Ther 54*:360–367 (1993).
13. E. Ben-Chetrit, J. M. Scherrmann, E. Zylber-Katz, and M. Levy. Colchicine disposition in patients with Familial Mediterranean Fever with renal impairment. *J Rheumatol 21*:710–713 (1994).
14. S. L. Wallace. Colchicine: clinical pharmacology in acute gouty arthritis. *Am J Med 30*:439 (1961).
15. J. I. Smallwood and S. E. Malawista. Colchicine, crystals and neutrophil tyrosine phosphorylation (editorial). *J Clin Invest 92*:1602–1603 (1993).
16. S. E. Malawista and K. G. Bensch. Human polymorphonuclear leukocytes: Demonstration of microtubules and effect of colchicine. *Science 156*(3774):521–522 (1967).
17. M. Bessis and J. Breton-Gorius. Rapports entre noyau et centrioles dans les granulocytes étalalés. Rúle des microtubules. *Nouvelle Revue Francaise d'Hématologie 7*:601–620 (1967).

18. S. E. Malawista. On the action of colchicine. The melanocyte model. *J Exp Med 122*:361–384 (1965).
19. S. E. Malawista. Colchicine: A common mechanism for its anti-inflammatory and anti-mitotic effects. *Arthritis Rheum 11*(2, pt. 1):191–197 (1968).
20. S. E. Malawista, K. G. Bensch, and H. Sato. Vinblastine and griseofulvim reversibily disrupt the living mitotic spindele. *Science 160*:770–772 (1968).
21. S. E. Malawista. Vinblastine: colchicine-like effects on human blood leukocytes during phagocytosis. *Blood 37*(5):519–529 (1971).
22. D. L. Sackett and J. K. Varma. Molecular mechanism of colchicine action: Induced local unfolding of â-tubulin. *Biochemistry 32*(49):13560–13565 (1993).
23. Vandecandelaere, S. R. Martin, and Y. Engelborghs. Response of microtubules to the addition of colchicine and tubulin-colchicine: evaluation of models for the interaction of drugs with microtubules. *Biochem J 323*:189–196 (1997).
24. R. B. Zurier, S. Hoffstein, and G. Weissmann. Mechanisms of lysosomal enzyme release from human leukocytes. I. Effect of cyclic nucleotides and colchicine. *J Cell Biol 58*:27–41 (1973).
25. D. G. Wright and S. E. Malawista. Mobilization and extracellular release of granular enzymes from human leukocytes during phagocytosis: Inhibition by colchicine and cortisol but not by salicylates. *Arthritis Rheum 16*(6):749–758 (1973).
26. S. A. Rudolph, P. Greengard, and S. E. Malawista. Effects of colchicine on cyclic AMP levels in human leukocytes. *Proc Natl Acad Sci USA 74*:3404–3408 (1977).
27. S. A. Rudolph, L. R. Hegstrand, P. Greengard, and S. E. Malawista. The interaction of colchicine with hormone-sensitive adenylate cyclase in human leukocytes. *Mol Pharm 16*:805–812 (1979).
28. J. I. Smallwood and S. E. Malawista. Misoprostol stimulates leukocyte adenosine 3':5' cyclic monophosphate production and synergizes with colchicine: Novel combination of established drugs may boost anti-inflammatory potential. *J Pharmacol Exp Ther 269*:1196–1204 (1994).
29. C. J. Roberge, M. Gaudry, R. De Medicis, A. Lussier, P. E. Poubelle, and P. H. Naccache. Crystal induced neutrophin activation. IV. Specific inhibition of tyrosine phosphorylation by colchicine. *J Clin Invest 92*:1722–1729 (1993).
30. C. J. Roberge, M. Gaudry, C. Gilbert, S. E. Malawista, R. de Mèdicis, A. Lussier, P. E. Poubelle, and P. H. Naccache. On the relationship between microtubules and stimulated tyrosine phosphorylation in human neutrophils: Paradoxical effects of colchicine on the activation of human neutrophils by chemotactic factors and inflammatory microcrystals. *J Leuk Biol 59*:864–871 (1996).
31. M. Paya, M. C. Terencio, M. L. Ferrandiz, and M. J. Alcaraz. Involvement of secretory phospholipase A2 activity in the zymosan air pouch model of inflammation. *Br J Pharmacol 117*:1773–1779 (1996).
32. P. H. Naccache, M. Grimard, C. J. Roberge, C. Gilbert, A. Lussier, R. De Medicis, and P. E. Poubelle. Crystal-induced neutrophil activation. I. Initiation and modulation of calcium mobilization and superoxide production by microcrystals. *Arthritis Rheum 34*(3):333–342 (1991).
33. F. S. di Giovine, S. E. Malawista, E. Thornton, and G. W. Duff. Urate crystals stimulate production of tumor necrosis factor alpha from human blood monocytes and

synovial cells. Cytokine mRNA and protein kinetics, and cellular distribution. *J Clin Invest 87*:1375–1381 (1991).

34. C. J. Roberge, J. Grassi, R. de Medicis, Y. Frobert, A. Lussier, P. H. Naccache, and P. E. Poubelle. Crystal-neutrophil interactions lead to interleukin-1 synthesis. *Agents and Actions 34*:38–41 (1991).
35. Z. Li, G. S. Davis, C. Mohr, M. Naim, and D. Gemsa. Inhibition of LPS-induced tumor necrosis factor-α production by colchicine and other microtubules disrupting drugs. *Immunobiol 195*:624–639 (1996).
36. A. H. Ding, F. Porteu, E. Sanchez, and C. F. Nathan. Downregulation of tumor necrosis factor receptors on macrophages and endothelial cells by mictotubule depolarizing agents. *J Exp Med 171*:715–727 (1990).
37. H. M. Burt and J. K. Jackson. The priming action of tumor necrosis factor-alpha (TNFα) and granulocyte-macrophage colony stimulating factor (GM-CSF) on neutrophils activated by inflammatory microcrystals. *Clin Exp Immunol 108*:432–437 (1997).
38. C. N. Serhan, U. Lundberg, G. Weissmann, and B. Samuelsson. Formation of leukotrienes and hydroxy acids from human neutrophils and platelets exposed to monosodium urate. *Prostaglandins 27*:503–581 (1984).
39. J. Reibman, K. A. Haines, A. M. Rich, P. Cristello, K. N. Giedd, and G. Weissmann. Colchicine inhibits ionophore-induced formation of leukotriene B4 by human neutrophils: The role of microtubules. *J Immunol 136*(3):1027–1932 (1986).
40. M. Ehrenfeld, M. Levy, M. Bar Eli, R. Gallily, and M. Eliakim. Effect of colchicine on polymorphonuclear leukocyte chemotaxis in human volunteers. *Br J Clin Pharmacol 10*:297–300 (1980).
41. P. Hambleton and P. Miller. Pharmacological investigation of acute cellular accumulation in immunological air pouch inflammation. *Agents and Actions 28*:73–77 (1989).
42. I. Spilberg and B. F. Mandell. Crystal-induced chemotactic factor. In: *Advances in Inflammation Research, Vol. 5* (G. Weissmann, ed.), Raven Press, New York, 57–65 (1983).
43. E. Gillespie, R. J. Levine, and S. E. Malawista. Histamine release from rat peritoneal mast cells: Inhibition by colchicine and potentiation by deuterium oxide. *J Pharmacol Exper Therap 164*:158–165 (1968).
44. S. E. Malawista, J. M. Oliver, and S. A. Rudolph. Microtubules and cyclic AMP in human leukocytes: On the order of things. *J Cell Biol 77*:881–886 (1978).
45. J. N. Fordham, J. Kirwan, J. Cason, and H. L. F. Currey. Prolonged reduction in polymorphonuclear adhesion following oral colchicine. *Ann Rheum Dis 40*:605–608 (1981).
46. H. Asako, P. Kubes, B. A. Baethge, R. E. Wolf, and D. N. Granger. Colchicine and methotrexate reduce leukocyte adherence and emigration in rat mesenteric venules. *Inflammation 16*(1):45–56 (1992).
47. C. F. Mojcik and E. M. Shevach. Adhesion molecules: a rheumatologic perspective. *Arth Rheum 40*:1005–1011 (1997).
48. B. N. Cronstein and G. Weissmann. The adhesion molecules of inflammation. *Arth Rheum 36*:147–157 (1993).

49. B. N. Cronstein, Y. Molad, J. Reibman, E. Balakhane, R. I. Levin, and G. Weissmann. Colchicine alters the quantitative and qualitative display of selectins on endothelial cells and neutrophils. *J Clin Invest 96*:994–1002 (1995).
50. M. Peters-Golden, R. W. McNish, J. A. Davis, R. A. Blackwood, T. G. Brock. Colchicine inhibits arachidonate release and 5-lipoxygenase action in alveolar macrophages. *Am J Physiol 271*:L1004–L1013 (1996).
51. Y. A. Mekori, D. Baram, A. Goldberg, and A. Klajman. Inhibition of delayed hypersensitivity reactions in mice by colchicine. *Cell Immunol 120*:330–340 (1989).
52. E. Gillepsie and L. M. Lichtenstein. Histamine release from human leukocytes; studies with deuterium oxide, colchicine and cytochalasine B. *J Clin Invest 51*:2941 (1972).
53. W. J. Malaisse, F. Malaisse-Lagae, E. Van Obbergen, G. Somers, G. Devis, M. Ravazzola, and L. Onci. Role of microtubules in the phasic pattern of insulin release. *Ann NY Acad Sci 253*:630 (1975).
54. E. P. Reaven and G. M. Reaven. A quantitative ultrastructural study of microtubule content and secretory granule accumulation in parathyroid glands of phosphate and colchicine treated rats. *J Clin Invest 56*:49 (1975).
55. E. Bonfoco, S. Ceccatelli, L. Manzo, and P. Nicotera. Colchicine induces apoptosis in cerebellar granule cells. *Exp Cell Res 218*:189–200 (1995).
56. B. T. Emmerson. The management of gout. *N Engl J Med 334*(7):445–451 (1996).
57. M. J. Ahern, C. Reid, T. P. Gordon, M. McCredie, P. M. Brooks, and M. Jones. Does colchicine work? The results of the first controlled study in acute gout. *Aust NZ J Med 17*:301–304 (1987).
58. W. N. Roberts, M. H. Liang, and S. H. Stern. Colchicine in acute gout. Reassessment of risks and benefits. *JAMA 257*(24):1920–1922 (1987).
59. S. L. Wallace and J. Z. Singer. Review: systemic toxicity associated with the intravenous administration of colchicine—guidelines for use. *J Rheumatol 15*:495–499 (1988).
60. M. G. Ellwood and G. H. Robb. Self-poisoning with colchicine. *Postgrad Med J 47*:129-131 (1971).
61. H. E. Paulus, L. H. Schlosstein, R. G. Godfrey, J. K. Klinenberg, and R. Bluestone. Prophylactic colchicine therapy of intercritical gout: a placebo-controlled study of probenecid-treated patients. *Arthritis Rheum 17*:609–614 (1974).
62. T. F. Yu and A. B. Gutman. Efficacy of colchicine prophylaxis in gout: prevention of recurrent gouty arthritis over a mean period of five years in 208 gouty subjects. *Ann Intern Med 55*:179–192 (1961).
63. T. F. Yu. The efficacy of colchicine prophylaxis in articular gout—a reappraisal after 20 years. *Semin Arthritis Rheum 12*:256–264 (1982).
64. E. Pascual and J. A. Castellano. Treatment with colchicine decreases white cell counts in synovial fluid of asymptomatic knees that contain monosodium urate crystals. *J Rheumatol 19*:600–603 (1992).
65. R. W. Kuncl, G. Duncan, D. Watson, K. Alderson, M. A. Rogawski, and M. Peper. Colchicine myopathy and neuropathy. *N Engl J Med 316*:1562–1568 (1987).
66. S. L. Wallace, J. Z. Singer, G. J. Duncan, F. M. Wigley, and R. W. Kuncl. Renal function predicts colchicine toxicity: guidelines for the prophylactic use of colchicine in gout. *J Rheumatol 18*:264–269 (1991).

67. D. Schiff and F. W. Drislane. Rapid-onset colchicine myoneuropathy. *Arthritis Rheum 35*:1535–1536 (1992).

68. M. Rochdi, A. Sabouraud, F. J. Baud, C. Bismuth, and J. M. Scherrmann. Toxicokinetics of colchicine in humans: analysis of tissue, plasma, and urine data in ten cases. *Hum Exp Toxicol 11*:510–516 (1992).

69. C. Putterman, E. Ben-Chetrit, Y. Caraco, and M. Levy. Colchicine intoxication: clinical pharmacology, risk factors, features, and management. *Semin Arthritis Rheum 21(3)*:143–155 (1991).

70. A. Ben-Chetrit, E. Ben-Chetrit, R. Nitzan, and M. Ron. Colchicine inhibits spermatozoal motility *in vitro. Int J Fert Menopausal Stud 38*(5):301–304 (1993).

71. P. P. De-Deyn, C. Ceuterick, V. Saxena, R. Crols, R. Chappel, and J. J. Martin. Chronic colchicine-induced myopathy and neuropathy. *Acta Neurol Belg 95*(1):29–32 (1995).

72. R. N. Hill, R. G. Spragg, M. K. Wedel, et al. Adult respiratory syndrome associated with colchicine intoxication. *Ann Intern Med 83*:523–524 (1975).

73. F. J. Baud, A. Sabouraud, E. Vicaut, P. Taboulet, J. Lang, C. Bismuth, J. M. Rouzioux, and J. M. Scherrmann. Brief report: treament of severe colchicine overdose with colchicine-specific Fab fragments. *N Engl J Med 332*(10):642–645 (1995).

15
Conditions Associated with Gout and Hyperuricemia

CHRISTIAN MOENS
Brussels, Belgium

PHILIPPE J. MOENS
St. Elisabeth Clinic, Brussels, Belgium

I. COMMON ASSOCIATED CONDITIONS

A. Diabetes Mellitus

Possible relationships between diabetes and gout have been investigated for many years. Hyperuricemia has been reported in 2–50% of patients with diabetes, whereas gouty arthritis has been reported from less than 0, 1–9% of diabetic individuals (1). Diabetes may affect the metabolism of uric acid in different ways. This may go from dietary habits of diabetic patients to a direct influence on the production of uric acid to a modification on the excretion of uric acid. Since the median amount of animal proteins consumed daily by diabetics is similar to that consumed by the nondiabetics, dietary habits should not play an important role. A disturbance in carbohydrate metabolism could cause an increase in uric acid production. Any interference with glycolysis could divert the metabolite flow through the hexose-monophosphate pathway and increase uric acid production. But the most important factor is a modification of excretion of uric acid. In newly diagnosed diabetics, the reduction in uric acid levels reaches significance, suggesting a definite association between diabetes and serum uric acid. Because the association is seen in newly diagnosed diabetics, it must be related to the disease and not the treatment (2).

When diabetes develops, serum uric acid levels fall and continue to decrease with increasing duration of disease. This may be due to a process involving the excretion of uric acid. Glucose is filtered by the glomeruli and is reabsorbed by the proximal tubules. At a critical concentration of blood glucose, complete reabsorption of glucose ceases and glycosuria results. Uric acid excretion is enhanced by hyperglycemia; this enhancement is independent of diuresis. It is possible that increasing glucose reabsorption may somehow impair tubular reabsorption of uric acid. Continued hyperexcretion of uric acid due to hyperglycemia could deplete the uric acid pool and gradually reduce uric acid levels. However, treatment of diabetes and the deterioration of renal function that accompanies longstanding diabetes might be expected to halt such lowering of uric acid levels, so low uric acid levels need not be a feature of clinical diabetes. Despite these observations, epidemiologic studies have not demonstrated a relationship between gout and diabetes or between serum urate and blood glucose concentrations. Hyperuricemia does occur in the presence of diabetic ketoacidosis, and the pathogenetic mechanism is well-explained on the basis of the probable inhibition of renal tubular excretion of uric acid by betahydroxybutyrate.

B. Obesity

The association of gout with obesity and overeating has been recognized for hundreds of years. A strong positive correlation between body weight and serum urate concentration has been documented, but the relationship is complex and multifactorial. In a large study of 7300 obese women, the women who were 85% above desirable body weight had gout 1.56 times more frequently than women weighing 10% above ideal body weight. In a group of male physicians studied prospectively, weight gain prior to age 35 appeared to be a determinant in the occurrence of gout. In another study, 52% of gouty patients were more than 20% over ideal body weight. The fact that 85% were hypertensive and 48% had abnormal glucose tolerance tests and hyperlipidemia points out the multiplicity of variables relating to obesity and its metabolic complications. Obesity has several effects on urate metabolism, including decreased renal urate clearance and increased uric acid production. Weight reduction is associated with a modest lowering of serum urate concentration and a decrease in the rate of purine synthesis de novo (3).

C. Hyperlipidemia

Hyperlipidemia has been associated with gout since 1955. A number of subsequent reports (4) have related gout with hypercholesterolemia, hypercholesterolemia combined with hypertriglyceridemia, and hypertriglyceridemia alone. This association between hyperuricemia and hyperlipidemia has been ascribed to the effects of external factors such as obesity, increased alcohol intake, and nutritional habits. However, results suggesting that external factors have no influence on this association have also been published.

In 1995, Tinahones et al. (5) showed that mixed and pure hyperuricemic hypertriglyceridemic patients exhibited increased levels of structural very low density lipoprotein (VLDL) components, decreased fractional excretion of uric acid and, increased apoCIII/CII ratios. The increased levels of structural VLDL components were negatively correlated with the fractional excretion of uric acid: this suggests a close biological relationship between the two parameters. Taking into account the role played by apoC and VLDL metabolism, the altered apoCIII/CII ratios found in hyperuricemic hypertriglyceridemic patients suggests that this apoprotein plays a central role in the physiopathology of the alterations observed. No change was observed in levels of serum urate or uric acid excretion when triglycerides were elevated in three gouty subjects receiving intravenous lipids. Although hypertriglyceridemia and hyperuricemia may coexist independent of other factors, a common metabolic defect remains elusive.

D. Hypertension

The association of hypertension with elevated uric acid has been noted for years. But since uric acid is often associated with other hypertension risk factors, such as obesity and triglycerides, it is difficult to evaluate its exact role. A strong independent association exists according to most of the authors. Others concluded that we are dealing with two separate disease processes. Hyperuricemia is reported in 22–38% of untreated hypertensive patients, and increased to 47–68% when patients with hypertension and renal disease are included.

The uric acid–hypertension association does not appear to be due to an effect of attained blood pressure level on uric acid metabolism at baseline. Rather, uric acid is either itself causally related to the development of hypertension or related to a still undetected factor. Uric acid level also has strong genetic determinants and it is possible that an increased uric acid level is a marker for a genetic susceptibility to developing hypertension. This genetic trait could, for example, influence renal function, altering both renal excretion and renin-angiotensin homeostasis or renal handling of sodium.

Hypertension may be associated with hyperuricemia in three ways apart from that due to concurrent diuretic therapy. First, hypertension reduces renal excretion of urate since renal urate clearances, which depend on tubular secretory and postsecretory reabsorption rates, are reported to be inappropriately low relative to glomerular filtration rates in adult and childhood essential hypertension. Second, renal damage from interstitial microtophi may lead to secondary hypertension. And third, excessive alcohol consumption may cause both hyperuricemia and hypertension (3, 6).

E. Alcohol

Alcohol consumption has traditionally been associated with hyperuricemia and, in susceptible persons, the precipitation of acute gouty arthritis. Early studies indicate that a decrease in the renal excretion of uric acid could account for the ethanol-induced hyperuricemia. The hyperuricemia and hypouricosuria were linked to ethanol-related elevations in blood lactate levels. Lactate competitively inhibits uric acid clearance by the proximal tubule and could diminish urate excretion. This was shown in studies where the blood ethanol levels were less than 150 per deciliter; a small uricosuric effect of ethanol was observed. Ethanol increases uric acid production. After ethanol infusion, levels of urinary oxypurines, which are precursors of uric acid, increase dramatically. It causes also a release of urate from the liver as calculated by arteriovenous differences. During ethanol infusion, the accelerated degradation of adenine nucleotides accounts for the increased production of uric acid and its precursors. A contribution to increased uric acid synthesis from de novo purine synthesis cannot be ruled out.

Pathways of ethanol metabolism indicate an additional mechanism for increased use of adenosine triphosphate. Ethanol is oxidized to form acetate, with the result that nicotinamide adenine dinucleotide (NAD) is converted to nicotinamide adenine dinucleotide hydroxide (NADH). Acetate then enters a stage of intermediary metabolism by initial conversion to acetylcoenzyme A. The energy for this latter reaction is provided by the conversion of adenosine triphosphate to adenosine monophosphate. This adenosine monophosphate may be recycled or degraded to form oxypurines and uric acid. Virtually all ethanol is converted to acetylcoenzyme A and oxidized to form carbon dioxide and water. This cycle represents a mechanism for massive turnover of adenosine triphosphate. Since adenosine triphosphate is converted to adenosine monophosphate, two moles of high-energy phosphate are consumed for each mole of ethanol that is metabolized. Therefore, if only a small proportion of the adenosine triphosphate that is turned over enters the pathway of purine nucleotide degradation, it could account for a substantial increase in uric acid synthesis. Ethanol ingestion decreases the excretion of uric acid and increases synthesis of urate (7). Beer may have a more potent effect on uric acid production as a result of its guanosine content.

II. LESS COMMON CONDITIONS

A. Gout and Carpal Tunnel Syndrome

Carpal tunnel syndrome caused by gout is rare. It is due to a tophaceous tenosynovitis of the transverse carpal ligament associated with gout. It may also be caused by deposits of uric acid on the median nerve causing compression of this nerve. Also, if during a carpal tunnel release operation, the surgeon observes white deposits in the flexor tendons and sheaths, he or she must keep in mind the possibility of gouty arthritis (8). The treatment should be medical, but some suggest that surgery is helpful for patients with poor drug compliance.

B. Musculoskeletal Conditions

1. Back Pain

Maybe the most common complaint that we hear as rheumatologists is back pain. It is usually caused by osteoarthritis of the spine or by an involvement of an intervertebral disc, or by more severe diseases such as metastasis. It may also be due to gout. This condition was recently reviewed by Fenton et al. (9). It is a rare condition and usually the patient reports a history of chronic peripheral polyarticular tophaceous gout. Among the 17 cases reviewed by Fenton et al., only three had no clinical evidence of tophi and no history of gout. So, if a patient is only complaining of low back pain, there is a very small chance that it is due to gout, but it is possible. X-rays show a disc space narrowing with ill-defined vertebral end-plate erosions and reactive vertebral sclerosis. A differential diagnosis must be made with discitis. According to Fenton et al., the diagnosis is best visualized on computed tomographic scans, as this technique makes it possible to determine if there are sodium urate deposits. They should have a radiographic attenuation density greater than that of the surrounding muscle, but less than that of bone. This is not a specific finding, because the attenuation density of clotted hemorrhage would be expected to be greater than that of muscle. Deposits of calcium pyrophosphate dihydrate can also occur within the substance of the ligamentum flavum, and it would be expected to have the high density of calcifications.

Gout of the spine presents in many different ways, with asymptomatic involvement being the least common and pain with neurological signs being the most usual. Of the 19 patients reviewed by Fenton, 9 were initially found to have tophi in the disc spaces with involvement of adjacent vertebral bodies, 4 had involvement of the osseous posterior ligaments, 3 had extradural soft-tissue involvement, and 3 had involvement of the bodies and the posterior elements of the affected vertebrae. The thoracic region appears to be the part of the spine that is the least affected by gout, but patients who had extradural deposits along segments of the thoracic spine that produced paraparesis have been described. The diagnosis was confirmed at the time of the operation, and the symptoms improved after the decompression. In our own experience, a patient presenting acute paravertebral pains at the level of the first thoracic vertebrae should have a dosage of uricemia. The cervical spine may also be involved. This can go from pain in the neck alone to neurological symptoms. Roentgenograms usually demonstrated erosions at the level of a disc as well as the level of the odontoid process. When percutaneous needle biopsies were performed, they revealed birefringent crystals.

2. Diffuse Idiopathic Skeletal Hyperostosis

In diffuse idiopathic skeletal hyperostosis (DISH), we must also look for a possible correlation with hyperuricemia. Vezyroglou et al. recently reviewed this problem (10).

DISH was first distinguished from ankylosing spondylitis by Forestier and Rotès-Querol (20). These pioneering studies were followed by extensive investigations that confirmed the high prevalence of the disease among diabetics and in the general population, increased frequency with age and duration of diabetes, and diverse localizations of DISH on the skeleton. In addition to diabetes mellitus, a high incidence of other common metabolic conditions such as dyslipidemia and hyperuricemia was found; associations were found in half these cases. In the study of Vezyroglou et al. (10) dyslipidemia and/or asymptomatic hyperuricemia and/or Type II diabetes mellitus were much more evident in the DISH group than in the age, sex, body mass index, and excess body weight matched group. Analysis of this finding showed that hyperuricemia and/or dyslipidemia, in association with or as a feature of diabetes mellitus, was exclusively represented within patients with DISH. Gout has also been associated or considered as the etiologic factor of avascular necrosis of the femoral head.

3. Muscle

It has been known since 1905 that a single bout of exhaustive exercise will cause an overproduction of uric acid. This event occurs in perfectly normal healthy individuals, as was demonstrated in a group of military recruits during intense training in the heat. There was no defect in purine metabolism other than the consequences of muscle cell injury and release of preformed purines that are subsequently converted to uric acid in the liver.

Aarflot et al. (11) looked for a relationship between musculoskeletal complaints and uric acid. They examined 737 men and 771 women. Both men and women with chronic musculoskeletal complaints had significantly higher uricemia than persons without such complaints. Moreover, the prevalence of chronic musculoskeletal complaints (gout excluded) changes significantly across increasing uricemic levels. Multivariate logistic regression analysis showed that the uricemia ratio for chronic complaints rose in a linear manner across these uricemia levels.

C. Hematopoietic Disorders

Many hematopoietic disorders in which there is excessive biosynthesis of uric acid and other purines resulting from increased formation and degradation of nucleic acid may have secondary gout as a complication. The pattern of overproduction of uric acid, as measured by the magnitude and rate of 15 N incorporation, is different from that in primary gout. In primary gout, there is an early peak enrichment of uric acid within 2–4 days of administration of the isotope. In secondary gout, the pattern is variable. In gout secondary to polycythemia vera, there is progressive enrichment of the isotope, with peak abundance at the end of the second week. In chronic granulocytic leukemia and myeloid metaplasia, a dysphasic pattern may be observed, with a prominent peak 2–3 days after isotope administration, and a second maximum at about 12 days. The initial peak is thought to represent biosynthesis de novo, without prior incorporation into nucleic acid. And the second peak, that of uric acid, is derived from the degradation of leukocyte nuclear purines. The familial incidence is low, as would be expected in secondary gout.

The sequelae of secondary gout, particularly renal calculi and uric acid nephropathy, contributed substantially to the morbidity and mortality of acute and chronic myeloproliferative disorders. Since the introduction of allopurinol, however, these major complications have been reduced significantly. Nevertheless, even with the availability of allopurinol, acute gouty arthritis, which often is atypical in presentation and frequently misdiagnosed, continues to be an accompaniment of myeloproliferative diseases (12).

D. Hyperuricemia and Endocrine Diseases

Since hyperuricemia is associated with certain endocrine diseases, its occurrence and interpretation with respect to clinical and laboratory parameters of these diseases needs to be delineated. This subject was extensively reviewed by Newcombe (13).

1. The Pituitary Gland

Only two disorders related to the pituitary gland, acromegaly and vasopressin-resistant diabetes insipidus, have been associated with alterations in uric acid metabolism. It has been stated that lesions exerting pressure on or near the hypothalamic area of the brain or acromegalic states may cause hyperuricemia. Whether these clinical observations represent reflections of the altered nitrogen metabolism seen in these disorders has not been determined. Certainly the occurrence of hyperuricemia and/or gouty arthritis in diseases of the pituitary gland is an uncommon clinical finding.

The association between hyperuricemia and congenital vasopressin-resistant diabetes insipidus was first recognized in 1962. In those patients there is a lowered clearance of urate, and the ratio of the clearance of urate to clearance of creatinine is lower than normal. But the 24-hr uric acid excretion is normal so the increased plasma concentration of urate is probably not the result of a defect in purine metabolism. It was suggested that the combination of a high plasma vasopressin concentration with water diuresis might, over a long period, result in an alteration in the capacity of the kidney tubule to handle uric acid. As the characteristic feature of congenital vasopressin-resistant diabetes insipidus is the dilatation of the renal collecting system, the possibility exists that this abnormality, resulting presumably from a constant high urinary flow rate, affects the renal tubular transport of urate (13). If diuretics are chosen as a treatment, the recognition of hyperuricemia and its appropriate treatment is important. Allopurinol administration to adults with this condition in conjunction with chlorothiazide for their vasopressin-resistant diabetes insipidus is a significant contribution to the prognosis and management of this disorder.

2. Hyperparathyroidism

The frequency of the coexistence of gout and hyperparathyroidism in patient populations varies widely, from 1.9 to 3.7% according to the series (13). The reasons for these discrepancies are not clear. Renal disease with the retention of nitrogenous waste products is associated with hyperuricemia, and the nephrocalcinosis of hyperparathyroidism provides a setting for this mechanism to be operative. But one cannot assume that the simple retention of urates resulting from uremia is the cause of gout because gout is a rare complication of uremia. Hyperuricemia and hyperparathyroidism have been diagnosed concurrently, and there has been no detectable renal disease suggesting either the existence of a subtle renal tubular lesion prior to the demonstration of clinical renal insufficiency or a lack of relationship between the uric concentration and the renal disease of hyperparathyroidism.

E. Systemic Diseases

1. Systemic Lupus Erythematosus (SLE)

The relatively rare co-occurrence of gout and SLE has been attributed to several causes. The clinicians miss the diagnosis. SLE is found in a higher frequency in young women, and gout is at a higher frequency in older men. During active SLE with low complement, the body may be less able to mount an inflammatory reaction to crystals. The steroids used often in the treatment of SLE depress or suppress the cytokine level elicited by the urate crystals. The uremia secondary to SLE may decrease the inflammation in a gouty joint in a patient with SLE by changing the specific balance of inflammatory and chemotactic cytokines. The multifactorial pathogenesis of gout may account for the decreased expression of gout in patients with SLE.

2. Rheumatoid Arthritis

Gout and rheumatoid arthritis (RA) may share a variety of manifestations. Although such an association has been emphasized on clinical grounds, there are only a few examples of the actual coexistence of both diseases. Possible reasons for the rare coexistence of gout and RA include a protective immunosuppressive effect of hyperuricemia, which may be related to the antioxidant properties of uric acid or to the inhibition of phagocytosis by urate, although other data have revealed the opposite and suggest an increase in the phlogistic effect of crystals with dissolved urate. Also, synovial hypocomplementemia and a decrease in the degree of inflammation in gout if crystals are coated with rheumatoid factor have been proposed. These and other findings that support impaired phagocytic functions of neutrophils in RA may explain the inhibition of the inflammatory response to urate crystals, but cannot explain the absence of urate deposition, a hallmark of gout, that may be inhibited by connective tissue abnormalities in RA (14).

F. Drug-Induced Hyperuricemia

Drug-induced hyperuricemia has for several years become a clinical problem. The study of this phenomenon has also produced some interesting information. In humans, it has been shown that hyperuricemia secondary to drugs results from their interference with excretion as well as their stimulation of production of uric acid (15).

1. Diuretics

Benzothiadiazines and other diuretics such as ethacrynic acid and fursemide cause hyperuricemia. This elevation is probably common in patients taking diuretics, although the level of uric acid will not necessarily rise above the normal range. A direct effect of these drugs upon the renal handling of uric acid is an important factor. A paradoxical dosage effect can be observed with diuretics comparable to that seen with drugs that are known to influence tubular transport of urate, low doses of which cause retention of urate and high doses cause uricosuria. The reduction of secretion is due to a suppression of the tubular secretion, and the uricosuric effect is due to the suppression of the tubular reabsorption. Organomercurial, triamterene, amiloride, and spironolactone do not cause hyperuricemia.

Action of the drugs upon renal tubular reabsorption and secretion is not the only mechanism. The diuretic-induced contraction of the extracellular fluid causes a decrease in the uric acid excretion. If urinary fluid loss is replaced with an isotonic saline solution, the excretion of uric acid is restored. If acute attacks of gout develop under diuretics, they should be treated with NSAIDs or colchicine. The incriminated diuretic should be changed for a diuretic not predisposing to hyperuricemia, or the hyperuricemia should be controlled by uricosuric agents (16).

2. Salicylates

The paradoxical effect of salicylates is well known. Sodium salicylate at a low dosage of less than 0.5 g daily has a hyperuricemic effect by blocking the urate tubular secretion. At doses above 2.5 g daily, there is a hypouricemic effect by blocking the reabsorption of uric acid at the tubular level. As the reabsorption predominates the secretion, the net effect is uricosuric. Salicylate at any dose inhibits the uricosuric effect of drugs such a probenecid and sulphinpyrazone.

3. Pyrazinamide

The antituberculous drug pyrazinamide reduces the renal excretion of uric acid. The clearance of uric acid may be diminished by over 80%. Pyrazinamide is metabolized to pyrazinoic acid. The hyperuricemic action is largely due to pyrazinoic acid, which is very potent in blocking excretion or urate. Acute attacks of gout have been described in patients taking pyrazinamide.

4. Ethambutol

Another antituberculous drug that can also raise the uric acid level by a renal effect is ethambutol. But the effect is not as clear as it with pyrazinamide.

5. Nicotinic Acid

Used in the treatment of schizophrenia and hypercholesterolemia, nicotinic acid may cause hyperuricemia and occasionally gout. The effect is probably largely due to impaired excretion of uric acid because there is a decrease in clearance of uric acid following the administration of nicotinic acid, but there may be an additional effect on urate formation as increased purine biosynthesis has been reported.

6. Fructose

Infusions of fructose leads to a rapid increase in serum and urinary urate concentrations. The phosphorylation of fructose leads to catabolic products with an increase in uric acid. There may also be a stimulation of purine biosynthesis, probably a secondary consequence of a reduced hepatic content of adenosine diphosphate. Chronic ingestion of fructose has no influence on serum or urinary uric acid levels.

7. Cytotoxic Agents

All the drugs causing a breakdown of cells, such as vincristine, busulfan, thiotepa, cytarabine, 6-mercaptopurine, and chlorambucil, will cause a nucleoprotein breakdown and increase the formation of uric acid and excretion of massive amounts of uric acid. Acute uric nephropathy may be the next step with urinary obstruction caused by extensive deposition of uric acid crystals in the collecting ducts and ureters. Allopurinol is the answer. It is recommended to start allopurinol before the cytotoxic therapy.

8. Liver Extracts

Liver extracts produce hyperuricemia and uricosuria when given to patients with pernicious anemia in relapse. The hyperuricemia corresponds with the onset of marked reticulocytosis. It is due to degradation of nucleic acid and soluble nucleotides, with subsequent oxidation of their purines to uric acid, associated with maturation of the megaloblastic marrow.

9. Cyclosporine

We have known since 1984 that cyclosporine may cause hyperuricemia. In a study by Burack (21), cyclosporine caused hyperuricemia in 72% of male and 81% of female patients. This was not correlated with cyclosporine level, presence of hypertension, or degree of renal insufficiency. In a study by Ben Hmida et al. (16), hyperuricemia and gout occurred in only 13% of cyclosporine-treated patients. What is the mechanism? Several potential mechanisms may contribute to the development of hyperuricemia and gout. First, cyclosporine-induced renal insufficiency causes the renal retention of urate by modifying steps in urate excretion. Hyper uricemia was concomitant with a clear decline of renal function, which emphasizes that hyperuricemia may be a consequence of renal insufficiency. Some studies have shown large urate pools with normal turnover rate but reduced urate clearance, supporting the notion that the hyperuricemia is a consequence of decreased urate clearance. Hypertension, a major side effect of cyclosporine therapy, may lead secondarily to hyperuricemia by reduction and redistribution of renal blood flow.

10. Azathioprine

The combination of allopurinol and azathioprine leads to a drug-drug interaction that increases hematological toxicity. The results of this combination may be fatal. It was first suggested to decrease azathioprine dosages during concomitant therapy with allopurinol. In transplant recipients, decreased immunosuppression could be dangerous after an acute rejection episode or in the early months after transplantation. Recently, Ippoliti et al. (17) suggested to not decrease the azathioprine dosage, but to use urate oxidase instead of allopurinol. Urate oxidase is an enzyme extracted from a selected strain of *Aspergillus flavus* that catalyses the conversion of uric acid to allantoin and that is lacking in man. Because this later substance is 100 times more soluble than uric acid, it is easily excreted by the kidney. When administered in man and other mammals, urate oxidase allows the conversion of uric acid into allantoin before renal filtration, as assessed by increased levels of allantoinuria.

In the treated patients, the administration of urate oxidase led to a complete normalization of uric acid levels and to the disappearance of acute clinical symptoms. There were no side effects. Given its enzymatic nature, cessation of this treatment obviously results in a return to xanthine oxidase pathways. After the last administration of the drug, the hypouricemic effect lasted about 20–30 days. Thereafter, levels of uric acid rose again. The administration of a second cycle of urate oxidase led to a good response. None of the patients complained of the intramuscular treatment.

G. Saturnine Gout

Lead nephropathy represents an important category of chronic renal disease associated with hypertension and gout. It is a very old story. The Romans made extensive use of lead. Roman wine was contaminated with lead due to the practice of simmering grape syrup in lead vessels to enhance the flavor. It has been speculated that the widespread consumption of lead-contaminated wine caused lead poisoning. Gout was common among patricians. The same occurred in England during the seventeenth and eighteenth centuries with the consumption of imported Portuguese wine, which was transported to England in containers with lead bars dipped in them to enhance flavor. Much of the English aristocracy also suffered from gout. A third epidemic again associated with gout and renal disease, the moonshine epidemic in the southern United States, was caused by distillation of illicit whiskey in kettles with lead-soldered joints.

Now our planet is heavily polluted from a myriad of uses of lead in all segments of contemporary life. But with the introduction of industrial exposure standards, nephropathy became a less obvious consequence of lead poisoning. Batuman (19) showed clearly that asymptomatic chronic lead poisoning is still present in today's society. This may cause a lead nephropathy that can be defined as a chronic tubulointerstitial nephritis. Clinically, it frequently presents with hypertension, hyperuricemia, and gout. Lead nephropathy should be suspected in patients who present with unexplained chronic tubulointerstitial disease, especially those with hypertension, gout, or both.

H. Inborn Errors of Metabolism

1. Lesch-Nyhan Syndrome

Lesch-Nyhan syndrome is an X-linked disorder that is fully expressed in males. Severe cellular deficiency of the purine salvage enzyme hypoxanthine guanine phosphoryl transferase (HPRT) is associated with primary purine overproduction, hyperuricemia, and gout, together with a neurological syndrome comprising choreoathetosis, spasticity, a variable degree of mental deficiency and striking behavioral disturbance characterized by self-mutilation. Severe familial X-linked gout with minor or absent neurological features may be associated with "partial" deficiency of HPRT.

2. Glycogeneses

Hyperuricemia and gout are known to occur in Type I glycogenesis, or von Gierke's disease, due to enhanced breakdown of adenosinetriphosphate (ATP) in the liver causing an overproduction of uric acid, and a decrease in its renal excretion due to lactic acidemia and ketonemia. It is associated with marked hyperuricemia from infancy.

Gouty arthritis may become a problem before the age of 10 years and chronic tophaceous gout with renal involvement can be a major factor of morbidity. Hyperuricemia has also developed in Type III glycogenesis, or Cori-Forbes disease, and in Type V, or McArdle's disease, suggesting an association of muscle glycogenesis and related disorders with hyperuricemia. In muscle phosphofructokinase deficiency, or Tarui disease, or Type VII glycogenesis, a unique genesis of hyperuricemia occurs, in which skeletal muscle is the primary site of impaired purine metabolism. Muscle glycogen is used as fuel for muscle exercise. In patients affected with Type VII glycogenesis, muscular exercise induces an increase of inosine and hypoxanthine, followed by a gradual increase in plasma uric acid levels. Urinary excretion of uric acid does not decrease during exercise. Overproduction of uric acid, rather than underexcretion, appears to be responsible for the elevation of plasma uric acid. The hyperuricemia and hyperuricosuria are improved by bed rest (18).

3. PPRPS

Primary purine overproduction is associated with structural enzyme mutation resulting in superactive PP-ribose-P synthetase (PPRPS). Affected males develop uric acid lithiasis or gouty arthritis in childhood or early adult life.

REFERENCES

1. W. N. Kelley, E. D. Harris, S. Ruddy, and C. Sledge. Textbook of Rheumatology (W. B. Saunders, ed.), 5th edition, 1997, p. 1318.
2. J. Herman and U. Goldbourt. Uric acid and diabetes: observations in a population study, *Lancet* 2:240 (1982).

3. W. J. Koopman. Arthritis and Allied Conditions, (Williams and Wilkins, ed.), 13th edition, 1997, p. 1318.
4. T. Gibson and R. Grahame. Gout and hyperlipidaemia, *Ann Rheum Dis 33*:298 (1974).
5. F. Tinahones, E. Collantes, F. Soriguer, A. Gonzalez-Ruiz, M. Pineda, J. Anon, and P. Sanchezguijo. Increased VLDL levels and diminished renal excretion of uric acid in hyperuricaemic-hypertriglyceridaemic patients, *Brit J Rheum 34*:920 (1995).
6. J. H. Klippel and P. A. Dieppe. Practical Rheumatology (Mosby, ed.), 1995, p. 255.
7. J. Faller and I. H. Fox. Ethanol-induced hyperuricemia, *New Engl J Med 307*:1598 (1982).
8. H. Chuang and C. Wong. Carpal tunnel syndrome induced by tophaceous deposits on the median nerve: case report, *Neurosurgery 34*:919 (1994).
9. P. Fenton, S. Young, and K. Prutis. Gout of the spine, *J Bone Joint Surg 5*:767 (1995).
10. G. Vezyroglou, A. Mitropoulos, N. Kyriazis, and C. Antoniadis. A metabolic syndrome in diffuse idiopathic skeletal hyperostosis: A controlled study, *J Rheum 23*:672 (1996).
11. T. Aarflot, E. Laerum, and D. Bruusgaard. Uric acid and chronic muskuloskeletal complaints, *Scand J Rheum 21*:277 (1992).
12. T. Yu, N. Weinreb, R. Wittman, and L. Wasserman. Secondary gout associated with myeloproliferative disorders, *Sem Arth and Rheum 8*:247 (1976).
13. D. Newcombe. Endocrinopathies and uric acid metabolism, *Sem Arth and Rheum 2*:281 (1972).
14. E. Martinez-Cordero, A. Bessudo-Babani, S. Trevino Perez, and E. Guillermo-Grajalez. Concomitant gout and rheumatoid arthritis, *J Rheum 15*:1307 (1988).
15. F. Demartini. Hyperuricemia induced by drugs, *Arth Rheum 8*:823 (1965).
16. M. Ben Hmida, J. Hachicha, Z. Bahloul, N. Kaddour, M. Kharrat, F. Jarraya, and A. Jarraya. Cyclosporine-Induced Hyperuricemia and Gout in Renal Transplants, Transplantation Proceedings 27:2722 (1995).
17. G. Ippoliti, M. Negri, C. Campana, and M. Vigano. Urate oxidase in hyperuricemic heart transplant recipients treated with azathioprine, *Transplantation 63*:1370 (1997).
18. A. Sato, T. Shirota, T. Shinoda, I. Komiya, T. Aizawa, Y. Takemura, T. Aizawa, Y. Takemura, and T. Yamada. Hyperuricemia in patients with hyperthyroidism due to Grave's disease, *Metabolism 2*:207 (1995).
19. V. Batuman. Lead nephropathy, gout and hypertension, *Am J Med Sci 305*:241 (1993).
20. J. Forestier, J. Rotès-Querol. Senile ankylosing hyperostosis of the spine, *Ann Rheum Dis 9*:321 (1950).
21. D. A. Burack, Bartley, P. Griffith, M. E. Thompson, L. E. Kahl. Hyperuricemia and gout among heart transplant recipients receiving cyclosporine, *Am J Med 92*:141 (1992).

16
Hypouricemic Drugs

A. TAREQ KHAWAJA and HERBERT S. DIAMOND
The Western Pennsylvania Hospital and University of Pittsburgh School of Medicine, Pittsburgh, Pennsylvania

I. INTRODUCTION

Hyperuricemia occurs as a result of increased production of uric acid and/or its underexcretion. The two main pharmacological approaches to therapy center on modifying these processes. Uricosuric agents increase the excretion of uric acid while blocking drugs, such as allopurinol, inhibit the synthesis of uric acid.

Therapy with a drug that lowers serum urate concentration should be considered when the following criteria are met (1):

1. The cause of the hyperuricemia cannot be corrected or if corrected does not lower the serum urate to less than 7.0 mg/dl.
2. The patient has had at least two definite attacks of gout or has tophi.
3. The patient has been convinced of the need to take medication regularly and permanently.

When the only indication for hypouricemic therapy is recurrence of acute gouty arthritis and episodes are infrequent, easily controlled by anti-inflammatory drugs, or prevented by colchicine prophylaxis, then hypouricemic therapy may be unnecessary.

II. ENHANCEMENT OF URATE EXCRETION

Uricosuric drugs facilitate urate excretion by the kidney with an increase in the urate clearance and the fractional excretion of filtered urate. This can result in an increase in the concentration of uric acid in the urine if the volume of the latter is not concomitantly increased. Many drugs with diverse chemical structures decrease the serum urate concentration in humans by enhancing the renal excretion of uric acid. This discussion will focus on those of clinical importance (Table 1).

Uric acid is normally handled in the kidney by filtration at the glomerulus and by secretion and reabsorption mechanisms in the renal tubules. Nearly 99% of filtered urate undergoes tubular reabsorption and additional urate enters the tubule through tubular secretion. Much of the secreted urate is also reabsorbed with the remainder being excreted in the urine. The secretory transport system is located at the basolateral membrane of the renal tube. When some uricosuric drugs are given at very low doses, the secretory transport system is inhibited and this results in a decrease in the renal excretion of uric acid. At higher doses, this effect is overridden as the reabsorptive process is inhibited. Most uricosuric agents (which are weak organic acids like uric acid) lower the serum uric acid by enhancing urate excretion through compet-

TABLE 1 Some Drugs with Uricosuric Activity

AA193	Glyceryl guaiacholate
Acetoheximide	Glycine
ACTH	Glycophyrrolate
Amflutizole	Halofenate (MK 185)
Ambroxol	Iodopyracet
Ascorbic acid	Iopanoic acid
Azapropazone	Meclofenamic acid
Azauridine	Meglumine iodipamide
Benzbromarone	Mersalyl
Benziodarone	Metiazininic acid
Calcitonin	Niridazole
Calcium ipodate	Orotic acid
Carinamide	Outdated tetracyclines
CGS12970	Phenolsulfonphthalein
Chloprothixine	Phenylbutazone
Cinchophen	Phenylindandione
Citrate	Phenoxylsobutyric acid
Dicumarol	Probenecid and metabolites
Diffumidone	Salicylates
Estrogens	Sodium diatrizoate
Ethyl biscoumacetate	Sulfaethylthiadiazole
Ethyl p-chlorophenoxy-isobutyric acid	Sulfinpyrazone
E5050	Ticrynafen
FK366	Zoxazolamine

TABLE 2 Indications for Uricosuric Agents

1. Hyperuricemia with decreased uric acid excretion
   a. Less than 800 mg urinary acid per 24 hours on a regular diet, or
   b. Less than 600 mg urinary uric acid per 24 hours on purine restricted diet
2. Satisfactory renal function (creatinine clearance greater than 50 ml/min)
3. No history of calculi

itive inhibition of the brush border transporter for the tubular reabsorption process for urate. Uricosuric drugs are indicated to correct hyperuricemia and treat gout when hyperuricemia is a result of defective renal excretion of urate and the patient understands that long-term treatment is required. These drugs are contraindicated in the presence of renal calculi, marked hyperuricosuria or a poor urine volume (<1 ml/min). They are often ineffective when the glomerular filtration rate is seriously impaired (Table 2).

A. Probenicid

Probenecid was the first uricosuric agent that gained widespread popularity and use (2,3). Its effects were noted during the late 1940s as part of the ongoing development of an organic acid inhibitor of the renal tubular secretion of penicillin. The predecessor of probenecid was carinamide, which was noted to have weak uricosuric activity. However, this agent was rapidly excreted and had a very short duration of action. Subsequent studies produced probenecid, which was longer acting and inhibited penicillin secretion more effectively (4).

Probenecid is a white, odorless, crystalline powder that is practically insoluble in water and dilute acid, but is soluble in alcohol, acetone, dilute alkali and chloraform (Figure 1).

The relatively long biologic half-life is explained by the lipid solubility and the pk of 3.4, which allows almost complete reabsorption by passive nonionic diffusion (6). Analogs of probenecid with substitution at the 2-nitro, 2-hydroxyl, and 2-chloro groups produce stronger acids that are up to 10 times more potent as uricosuric agents. The reason underlying this difference in potency is unknown (6).

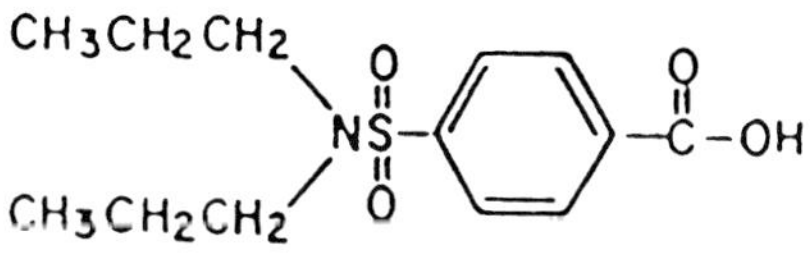

FIGURE 1 Structure of probenecid.

Probenecid is absorbed rapidly following oral administration in man (9). Peak serum concentrations occur in two to three hours following an oral dose of 1 gram. The plasma half-life is variable and dose dependent, ranging from 4 to 12 hr, probably due to metabolic pathway saturation or hepatic uptake (7). Elimination is predominantly by metabolism because probenecid is almost completely reabsorbed by nonionic diffusion in acid urine. Only 4–13% is excreted unchanged and the major metabolic product excreted in the urine is probenecid monoacyl glucuronide (34–47%). Probenecid and its conjugated metabolites are excreted in the bile and may undergo enterohepatic circulation (6).

Plasma protein binding is extensive (89–94%) and the volume of distribution limited mainly to extracellular fluid. Probenecid can cross both the blood brain barrier and placental barrier. By alkalinizing the urine, renal excretion can be greatly increased. This is a result of the inhibition of passive nonionic reabsorption resulting in net tubular secretion. The increased secretion is associated with an increase in uricosuric effect. The response to probenecid appears promptly after intravenous administration and is evident within 30–40 min after oral administration. It has been demonstrated that serum urate can be satisfactorily controlled on 1 g or less of probenecid in 50% of patients and on 2 g or less in 85% of patients (8). The initial starting dose is 250 mg twice daily, and, following observation of the uricosuric effect and measurement of serum urate, the dose is increased at weekly intervals (by 500 mg/day in divided doses) until a satisfactory therapeutic response is achieved. The uricosuric effect of probenecid is reduced as glomerular function declines and the drug has little effect in patients with a creatinine clearance of less than 50–60 ml/min.

1. Toxicity

Acute toxicity from overdosage produces vomiting, muscle twitching, hyperactive tendon reflexes, coma, and seizures (9). The frequency of side effects of probenecid has been extensively documented. In one large series (10), gastrointestinal side effects were noted in approximately 20% of patients. Furthermore, 5% developed rash or other hypersensitivity reactions. Serious toxicity is very rare. Hepatic necrosis has been reported in one patient and nephrotic syndrome in two others (10). Autoimmune hemolytic anemia has also been reported with probenecid therapy. Other complications of probenecid therapy are precipitation of acute attacks of gout and urolithiasis. Both of these complications are common to all uricosuric drugs and are largely preventable. The incidence of acute gout following uricosuric therapy can be greatly reduced by concomitant low-dose colchicine prophylaxis. The incidence of renal stones can be reduced by gradual introduction of uricosuric therapy, maintenance of a large urine volume, and alkalinization of the urine.

2. Drug Interactions

As mentioned earlier, probenecid alters the transport of other organic acids across cell membranes. This results in a number of drug interactions that are of clinical importance. The renal excretion of salicylic acid and its glucuronide derivatives is delayed by probenecid and acetyl salicylate completely blocks the uricosuric effect of probenecid and other uricosuric agents. Dapsone and indomethacin should be used at lower doses when combined with probenecid. Subtherapeutic doses of heparin may have profound anticoagulant effects on patients receiving probenecid (11). The half-life of penicillin and amipicillin is prolonged by probenecid due to the inhibition of renal excretion of these agents. Additionally, the hepatic uptake of rifampin is impaired by probenecid, and this effect has been shown to be therapeutically useful (12). Allopurinol lengthens the half-life of probenecid and potentiates its uricosuric effect. Conversely, uricosuric drugs increase the clearance of oxypurinol in humans (13). This diminishes the degree of xanthine dehydrogenase inhibition. With these observations in mind, one might expect probenecid to be required in smaller doses and allopurinol in a larger dose when used together. However, these drugs are tolerated very well and there is no need to alter the usual dose of either drug (10) (Table 3).

TABLE 3 The Effects of Probenecid on Metabolism of Other Agents

Decreased Renal Excretion
p-Aminohippuric acid
Phenosulfonphtalein
Salicylic acid and its acyl and phenolic glucuronides
Phlorizin and its glucuronide
Acetazolamide
Dapsone and its metabolites
Sulfinpyrazone and its parahydroxyl metabolite
Indomethacin
Ampicillin
Penicillin
Cephradine
Reduced Volume of Distribution
Ampicillin
Ancillin
Nafcillin
Cephaloridine
Delayed Metabolism
Heparin
Impairment of Hepatic Uptake
Bromsulfonphthalein
Indocyanin green
Rifampicin

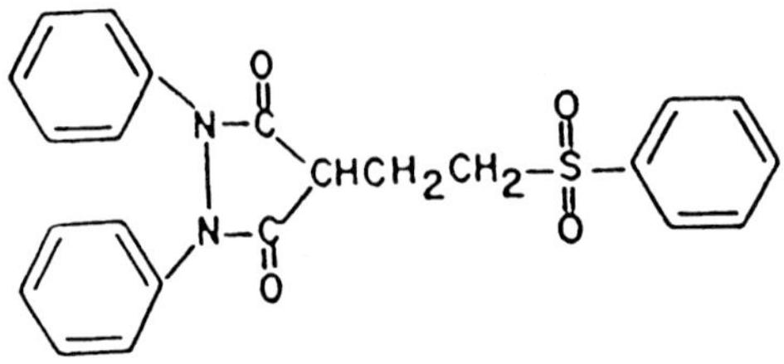

FIGURE 2 Structure of sulfinpyrazone.

B. Sulfinpyrazone

Sulfinpyrazone (1,2 diphenyl 4-2, phenylsulfinethyl 3,5 pyrazolidinedione) was first isolated from urine as the sulfoxide metabolite of the phenyl thioethyl analog of phenylbutazone (Figure 2).

Structure activity relationships of the pyrazolidinediones were reviewed by Gutman (14). Uricosuric potency varies inversely with pKa. Maximum uricosuria is attained at a pKa of approximately 3 (the pKa of sulphinpyrazone is 2.8) with no further increment in uricosuric activity with more acidic analogs (6). The rate of excretion also varies inversely with pKa, indicating that reabsorption is attributable to nonionic back diffusion. The potency correlates directly with excretion rate and, therefore, with concentration in the renal tubule. There appears to be no correlation between potency and lipid solubility, plasma protein binding, or plasma half-life (14). Unlike phenylbutazone, sulphinpyrasone has no analgesic or anti-inflammatory properties.

1. Pharmocokinetics

Sulphinpyrazone is rapidly and completely absorbed from the gastrointestinal tract as evidenced by 14-carbon labeled sulphinpyrazone studies (19). The plasma concentration reaches a peak after approximately 1 hr and the half-life after an oral dose is approximately 1–3 hr. Up to 98% of the agent is plasma protein bound and is mainly confined to the extracellular fluid. Renal excretion, therefore, is by tubular secretion. Between 20% and 40% of the drug is excreted unchanged in 24 hr (6). The major urinary metabolite is the glucuronide of sulphinpyrazone. Approximately 8% is excreted as the parahydroxyl metabolite, which itself may contribute to the uricosuric activity of the parent compound (15).

2. Biological Effects

Sulphinpyrazone is three to six times more potent that probenecid on a weight-for-weight basis and more effective than probenecid in patients with renal disease (16). Its uricosuric effect is neutralized by salicylates and pyrazinamide (6). It has an additional effect of reducing platelet adhesion. It also prolongs platelet survival and reduces the tendency to thromobsis in AV shunts and mechanical intravascular devices. In the treatment of gout, the initial dose is 50 mg twice daily increasing to 100 mg and then 200 mg twice daily. Hyperuricemia can be controlled in most patients on 200–400 mg per day in divided doses. The drug is well tolerated, but the uricosuric potency of sulphinpyrazone can be a problem because of the increased risk of uric acid crystalluria and renal failure. Precautions to prevent these complications are the same as for probenecid. Gastrointestinal (GI) toxicity is found in 10–15% of patients, with skin rash occurring in less than 3%. Bone marrow suppression has also been reported (14). Sulphinpyrazone may potentiate the activity of oral hypoglycemic agents and sulfa drugs.

C. Benzbromarone

Benzbromarone, a benzofuran derivative, is a potent uricosuric agent that has been used extensively in Europe. It is not available in the United States. A closely related agent, bensiaderone, was withdrawn due to toxicity related to its iodine content (Figure 3).

Benzbromarone is essentially insoluble in water. Following oral administration, the absorption from the gastrointestinal tract is variable, but with the micronized preparation a peak serum concentration occurs within 4 hr. Its metabolites, mostly notably benzarone, also have uricosuric effects (17). Renal excretion is slow with biliary excretion being the major route or elimination (up to 60%). The time of peak uricosuric response varies among individuals, but does not correlate with benzbromarone blood levels. In fact, the correlation appears better with plasma concentrations of the metabolites of benzbromarone.

Benzbromarone does not interfere with the urinary excretion of penicillin and has no clinically significant anti-inflammatory or antiplatelet aggregatory effect. It is a potent uricosuric agent with 100 md/day (micronized) giving a urico-

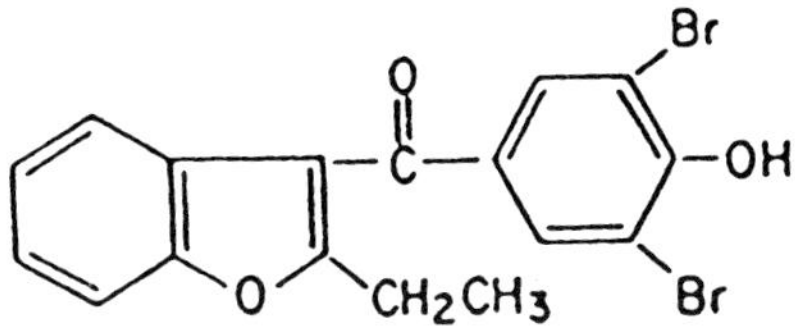

FIGURE 3 Structure of benzobromarone.

suric response equivalent to 1 g per day of probenecid (6). Although there is some in vitro evidence of xanthine oxidase inhibition, it seems unlikely that this phenomenon is of any clinical significance in vivo, since there is no increase in urine oxypurine levels following administration.

Benzbromarone is given in single daily doses with a maximum of 80 mg/day in the micronized form. It is effective in the presence of renal insufficiency and appears to be useful therapy in patients unable to tolerate probenecid, allopurinol, or prophylactic colchicine. Precautions to prevent acute attacks of gout, tubular deposition of urate, and stone formation are the same as previously mentioned for other uricosuric agents. The uricosuric effect is antagonized by pyrazinimide and salicylate, but benzbromarone retains significant uricosuric activity during salicylate administration.

The most commonly reported side effects are gastrointestinal disturbance, particularly diarrhea, with hypersensitivity and rash occurring much less frequently. Mertz and Loewer (18) proposed using combined uricosuric and uricostatic therapy with a fixed ration of 100 mg of allopurinol to 20 mg of benzbromarone for the treatment of gout and hyperuricemia. They believe this would reduce the risk of adverse effects of either drug used alone. Muller et al. (19) studied the effects of benzbromarone on allopurinol-oxypuyrinol kinetics in 14 men using an open, randomized cross-over study. The results confirmed that benzbromarone lowered plasma oxypurinol concentrations, but did not affect plasma allopurinol concentration. Despite this effect, the combination drug (Allomarin) was superior to allopurinol alone in lowering serum uric acid.

D. Zoxazolamine

In 1958, Reed et al. (20) described zoxazolamine, a potent uricosuric agent. Unfortunately, this agent is now only of historical interest, since its use has largely been abandoned due to unacceptable hepatic and bone marrow toxicity.

E. Diflunisal

Diflunisal is a fluorinated salicylate that retains the salicylate uricosuric effect and that can usually lower the serum urate concentration during long-term therapy (24). In normal volunteers, an increase in the renal clearance of uric acid and the decrease in serum uric acid was observed when diflunisal was administered at 500 or 750 mg daily in divided doses. Patients on long-term therapy taking 500–1000 mg per day showed a prompt and consistent reduction across studies in mean serum uric acid levels, which were lowered as much as 1.4 mg %. It is not known whether diflunisal interferes with the activity of other uricosuric agents.

F. Aspirin

Aspirin or salicylates in doses of 5 g per day with sodium bicarbonate 5 g per day are effective uricosurics. However, most patients are unable to tolerate such high doses. At low doses (less than 2.4 g per day), aspirin or salicylates inhibit the renal tubular secretion of uric acid, leading to hyperuricemia (22).

G. Tienilic Acid

Tienilic acid (2,3, dichloro 4,2 thienyle carbomyle phenoxy acetic acid) is a diuretic chemically related to ethacrynic acid. Unlike thiazide diuretics, it is a potent uricosuric agent in man following oral administration (17). Diuretic activity has also been demonstrated in many animal species and based on these studies it is thought that the proximal tubule is the site for the uricosuric effect (23) (Figure 4).

Tienilic acid is extensively bound to plasma proteins and metabolism is via reduction or oxidation. Plasma levels reach a peak value after 3–4 hr. Its uricosuric potency is similar to other agents, but the marked volume depletion that results from daily use has limited its role. The risk of tubular deposition of urate or renal stone formation is similar to other uricosuric agents. Increases in serum uric acid occur upon discontinuation, which is accounted for by the diuretic-induced volume depletion. The diuretic effect may also result in hyponatremia, hypokalemia, hypochloremic alkalosis, and elevation of blood urea nitrogen and creatinine.

Tienilic acid has found no clinical role at present; however, it has prompted research into related compounds that may be of benefit in the future.

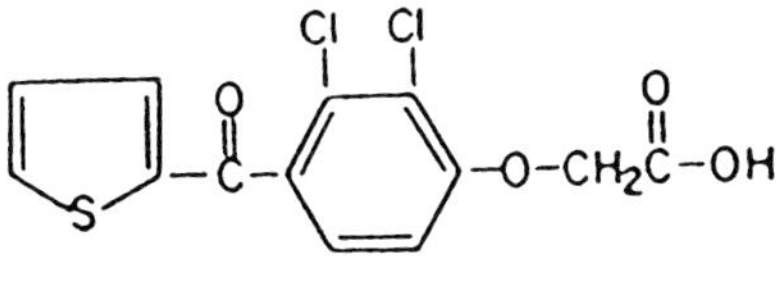

FIGURE 4 Structure of tienilic acid.

III. INHIBITION OF URATE SYNTHESIS: XANTHINE OXIDASE INHIBITORS—ALLOPURINOL

Uric acid production may be inhibited at a number of different enzymatic steps. Agents such as diazo-oxo-norleucine and azaserine certainly block the early steps of purine biosynthesis but, unfortunately, also interfere with nucleic acid synthesis and are, therefore, cytotoxic (24).

Patients with congenital xanthinuria lack xanthine oxidase, but can still convert inosinate to xanthylate via the enzyme inosinate dehydrogenase (25). This finding originally focused attention on the importance of xanthine oxidase in uric acid production. In the 1950s, studies with carbonyl reagents succeeded in inhibiting xanthine oxidase in rats, but only at toxic levels (36). Successful in vitro agents such as pteridine failed to give any inhibition in vivo. The ideal drug for the treatment of hyperuricemia reduces uric acid synthesis without interfering with important anabolic pathways or normal regulatory functions. Allopurinol [4 hydroxy pyrazolol (3,4, d) pyrimidine] was chosen for in vivo studies because it was found to be a potent inhibitor of xanthine oxidase in vitro. More importantly, it did not appear to interfere with anabolic processes within the cell (28). Allopurinol, a structural analog of hypoxanthine, is both a substrate and a potent inhibitor of xanthine oxidase (Figure 5).

The enzymatic oxidation of allopurinol produces the xanthine analog oxypurinol [4,6 dihydroxy pyrazolo (3,4d) pyrimidine]. The success of allopurinol as a xanthine oxidase inhibitor in vivo is undoubtedly due in large part to the properties of oxypurinol as an enzyme inhibitor and to its persistence in body fluids. Approximately 60–70% of allopurinol is metabolized to oxypurinol, which itself has a much longer half-life of 14–26 hrs as a result of renal tubular absorption (29). Oxypurinol is renally excreted in direct proportion to the creatinine clearance and will accumulate in renal impairment.

The first evidence that allopurinol was an inhibitor of xanthine oxidase in vivo was demonstrated in the early 1960s with its ability to prevent the oxi-

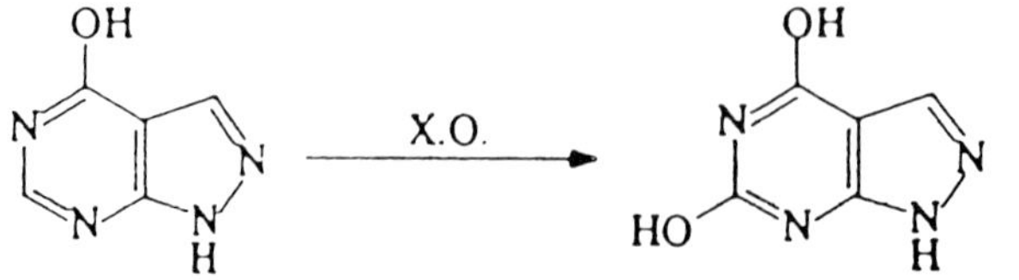

FIGURE 5 Structure of allopurinol.

dation of 6 mercaptopurine to 6 thiouric acid in mice (30). This conversion is mediated by xanthine oxidase and is a major catabolic pathway in the metabolism of 6 mercaptopurine. The inhibition achieved with allopurinol also results in potentiation of the antitumor, immunosuppressive effect and toxicity of 6 mercaptopurine.

Reduction of uric acid levels in serum and urine arises as a result of the ability of allopurinol to inhibit the oxidation of endogenous purines by xanthine oxidase. This results in a concomitant increase in the urinary excretion of hypoxanthine and xanthine. These features have made allopurinol an excellent agent in the treatment of primary and secondary hyperuricemia. The uric acid lowering effect is dose related. When serum urate levels are maintained below the saturation level of sodium urate, crystalline deposits of urate dissolve and tophi decrease in size. There is also an improvement in destructive arthritis, gouty nephropathy appears to be halted, and acute attacks become less frequent. Long-term use produces a constant degree of xanthine oxidase inhibition with no induction of the enzyme. Hence, increased doses of allopurinol are not required for prolonged periods of treatment (31).

The immediate precursors of uric acid are hypoxanthine and xanthine. One might expect these precursors to accumulate when xanthine oxidase is inhibited, however, these oxpurines are cleared rapidly by the kidney at a rate close to the glomerular filtration rate (GFR) (32), which results in a minimal rise in the serum oxypurine level.

Elevated levels of oxypurine appear in the urine during allopurinol therapy. However, this increase is not as great as the decrease in uric acid production. The reason underlying this phenomenon is the reutilization of hypoxanthine and xanthine for nucleic acid synthesis. The nucleotides, adenylic acid, and guanylic acid produced by this process act as feedback inhibitors or the enzyme glutamine phosphoribosyl pyrophosphate amidotransferase, the first enzyme of purine biosynthesis.

The enzyme hypoxanthine guanine phosphoribosyl transferase (HGPRT) is essential to the reutilization of oxypurines. Patients with Lesch-Nyhan syndrome are deficient in this enzyme and the amount of oxypurine excreted in the urine exactly matches the decrease in uric acid production caused by allopurinol. These patients may produce xanthine precipitates in the urine when aggressively treated with allopurinol. Overall, the number of reported cases of xanthine stones is small. Other than in this group of patients, allopurinol reduces total purine production by utilizing HGPRT and the high energy phosphate compound, phosphoribosyl pyrophosphate (PRPP) both of which are necessary for de novo purine synthesis.

Orotic aciduria and orotidinuria may also occur during allopurinol therapy. This is related to inhibition of de novo pyrimidine synthesis of orotidylic decarboxylase by allopurinol and oxypurinol ribonucleotide (13).

A. Pharmacokinetics

Allopurinol is rapidly absorbed from the gastrointestinal tract. Peak plasma levels in humans occur at 30–60 min after ingestion (31). The half-life of allopurinol ranges from 40 min to 2 hr. Approximately 20% of ingested allopurinol is excreted in the feces (33). However, most of the drug is rapidly converted to its principle metabolite, oxypurinol, with small amounts being converted to the riboside and ribotide of allopurinol. Despite the fact that allopurinol has a short half-life, xanthine oxidase inhibition can be maintained at a steady state with a single daily dose. This results from the prolonged half-life of oxypurinol (14–28 hr) (34). The long plasma half-life is not due to either plasma protein binding or concentration in tissues; both allopurinol and oxypurinol show no binding to plasma proteins and are freely diffusable and distributed in total body water. Whereas allopurinol is cleared mainly by glomerular filtration, oxypurinol is rabsorbed in the kidney tubules in a similar fashion to the absorption of uric acid. Allopurinol is cleared by the kidney at a rate of 14–20 ml/min (10), whereas oxypurinol is cleared more slowly (23–31 ml/min). Overall, oxypurinol is poorly absorbed from the gastrointestinal tract and has a relatively poor solubility. This limits its usefulness as a therapeutic agent. The prolonged half-life of oxypurinol can be even longer for protein malnourished patients (up to 50 hr) (35), which means the dose should be reduced in such cases.

Both allopurinol and oxypurinol are dialysable. Patients who have hyperuricemia require a dose of only 300 mg of allopurinol after each dialysis to maintain an adequate oxypurinol concentration between dialyses (36).

Uricosuric drugs increase the excretion of oxypurinol whereas renal insufficiency reduces its excretion. Thus, dose adjustments are required to compensate for these clinical situations. Occasionally uricosurics and allopurinol may need to be combined, and there is a theoretical possibility of a drug interaction resulting in an increase clearance of oxypurinol. Clinically, this has not been a major problem and there is no need to alter the usual dosages of either drug.

B. Metabolism

Allopurinol undergoes three pathways of metabolism. It may be converted to a necleotide 5′-monophosphate derivative. This can be dephosphorylated to a necleoside derivative. The latter compound can also be formed directly from allopurinol by the reaction of purine nucleoside phosphorylase. The major pathway of metabolism is clearly oxidation to oxipurinol.

Oxipurinol, a structural analog of xanthine, has four different pathways of metabolism. Xanthine is a substrate for HGPRT and purine nucleoside phosphorylase (PRPP). These metabolic pathways result in the purine nucleoside and nucleotide derivatives. Additionally, oxipurinol is also a substrate or orotate

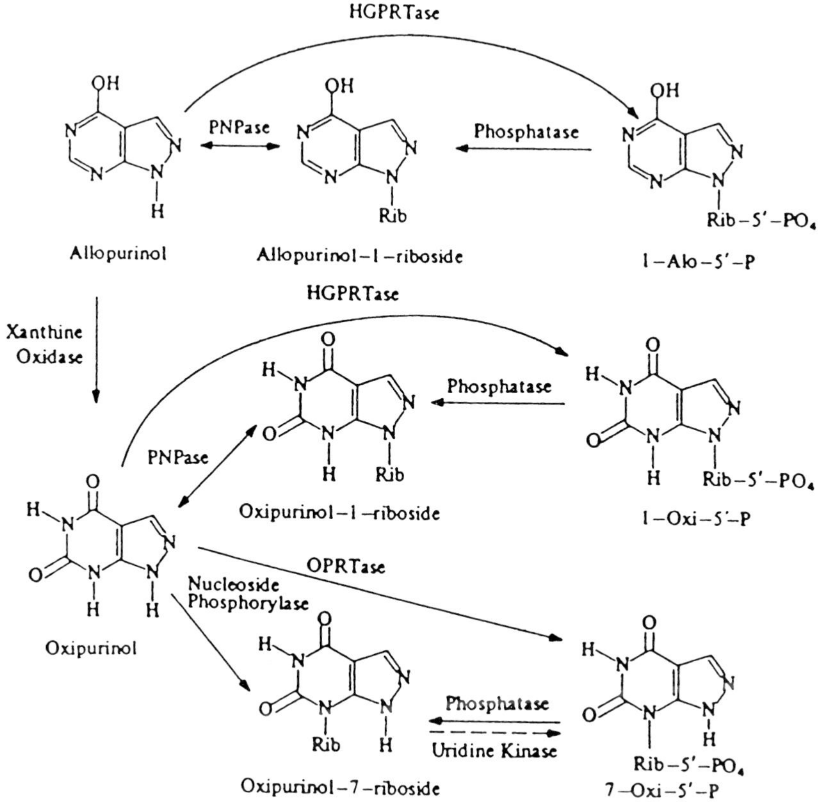

FIGURE 6 Metabolic transformation of allopurinol and oxpurinol.

phosphoribosyl transferase and pyrimidine nucleoside phosphorylase (PNP). The compounds formed are 7N (5′-phosphoribosyl oxipurinol) and 7N5′-ribosyl oxipurinol derivatives (Figure 6).

C. Drug Interactions

There are several clinically important drug interactions. Since azathioprine and mercaptopurine are normally inactivated by xanthine oxidase, inhibition of this enzyme by allopurinol increases the toxic effect of the other two drugs (37). For this reason, the dose of these drugs should be reduced to 25% of the standard dose if the patient is already receiving allopurinol. There is an increased incidence of bone marrow suppression in patients already receiving cyclophosphamide, although the mechanism is not clear (38). The use of ampicillin in

TABLE 4 Indications for Allopurinol in Patients with Hyperuricemia

1. Hyperuricemia with increased uric acid production and/or normal to increased uric acid excretion.
   a. Greater than 800 mg of urinary uric acid for 24 hours on a regular diet, or
   b. Greater than 600 mg of urinary uric acid per 24 hours on purine restricted diet
2. Hypoxanthine guanine phoso ribosyl transferase deficiency (HGRPT)
3. PP ribose synthetase overactivity
4. Nephrolithiasis
5. Uric acid nephropathy
6. Tophaceous deposits
7. Renal insufficiency (creatinine clearance less than 50 ml/min)
8. Allergy or intolerance uricosurics
9. Uricosuric ineffective in controlling hyperuricemia
10. Recurrent attacks of gout not effectively prevented by colchicine prophylaxis
11. Other indications: Prophylaxis prior to chemotherapy

patients already receiving allopurinol has reportedly been shown to produce a tenfold increase in the incidence of skin rash (39). Allopurinol has also been shown to reduce the activity of hepatic microsomal drug metabolizing enzymes and therby prolong the half-lives of antipyrene, aminophenozone, theophylline, dicoumerol, and warfarin (40) (Table 4).

D. Therapeutic Effects

Allopurinol, when given to patients with normal renal function, produces a decrease in serum and urinary uric acid values within 24–48 hr. The maximum effect is seen between 4 and 14 days, and serum urate levels then stay relatively constant over a prolonged time course. If allopurinol is withdrawn, the serum level of urate usually rises over 2–3 days. Once antihyperuricemic therapy is started for an appropriate indication, it should be continued indefinitely if possible. It has been shown that intermittent administration of allopurinol is less effective that continuous therapy in controlling gout symptoms. After 3–6 months of normal serum urate levels, a reduction in the frequency of gouty attacks may be expected. Allopurinol administration results in depletion of PRPP from cells, which is also necessary for de novo purine synthesis. The increased concentrations of hypoxanthine in serum urate is rarely a problem because they remain well below their solubility limits. Tophi resolve in 6–12 months with maintenance of normal serum urate levels (10) and destructive arthritis improves in most patients. Gottlieb et al. (41) have reported an interesting phenomenon of allopurinol associated hand-and-foot deformities in patients with chronic topha-

TABLE 5 Glomerular Filtration Rate and Dosage Adjustment of Allopurinol

GFR, ml/min	Dose, milligrams
100	300
60	200
20	100
0	100 q 3days

ceous gout. With renal insufficiency, there appears to be a slower course in improvement, but gouty nephropathy appears to be halted.

Allopurinol is available in 100 mg and 300 mg tablets. The dose, given once a day, is adjusted to bring serum urate levels to less than 6.7 mg/dl (0.4 mmol/l). Only rarely is a dose greater than 300 mg required, and under these circumstances one should strive to look for any additional correctable factors contributing to the hyperuricemia. Measurement of plasma oxipurinol may be of considerable value in this situation. Oxipurinol is excreted principally by the kidney and may have a prolonged half-life in patients with renal impairment as mentioned earlier. Thus, in patients with renal insufficiency the dosages should be adjusted in accordance to the reduced glomerular filtration rate (Table 5).

For those patients who are unable to ingest oral medication, parental and rectal administration may be an alternative. However, it should be remembered that drug absorption may be limited by poor solubility.

E. Adverse Reactions

Initiation of allopurinol therapy has been shown to precipitate gout attacks with serum urate levels of only 2 mg/100 mls and a low urinary urate excretion (42). The use of daily colchicine has been advocated during the first 6–12 months of therapy with allopurinol to minimize such recurrent acute attacks (10). As mentioned previously, the urinary excretion of xanthine increases during allopurinol therapy to the level of xanthine excretion observed in hereditary xanthinuria. Patients with this disorder produce urinary xanthine stones. However, other than in patients with partial deficiency of HGPRT, development of xanthine crystalluria or stones is rarely seen as a complication of allopurinol therapy (43).

Xanthine stone formation with allopurinol therapy has also been reported in patients with Lesch-Nyhan syndrome, lymphosarcoma, or Burkitt's lymphoma.

F. Toxicity

Up to 5% of normal subjects are unable to tolerate allopurinol because of adverse reactions (44). Minor gastrointestinal disturbance is common, but is usually minimized by administering the medication with food. More serious toxicity may occur, but is rare. Some adverse reactions to allopurinol may be mediated by lymphocyte reactivity to oxipurinol, which may represent a delayed type hypersensitivity reaction. The major adverse effect is a sensitivity reaction, which may range from an erythematous skin rash (occasionally with fever) to a considerable eosinophilia, abnormal liver function tests, and worsening renal function characterized by chronic interstitial nephritis and severe jaundice. The incidence of side effects overall may be up to 20%. As long as there is no evidence of laryngeal edema or anaphylactic reaction, the patient may be treated with antihistamine for symptomatic relief of pruritus. After a few weeks of therapy it may be possible to continue the allopurinol and withdraw the antihistamine without difficulty. Reducing the dose, particularly in patients with renal insufficiency, may also be of benefit in improving skin lesions.

Desensitization has been utilized in patients with less severe cases of hypersensitivity with some success. Very low doses (0.05 mg) of allopurinol have been given by mouth with gradual increasing amounts over a period of days (45). In patients where the oral desensitization has failed, intravenous desensitization has been successfully used (46).

Allopurinol hypersensitivity syndrome (AHS) is an infrequent but life-threatening condition. The incidence is low, with around 100 cases having been described in the literature. Criteria used for establishing the diagnosis is outlined in Table 6 and was originally proposed by Singer and Wallace (47).

It appears the mechanisms, though still uncertain, probably involve the accumulation of allopurinol/oxipurinol in patients with renal insufficiency, im-

TABLE 6 Criteria for Diagnosis of Allopurinol Hypersensitivity Syndrome

1. History of exposure to allopurinol
2. At least two of the following:
   a. Worsening renal function
   b. Acute hepatocellular injury
   c. Rash including toxic epidermal necrolysis, erythema multiforme, or diffuse maculopapular or exfoliative dermatitis
   d. One of the above, plus one of the following:
      - Fever
      - Eosinophilia
      - Leukosytosis
3. Lack of exposure to any drug that might produce a similar clinical picture.

munological factors revolving around Type 3 and Type 4 hypersensitivity reactions, and possible genetic predesposition (48).

Mortality from this syndrome is in the range of 30% and current management consists of early recognition, withdrawal of the drug, and appropriate supportive therapy. There is still controversy over the use of corticosteroids with some authors recommending the use of 40–200 mg per day for treating AHS, while others consider this drug to be of no use. The review by Arellano and Sacristan (48) reveals that 66 of patients were treated with corticosteroids whereas 22 were not. Thirty percent of those receiving steroids died, compared with only 2% who did not receive corticosteroids. The higher mortality rate may simply reflect the greater severity of disease in these patients.

These findings illustrate the importance of reducing the dose of allopurinol in patients with renal insufficiency and restricting its use to those patients in whom it is clearly indicated.

Oxipurinol, the active metabolic product of allopurinol, it not commercially available in the United States but can be obtained on a compassionate use basis. A direct comparison of the two agents given orally suggest that allopurinol is more effective (due the superior absorption from the gastrointestinal tract) (10) compared to enteric coated mircotablets of oxipurinol in a small group of healthy individuals.

The use of oxipurinol has been proposed for individuals who are sensitive to allopurinol. However, due to their structural similarities, toxic reactions identical to allopurinol have been observed in 30% of patients treated with oxipurinol.

Clearly this remains a difficult problem to overcome and oxipurinol will continue to have a very limited role.

IV. NEW DEVELOPMENTS

It has been reported that a newly synthesized compound, E5050, is able to induce uricosuria in humans via inhibition of the postsecretory reabsorption of urate. This compound is derivative of ethanolamine and its effects were examined in rats loaded with oxonate. When compared to trichlormethiazide and probenicid, the E5050 (administered I,P) increases the urinary excretion of urate and the ratio of urate clearance to insulin clearance in a dose-dependent manner, while the urine volume increased only slightly. The glomerular filtration rate and plasma urate level were not changed (49).

FK366 is an aldose reductase inhibitor whose uricosuric activities have been studied at doses ranging from 150 mg to 600 mg in healthy volunteers (50). Serum uric acid decreased dose dependently, with a minimum concentration of 4 mg/dl 8 hr after receiving 600 mg of FK366. With multiple dosing, the serum uric acid declined rapidly and remained at a concentration of 3.1 mg/dl until the end of the study (day 8). Urinary excretion of uric acid was high on day 1, but decreased significantly and stabilized by day 2. As FK366 falls under the category of a carboxilic acid, the authors suggest that its mechanism of action involves the inhibition of reabsorption of uric in the renal tubules, resulting in increased urinary excretion.

CGS12970 [3 methyl 1-,2-(3 pyridyl)-1-, indole octanoic acid] is a reversable thromboxane synthase inhibitor that was noted to lower serum uric acid during preliminary trials in humans. Saris et al. (51) have reported a small human study using 20 health male volunteers. The subjects received two doses of CGS12970 12 hr apart and the serum uric acid concentration decreased between 34% and 47%. Based on further testing of the agent in vitro, the author postulates that the uricosuric effect may be attributable to the acidic properties of CGS 12970 rather than its inhibition of thromboxane synthase.

Ambroxol, an expectorant that promotes bronchial secretions, has been noted to reduce plasma uric acid concentration in high doses. Using a placebo-controlled double-blind parallel study of health volunteers, Oosterhuis et al. (52) have shown that ambroxol can produce a significant, dose-dependent reduction in plasma uric acid. Doses of 250–500 mg twice daily were well tolerated and produced a 20–30% reduction in plasma uric acid. There appeared to be no notable effect on creatinine clearance and plasma hypoxanthine levels were not affected. The authors conclude that ambroxol enhances renal excretion of uric acid at the tubular level based on their study findings.

Another new class of uricosuric is AA193 [5 chloro-7,8-Dihydro-3-phenyl furol (2,3 G)-1,2-bensizoxazole]. Oral administration of this drug increases uric acid excretion in normal rats, mice, and cebus monkeys. Using the hyperuricemic rat model (oxonate fed rats), Dan et al. (53) showed that administration of AA193 for 7 days increased urate excretion and decreased plasma urate level.

V. URATE DEGRADATION

Another new approach to the treatment of hyperuricemia involves the enzymatic destruction of urate. Uricase (urate oxidase) degrades uric acid to allantoin and carbon dioxide. The clinical usefulness of this agent has been described in a patient with non-Hodgkin's lymphoma where the serum urate concentration was lowered from 15.3 to 3.2 mg/dl over 30 hr with a 3 ml/kg IM dose (54). Uricase is not available for clinical use in the United States, but is available in France and Italy under the trade name Uricozyme. The enzyme is obtained from extracts of *asperigillus flavus* and other fungal species. The drug must be administered IV or IM. Reports have been published utilizing this agent in clyclosporin-induced hyperuricemia in renal transport patients (55) as well as in treatment of tophaceous gout in heart transplant patients (56). There is a risk of anaphylaxis, bronchospasm, and hemolytic anemia, which is significantly reduced with polyethylene glycol modification (57).

This agent appears to be attractive in managing severe gout in this patient group as well as in those patients where treatment with allopurinol is indicated but toxic effects preclude its use. Clearly, further research is required before this drug gains more widespread usage.

The hypouricemic drugs that are currently available may be utilized to successfully treat the majority of patients in whom treatment is indicated. However, a small minority of patients, particularly those with gouty nephropathy and intolerance or hypersensitivity to existing agents, continue to pose significant therapeutic difficulties for clinicians.

ACKNOWLEDGMENT

The authors would like to thank Ms. Gina Ohm for her excellent typing skills.

REFERENCES

1. B. T. Emmerson. The management of gout, *NEJM 7*:443–445 (1996).
2. J. H. Talbott, B. M. Norcross, and L. M. Lockje. The clinical and metabolic effects of Benemid in patients with gout. *Trans Amer Assn Phys 14*:372 (1951).
3. A. B. Gutman and T. F. Yu. Benemid as a uricosuric agent in gouty arthritis. *Trans Amer Assn Phys, 64*:279 (1951).
4. K. H. Beyer, H. F. Russo, E. K. Tillson, A. K. Miller, W. F. Verwey, and Gass Sr. Benemid, p-(di-N-propyl-sulfamyl)-benzoic acid: Its renal affinity and elimination. *Am J Physiol 166*:625 (1951).
5. I. M. Weiner, K. C. Blanchard, and G. H. Mudge. Factors influencing renal excretion of foreign organic acids. *Am J Physiol 207*:953 (1964).
6. H. S. Diamond. Uricosuric drugs in uric acid, In: Handbook of Experimental Pharmacology, (W. N. Kelley and I. M. Weiner, eds.), Vol. 51, Springer Verlag, Berlin, Germany, 1977, p. 459.
7. P. G. Dayton and J. M. Perel. The metabolism of probenecid in man. *Ann NY Acad Sci 179*:229 (1971).
8. A. B. Gutman and T. F. Yu. Protracted uricosuric therapy in tophaceous gout. *Lancet IIIb*:1258 (1957).
9. V. I. Rizzuto, T. Inglesby, and W. J. Grave. Probenecid (Benecid) intoxication with status epilepticus. *Am J Med 38*:646 (1965).
10. I. H. Fox. Antiphyperuricemic drugs, In: Textbook of Rheumatology, 4th Ed., (W. N. Kelley, E. D. Harris, S. Ruddy, C. B. Sledge, eds.), W.B. Saunders and Company, Philadelphia, PA, Vol. I, Chap. 50, 822–830, 1993.

11. G. Sanchez. Enhancement of heparin effect by probenecid. *N Eng J Med 292*:48 (1975).
12. S. Kenwright and A. J. Levi. Impairment of hepatic uptake of Rifamycin antibiotics by probenecid and its therapeutic implications. *Lancet II*:1401 (1973).
13. G. B. Elion, T. F. Yu, and A. B. Gutman. Renal clearance of oxipurinol, the chief metabolite of allopurinol. *Am J Med 45*:69 (1968).
14. A. B. Gutman. Uricosuric drugs, with special reference to probenecid and sulfinpyrazone. *Advan Pharmacol 4*:91 (1966).
15. P. C. Dytonm, L. E. Sicam, M. Landrau, and J. J. Burns. Metabolism of sulfinpyrazone (anturane) and other thioanalgogues of phenylbutazone in man. *J Pharmacol Exp Ther 132*:286 (1961).
16. B. T. Emmerson. A comparison of uricosuric agents in gout with special reference to sulfinpyrazone. *Med J Aust 1*:839 (1963).
17. A. Masternard and C. P. Giudicelli. Etude clinique de l'action antihypertensive de l'acide chloro 2.3 (tienil-2-ceto)-phenoxy acetique en administration pronlangee. *Lyon Med 232*:165 (1974).
18. D. P. Mertz and H. Loewer. Wirkungsprofil der Harnsaurenskung bei Hoheerdosieerung von Allopurinol. *Dtsch Med Wochenshr 104*:324 (1979).
19. F. O. Muller, F. Shall, G. Groenewoud, H. K. L. Hundt, J. C. Van der Merwe and M. Van Dyk. The effects of benzbromarone on allopurinol/oxypurinol kinetics in patients with gout, *Eur J Clin Pharmacol 44*:69 (1993).
20. E. B. Reed, T. V. Feichtmeir, and F. M. Willett. Zoxaxolamine: A potent uricosuric agent, a preliminary report. *New Engl J Med 258*:394 (1958).
21. B. T. Emmerson, R. A. Hazelton, and J. M. Whyte. Comparison of the urate lowering effects of allopurinol and diflunisal. *J Rheumatol 14*:335 (1987).
22. T. F. Yu and A. B. Gutman. Paradoxical retention of uric acid by uricosuric drugs in low dosage. *Proc Soc Exp Biol (NY) 90*:542 (1955).
23. G. Lemieux, A. Kiss, P. Vinay, and A. Gougoux. Nature of the uricosuric effect of tienilic acid, a new diuretic. *Kidney Int 12*:104 (1977).
24. A. Grayzel, J. E. Seegmiller, and E. Lane. Suppression of uric acid synthesis in the gouty human by the use of 6-diazo-5-oxo-L-norlleucine. *J Clin Invest 39*:447 (1960).
25. R. W. E. Watts, K. Engelman, J. R. Klineberg, and A. Sjoerdsma. Seegmiller, JE. Enzyme defect in a case of xanthinuria. *Nature (Lon) 201*:395 (1964).
26. W. W. Westerfield, D. A. Richert, and R. J. Bloom. Inhibition of xanthine and succinic oxidases by carbonyl reagents. *J Biol Chem 234*:1889 (1959).
27. S. O. Byers. Xanthine oxidase studies. *J Amer Pharm Ass Sci Ed 41*:611 (1952).
28. G. B. Elion, S. Gallahan, H. Nathan, S. Bieber, R. W. Rundles, and G. H. Hitchings. Potentiation by inhibition of drugs degradation: 6 substituted purines and xanthine oxidase. *Biochem Pharmacol 12*:85 (1963).
29. K. B. Hande, R.M. Noone, W. J. Stone. Severe allopurinol toxicity. Description and guidelines for prevention in patients with renal insufficiency. *Am J Med 76*:47 (1984).
30. G. B. Elion, S. W. Callahan, G. H. Hitchings, R. W. Rundles, and J. Laszlo. Experimental, clinical and metabolic studies of thiopurines. *Cancer Chemother Rep 16*:197 (1962).

31. G. B. Elion. Allopurinol and other inhibitors of urate synthesis in uric acid, In: *Handbook of Experimental Pharmacology*, 51, Chap. 21, 485: Springer Verlag, Berlin, Germany, 1977.
32. S. Goldfinger, J. R. Klineberg, and J. E. Seegmiller. The renal excretion of oxypurine. *J Clin Invest 44*:623 (1965).
33. G. E. Elion, A. Kovensky, G. H. Hutchings, E. Metz, and R. W. Rundles. Metabolic studies of allopurinol, an inhibitor of xanthine oxidase. *Biochem. Pharm 15*:863 (1966).
34. G. P. Rodnan, J. A. Robin, S. F. Tolchin, and G. B. Elion. Allopurinol and gouty hyperuricemia: Efficacy of a single daily dose. *JAMA 231*:1143 (1975).
35. W. G. Berlinger, G. D. Park and R. Spector. The effect of dietary protein on the clearance of allopurinol and oxypurinol. *NEJM 313*:771 (1985).
36. R. W. Rundles. Allopurinol in gouty nephropathy and renal dialysis. *Ann Rheum Dis 25*: 694 (1966).
37. G. Venkat Raman, V. I. Sharman, and H. A. Lee. Azathioprine and allopurinol: A potentially dangerous combination. *J Int Med 228*: 69 (1990).
38. J. H. Fox, and W. N. Kelly. Management of gout. *JAMA 242*:261 (1979).
39. Boston Collaborative Drug Surveillance Program. Excess of amipcillin rashes associated with allopurinol or hyperuricemia. *NEJM 286*: 505 (1972).
40. M. Barry and J. Freely. Allopurinol influences aminophenazone elimination. *Clin Pharmacokin 19*: 167 (1990).
41. N. L. Gottlieb and R. G. Gray. Allopurinol associated hand and foot deformities in chronic tophaceous gout. *JAMA 238*: 1663 (1997).
42. T. F. Yu and A. B. Gutman. Effect of allopurinol (4-hydroxypyrazolo (3,4-d) pyrimidine) on serum and urinary uric acid in primary and secondary gout. *Am J Med 37*:885 (1964).
43. W. N. Kelley and I. H. Fox. Antihyperuricemic drugs, In: Textbook of Rheumatology, 3rd Ed. W. B. Saunders Philadelphia, PA, 1989, p. 889.
44. B. T. Emmerson. Pharmacological approaches: Antihyperuricemic 15. 1–6. In: Rheumatology, (J. H. Klippel, and P. A. Dieppe, eds.), Times Mirror International Publishers Ltd Mosby, 1994.
45. J. MacDonald, A. G. Fam, T. Paton, and J. Senn. Allopurinol hypersensitivity in patient with coexistent systemic lupus erythematosus and tophaceous gout. *J Rheumatol 15*:865 (1988).
46. S. A. Walz Leblanc, W. J. Reynolds, and D. K. MacFadden. Allopurinol sensitivity in a patient with chronic tophaceous gout: Success of intravenous desensitization after failure of oral desinsitization. *Arth Rheum 34*(10):1329 (1991).
47. J. Z. Singer and S. L. Wallace. The allopurinol hypersensitivity syndrome: Unnecessary morbidity and mortality. *Arth Rheum 29*: 82 (1986).
48. F. Arellano and J. Sacristan. Allopurinol Hypersensitivity Syndrome: A review. *Ann Pharmacother 27*:337 (1993).
49. H. Sugino and H. Shimada. The uricosuric effect in rats of E5050, a new derivative of ethanolamine, involves inhibition of the tubular post secretory reabsorption of urate. *Jpn J Pharmcol 68*:297 (1995).
50. M. Kanamaru, T. Vematsu, S. Nagashima, A. Mizuno, M. Terakawa, A. Sugiyama

and M. Nakashima. Aldose reductase inhibitory and uricosuric activities of FK366 in healthy volunteers. *J Clin Pharmocol 33*:1122 (1993).

51. S. Savis, A. J. Piraino, J. M. Morgan, W. L. Hirschhorn, E. Miedl, and A. V. Schaffer. Uricosuric effect of CGS 12970, a new thromboxane synthase inhibitor. *Clin Pharm Ther 54*(1):65 (1993).
52. B. Oosterhuis, G. Storm, P. J. G. Cornelissen, C. A. P. Su, E. A. E. Sollie, and J. H. G. Jonkman. Dose dependent uricosuric effect of ambroxol. *Eur J Clin Pharm 44*:237 (1993).
53. T. Dan, T. Yoneya, E. Onoma, and Ozawak. Hypocuricemic and uricosuric actions of AA-193 in a hyperuricemia rat model. *Metabolism 43*(1):123 (1994).
54. C. C. Chua, M. I. Greenberg, A. T. Viau, M. Nucci, W. D. Brenshman, and M. S. Hershfield. Use of polyethylene glycol-modified uricase (PEG uricase) to treat hyperuicemia in a patient with non-Hodgkin's lymphoma. *Ann Int Med 109*:114 (1988).

17

Gout and Renal Disease

BRYAN T. EMMERSON
University of Queensland at the Princess Alexandra Hospital, Brisbane, Queensland, Australia

I. INTRODUCTION

The kidney is so important in urate metabolism that it would be expected that kidney disease would have an effect on urate homeostasis (1). In addition to its excretory function, the kidney is also a major organ for concentration, affecting urate as well as sodium and urea. Because urate is relatively insoluble, it would be expected that there would be times when the kidney would be particularly susceptible to deposition of urate and/or uric acid crystals with resultant tissue reactions to such deposition.

Accordingly, it is important, when a patient is seen with both gout and kidney disease, to consider whether the primary problem is intrinsic renal disease with a secondary disturbance of urate metabolism or whether the primary problem is the disorder of urate metabolism having deleterious effects upon the kidney and thereby causing secondary renal disease. This distinction can be made easily if there is a clear history that one preceded the other, i.e., that a patient is known to have had renal disease prior to the first attack of gout or a patient with gout was known to have had normal renal function at one time and later developed renal disease. The distinction is sometimes more difficult if evidence is inadequate. However, the clinical pattern of the two sequences is different (Table 1) and patients with renal disease due to gout have usually suffered numerous attacks of severe gout over many years prior to developing renal disease and will usually have developed tophi. By contrast, patients with primary renal disease who develop gout tend to have had fewer, less severe attacks of gout. In such patients, the renal

TABLE I Clinical Findings in Patients with both Renal Disease and Gout

Feature	Renal disease antedating gout	Gout antedating renal disease
M:F	35:65	75:25
Onset of gout	40 years	40 years
Onset of renal disease	30 years	50 years
Gout antedating renal disease	—	10 years, 20+ attacks
Renal disease prior to gout	10 years	—
Attacks of gout	3	>50
Tophi present	5–10%	50%
Gout affecting upper limbs	10%	75%

disease has often been of a particularly chronic and slowly progressive variety. Fewer such patients develop tophi (2).

The differentiation between these two patterns is further complicated by two common associations of primary gout, namely, hypertension and hyperlipidemia. Both of these promote vascular disease and this can have adverse effects upon kidney structure and function. Since both gout and renal disease are very chronic conditions, it may be particularly difficult to elucidate the most important factor contributing to the renal disease in a particular patient. Several factors may be operating simultaneously. Nonetheless, if one is to understand a patient's problem and manage the patient rationally, it is important to decide whether primary gout or primary renal disease is the basic problem. Each of these possibilities will be considered in detail.

II. GOUT SECONDARY TO RENAL DISEASE

A. The Effect of Renal Disease on Urate Homeostasis

The serum urate in any individual at any particular time is determined by an interaction of genetic and environmental factors, the principal genetic factors being purine nucleotide degradation and the renal clearance of urate and the principal environmental determinants including the diet, alcohol consumption, adiposity, muscularity, and blood pressure (3).

A moderate degree of hyperuricemia is usually seen in the early stages of most chronic renal disease, although the rise is less than would be expected from the fall in the glomerular filtration rate (GFR) and less than that seen with other nitrogenous breakdown products. As the number of residual functional nephrons falls, there is a compensatory rise in the urate excretion per residual nephron and this minimizes the resultant hyperuricemia (1). Despite this, the total urate excretion by the kidney (which is normally two-thirds of the urate produced) falls as the glomerular filtration rate falls.

Active excretion of urate in the alimentary secretions is normally important in urate homeostasis and, as the renal route becomes less able to eliminate urate, excretion via the alimentary tract increases and may rise from the usual one-third until two-thirds of produced urate is eliminated by this route. When urate passes from the small bowel into the colon, it is degraded by colonic bacteria to CO_2 and ammonium (4). The effect of progressive renal disease on urate production has not been frequently documented; some results suggest that there is no change and others suggest that there is a modest fall. However, the important outcome is that, in most cases, the serum urate becomes only moderately increased as renal function deteriorates, and is rarely greater than 0.6 mmols/l (10 mg/dl) in chronic renal disease unless additional factors are operating.

With only a moderate degree of hyperuricemia occurring in most uncomplicated renal failure, the risk of gout will ultimately depend upon the severity of the hyperuricemia and its duration. Acute gout is not commonly a problem in patients with advanced chronic renal insufficiency. A study of patients on hemodialysis showed that only 7% had suffered from gout prior to the onset of renal disease and that gout was not a recurring problem during dialysis, despite only intermittent control of hyperuricemia (5). However, while there is little if any increase in the incidence of gout in chronic renal disease patients on dialysis in whom inflammatory responses might be expected to be diminished, the pattern is rather different when renal insufficiency is mild, as in some chronic nephropathies that are only very slowly progressive. Several of these have been associated with both disproportionate hyperuricemia and an increased prevalence of gout. In considering whether any hyperuricemia is disproportionate, it is important to realize that any plasma urate levels, particularly in the presence of renal disease, will be modified by the purine content of the diet, urine flow rate, blood pressure, plasma volume, and drug therapy. Gout may also be more common at an early rather than late stage of renal insufficiency. Each of these chronic nephropathies will be considered separately and the adequacy of the evidence supporting an etiological association will be discussed.

B. Primary Renal Disease Associated with an Increased Frequency of Hyperuricemia and Gout

1. Chronic Lead Nephropathy and Saturnine Gout

The best documented situation in which gout develops in patients with pre-existing renal disease occurs in chronic lead nephropathy where the gout is often referred to as saturnine gout. For any particular level of glomerular filtration, the serum urate in chronic lead nephropathy is higher than in other varieties of chronic renal disease of comparable severity (6). This prolonged hyperuricemia results in an increased frequency of gout so that half of the patients with chronic lead nephropathy ultimately develop recurrent acute gouty arthritis, sometimes with tophi. It is particularly important to emphasize that this type of renal disease results from a longstanding exposure to lead and not from an acute exposure of short duration. In addition, the renal disease that occurs is relatively stable and either nonprogressive or very slowly progressive, in part because of the lack of association with severe hypertension. The clinical pattern is almost as if a number of the nephrons had been lost in the episode of acute lead poisoning and the remaining nephrons had hypertrophied to adapt to the reduced numbers. In such a situation, the patient's renal function would have stabilized with this reduced number of nephrons. Studies of urate handling in such patients have shown a consistent reduction in the urate clearance of sufficient degree to account for the hyperuricemia. More detailed studies of the renal handling of urate by these kidneys have suggested that this is caused by an increased tubular reabsorption of urate. In those in whom the acute lead exposure occurred in childhood, the patients have often survived for up to 50 years after the original nephrotoxic episode, the duration of survival being in proportion to the degree of nephron loss (6).

In establishing a distinctive entity of chronic lead nephropathy, adequate documentation and epidemiological studies were necessary to demonstrate that the lead was etiological in the development of the renal disease and not merely an associated finding (7). Such documentation has been completed in relation to the chronic lead nephropathy that developed in children in Queensland, Australia, and also in relation to moonshine drinkers in the southern states of the United States (8). Suggestive similar data are being collected in relation to industrial exposure to lead (9).

In the 1890s, a large number of children in Queensland were diagnosed as suffering from acute lead poisoning, with the characteristic features of encephalopathy, neuropathy, and anemia with basophilic stippling and sometimes with encephalopathy. In the same community between 1910 and 1930, an increase was noted in the death rate from chronic renal failure in adolescents (7). These two observations were connected and the suggestion was made that the acute lead poisoning had produced renal damage, which became critical some 15–30 years later. In this particular community, which is subtropical, most of the houses had verandas surrounded by railings painted with lead paint where children would commonly play. The lead in the paint on these railings was therefore particularly accessible to children, who could inadvertently swallow the powdering paint or lick the moist paint after rain. Suggestive evidence that the acute lead poisoning was subsequently causing the chronic nephritis was backed up when legislation enacted in 1922 to exclude the use of lead paint in areas accessible to children was followed by a reduction in the frequency of lead poisoning.

Subsequently, the relationship was established unequivocally by a series of studies, the first of which followed up children who had been admitted to hospital with childhood lead poisoning, revealing a greatly increased mortality from chronic renal disease and hypertension (7). In addition, an increased mortality from "chronic nephritis" in the State of Queensland was demonstrated and shown to be attributable to a nephropathy in which the kidneys were granular and equally contracted, though without a specific pathology. In patients with these granular contracted kidneys, a regular association was established with an increased lead concentration in bone, leading to the reasonable deduction that lead was the etiological factor in this type of chronic renal disease (7). When the patients were seen at the stage of chronic renal disease, no lead exposure had occurred for 10 to 20 or more years and there were no residual signs of lead intoxication. However, there was an increase in the lead content of bone, which is in equilibrium with lead in soft tissues where it is accessible to chelation by ethylene-diamine-tetra-acetate (EDTA). Thus, despite the absence of continuing signs of lead intoxication, an increase in lead excretion after EDTA was able to demonstrate that remote but excessive past lead absorption had occurred (6).

A somewhat similar situation has been observed in the southern United States except that the lead ingestion there originated in illicit stills used for the production of "moonshine." Those who consumed the lead-contaminated moonshine would develop a chronic nephropathy with a high association with gout, the major difference from the Queensland situation being that there were continuing signs of lead intoxication in the form of disordered porphyrin metabolism and increased blood lead concentrations. Again, there was disproportionate hyperuricemia due to impaired renal elimination of urate resulting in a similar association with gout (8).

Lead exposure and absorption have long been a problem in the lead industries. Studies in lead workers in Paris in the 1960s frequently showed a chronic renal lesion, usually associated with hypertension and gout due to impaired renal excretion of urate. Adults are less susceptible to lead intoxication than children, and in this case the lead workers were often relatively asymptomatic despite their long continued but moderate degrees of excessive absorption of lead. In these cases, there was less opportunity for epidemiological follow-up to establish that lead was etiological. However, by analogy with the Queensland experience and the well-described situation with moonshine drinkers, there must be a strong suspicion that sufficient lead absorption in adult life may also lead to chronic renal disease and gout. In this case, it was rather more difficult to establish that the increased lead in the tissues was actually the cause of the associated renal disease. Excessive past lead absorption in lead workers, confirmed by the increase in lead excretion after EDTA, has provided further support for a relationship with subsequent chronic renal disease and gout (9). The renal histopathology is not pathognomonic, however, and exclusion of other varieties of chronic renal disease is necessary for diagnosis. Moreover, lead exposure in an industrially advanced country like the United States is usually much less than that seen in less-developed countries. In such countries with increased lead exposure and less close industrial supervision, there may well continue to be sufficient lead exposure to establish a connection between industrial lead exposure and chronic renal disease and gout.

2. Cystic Disease of the Kidneys

There are two varieties of inherited cystic disease of the kidney, commonly referred to as medullary cystic disease and polycystic disease of the kidneys, which have been reported to be associated with an increased degree of hyperuricemia and an increased prevalence of gout.

a. Medullary Cystic Disease

There have been several reports of families with gout and medullary cystic disease (nephronophthisis) with characteristic pathology. From these it is clear that renal glomerular function may be normal when there are histological changes of medullary cystic disease, and also that hyperuricemia and gout may antedate by several years clinical evidence of renal disease in the form of proteinuria and nitrogen retention (10). Thus, in choosing whether renal disease is a primary or secondary phenomenon in a particular patient, the decision may depend upon how hard one searches. The underlying condition progresses at the same rate whether or not gout develops. Thus, there is need for caution in patients with gout and renal disease in attributing the renal disease to gout when a specific alternative diagnosis cannot be established with certainty.

b. Polycystic Disease of the Kidneys

Gout has been reported in between 20% and 25% of two groups of patients with polycystic kidney disease (11). However, these were selected groups each of less than 20 patients and the overall prevalence of gout has not been documented in a larger group. Since hyperuricemia and gout may be more troublesome at a stage when renal insufficiency is mild rather than when it is severe, only a specific search for a past history of gout would give reliable information concerning the true prevalence.

However, an extensive study of urate handling in over 100 patients with adult polycystic disease did not demonstrate any difference in renal urate handling between patients with adult polycystic kidney disease and their relatives with comparable glomerular function when the creatinine clearance was greater than 80 mls per minute. The authors concluded that urate homeostasis was normal while renal function was normal, but that hyperuricemia due to reduced renal excretion of urate may develop as renal function worsens (12). This was similar to that seen in their control subjects. However, the authors did not record whether the patients with polycystic kidney disease had actually suffered from gouty arthritis. Accordingly, this large group does not throw further light upon the validity of the reported association of an increased prevalence of gout in patients with polycystic kidney disease.

3. Familial Nephropathies

There are now numerous reports from all continents of families with a primary tubulointerstitial type of nephritis with a dominant inheritance that is associated with an increased prevalence of hyperuricemia and gout. The frequency of these reports is now sufficient to provide clear evidence of a familial type of interstitial nephritis with gout comprising a distinct entity. As is common in all varieties of gout secondary to primary renal disease, there is a higher proportion of female involvement and a higher incidence in younger patients than is found in primary gout (13). Reports generally indicate that proteinuria is minimal, that hypertension is not a major feature and that the earliest manifestation of renal disease is loss of urine concentrating power. In most of these patients, the earliest symptom is of gout occurring at a young age at a time when renal insufficiency is only mild in degree. The renal disease could be overlooked unless sought and identified with care. The variety of these reports suggests that the renal disease may not be genetically or pathologically homogenous. However, there are sufficient similarities for them to constitute an important syndrome. Their frequency is such that they cannot be regarded as rare. In most of these families, the progression of the renal insufficiency is that of the underlying renal disease. Some have suggested that the rate of progression may be ameliorated by correction of the hyperuricemia, but this has not been the common experience.

4. Other Varieties of Tubulointerstitial Nephritis

There are other reports of renal disease associated with increased hyperuricemia and gout. Renal amyloidosis has been reported to be associated with gout, and in fact the extensive publication on the gouty kidney by Talbott and Terplan (14) included four patients with amyloid deposits in the glomeruli. This brings up the question of which came first. Other less well documented associations between gout and renal disease are with cystinuria, with bilateral hydronephrosis, and with analgesic nephropathy. What is common about these different varieties of renal disease is that they principally affect the renal tubule and are often categorized as tubulointerstitial varieties of renal disease.

C. Summary

Disproportionate hyperuricemia may be an early association of many varieties of tubulointerstitial renal disease, sometimes at a time when there is no clinical evidence of renal insufficiency. In most cases, it can be shown that the hyperuricemia is due to defective tubular excretion of uric acid. The resulting persistent hyperuricemia may, if it is of sufficient degree and duration, lead to the development of gout. In comparison with primary gout, gout secondary to renal disease is more common in the young and in females and usually shows only a mild degree of proteinuria and impairment of concentrating power as one of the first manifestations. The progression of the renal disease is usually quite slow, but it is the same whether the gout is present or not. Although the associated hyperuricemia and gout may be corrected by the administration of allopurinol, this does not usually alter the rate of progression of the renal disease. Thus, in any patient with both gout and renal disease, it is important to consider the possibility that renal disease may be the primary lesion and the gout a secondary development. The history may be helpful in determining which is the primary disease, but detailed investigation of renal structure and function may be necessary to demonstrate the early changes of some varieties of primary renal disease.

III. KIDNEY DISEASE SECONDARY TO GOUT

Gout is a clinical syndrome due to the acute inflammatory response to the formation of monosodium urate monohydrate (MSUM, or urate) crystals. While hyperuricemia is almost invariably present in gout, no pathological or clinical features have been shown to be secondary to hyperuricemia unless urate crystals have been formed. Supersaturation of urate exists at the site of crystal formation, and the adverse effects of hyperuricemia occur only if urate (MSUM) crystals form. We must now examine whether these general observations apply specifically to relationships between gout and the kidney.

The factors which cause hyperuricemia in any individual vary considerably, with different factors operating to different degrees in different patients (3). The serum urate always represents a balance between the production of urate and its elimination from the body. The amount of urate produced in the body depends upon nucleic acid turnover. In particular, the degradation of adenine nucleotides, which normally undergo a dynamic process of utilization and regeneration, is an important contributor to the amount of urate that is produced by the body. In comparison, urate excretion by the kidney also ranges widely and the urate clearance in normal subjects can range between 6 and 15 mls per minute. The renal handling of urate has a high degree of heritability (15) and the ultimate urate concentration in the plasma (and accordingly in the tissues) will reflect the balance between production and renal elimination. Thus, patients who have principally a defect in control of urate production and are thereby overproducers of urate will tend to have very high concentrations of urate in the urine, whereas those whose hyperuricemia is principally due to a defect in elimination of urate by an otherwise healthy kidney will tend to have low urate concentrations in the urine (16). Most gouty patients will have the combination of a high contribution to urate production from dietary purines and a poor renal ability to eliminate urate.

At any particular site, the tendency for urate to crystallize will depend upon local factors. Accordingly, the concentration of urate at a particular site in the kidney will be important in determining the tendency for urate crystallization at that site. Urate is more soluble in an alkaline fluid. However, at a pH of 5.5, as occurs in the collecting ducts, half of the urate is present in the form of uric acid. As the urine becomes increasingly acidic and concentrated, there is an increasing risk of formation of crystals of uric acid within the tubular fluid (Figure 1). The kidney is the only place in the body where the pH is sufficiently low for crystals of uric acid to form. It is important to note that the increasing concentration gradient of sodium, water, and urea towards the renal papilla also applies to urate concentrations, so that the concentration of urate in the papilla is considerably higher than that in the cortex. Thus, crystals of both urate (acicular in shape) and of uric acid (amorphous in shape) may

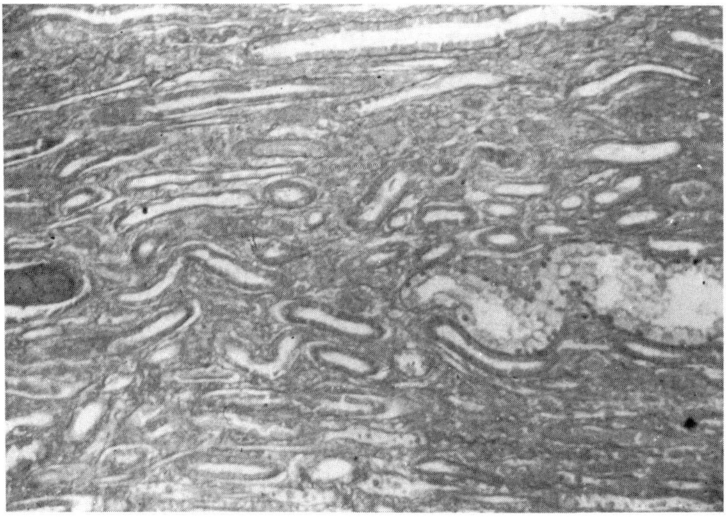

FIGURE 1 Renal medulla from a patient with renal disease caused by primary urate overproduction due to HGPRT deficiency. An intraluminal cast, stained black for uric acid, appears to be filling a collecting duct.

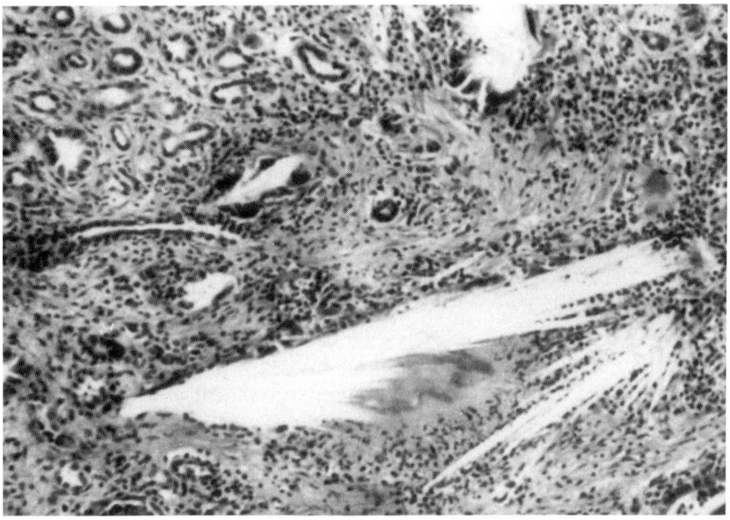

FIGURE 2 Acicular urate crystals with surrounding giant cell reaction forming an interstitial microtophus in the kidney of the same patient with primary urate overproduction due to HGPRT deficiency.

be demonstrated within the kidney and each may contribute to the pathology (17). Urate crystals characteristically form interstitial microtophi and these may develop insidiously depending upon local factors including the urate concentration (Figure 2). Uric acid crystals, by contrast, characteristically develop acutely in an intraluminal site where they may cause tubular obstruction, which is potentially reversible (16,18). There is also a strong suggestion that tubular lining cells may phagocytose these crystals (18) and that some crystals may also pass through the tubular epithelium where they can form a nidus for microtophus formation.

Patients with gout will have different degrees of hyperuricemia and it should not be expected that a uniform pattern of renal disease will be seen in patients who have suffered at some time from an attack of gout. It is also important to remember that the same varieties of renal disease can develop in patients with gout as develop in patients who have never suffered from gout. However, this chapter will particularly emphasize any renal consequences due to gout rather than only associated with it.

B. The Association Between Gout and Renal Disease over the Centuries

Just as the frequency and severity of gout in populations has changed over the years, so has the frequency of association between gout and renal disease. Eighteenth century reports include those of Scudamore, who emphasized the frequency of proteinuria in gouty patients, and of Castelneau, who described uric acid deposits within the kidney parenchyma similar to those seen in the joints. The "gouty kidney" was described by Todd in 1857 as "a contracted state of the kidney particularly apt to be developed in the inveterate gouty diathesis." He reported the "opaque streaks of lithate of soda, taking the directions of the tubules," whereas Charcot and Cornil reported the deposition between the tubules of needle-shaped crystals, as well as the presence of amorphous urates producing obstruction within the tubules. Garrod in 1876 regarded the interstitial crystalline deposits of urate as specific for gout and reported their presence in the uniformally contracted kidneys of "all cases of chronic chalk gout when the opportunity of making the examination was afforded."

In the first half of this century, renal disease was reportedly common in gout, affecting 30–50% of patients. One of the earliest signs of renal damage was the inability to concentrate the urine. In addition, hypertension was noted in up to half of the patients at a time when renal impairment was only moderate in degree. Medullary urate deposits, together with a foreign body giant cell reaction, were a common finding. There were also features of vascular nephrosclerosis. In some, advanced renal failure would develop. The most extensive pathological survey of the kidney in patients with gout was reported in 1960 by Talbott and Terplan, who regarded the formation of urate crystals and the surrounding giant cell inflammatory reaction as the distinctive pathological feature (14).

At about this time, effective drug treatment for hyperuricemia became available, which enabled the underlying hyperuricemia to be corrected and reduced the tendency to urate crystal deposition. In patients who were able to be rendered normouricemic, the pattern of the disease changed quite markedly, with the pathological changes being found only at later ages and then consisting principally of vascular and hypertensive disease. However, even as late as 1970, Graham and Scott reported renal insufficiency in 25% of a large group and hypertension in 50% (19). In particular, they found a positive correlation between the presence of tophi and impairment of renal function, and this is consistent with a role for urate crystals and renal tophi in the formation of the associated nephropathy. By this time, critical renal insufficiency was rarely seen until after middle age and was uncommon in patients with gout in countries with advanced systems of medical care. Such patients also commonly exhibited Type IV hyperlipoproteinemia, hypertension, and obesity, all of which can also be risk factors for vascular disease that can cause renal insufficiency.

Extensive studies of renal function in gouty patients were undertaken by Yu and Berger between 1960 and 1982 in New York (20). They found little adverse effect from gout on renal function except in fulminant cases or neglected cases with long standing extensive tophaceous deposits. They also confirmed a correlation between the presence of tophi and reduced glomular filtration rate. In this large group of patients, they attributed most of the renal disease to the association with vascular disease and hypertension or with calculi and pyelonephritis. Fessel (21) also followed patients in the United States and confirmed that renal insufficiency was rarely a problem in gout unless hyperuricemia was persistently severe (>10–13 mg/dl).

However, recent reports from areas with less sophisticated medical care have confirmed that, when a group with gout is compared with a nongouty control group, renal function may still be impaired and more severely impaired in patients with clinical tophi (22). A high incidence of associated hypertension and a further decline in renal function in those gouty patients who also suffered from hypertension was also noted in these Taiwanese patients. As far as the nature of the underlying renal insufficiency is concerned, they found, in almost all of their patients with tophaceous gout, the presence of kidneys of reduced size containing highly echogenic lesions scattered in the corticomedullary junctions of both kidneys consistent with the pathology that they found, namely the presence of crystals surrounded by a urate granuloma with foreign body giant cells, together with interstitial fibrosis and vascular changes.

The possibility needs to be considered that hypertension may be an early manifestation of an adverse effect on the kidney from gout, but idiopathic hypertension is so common that it has not been possible to demonstrate any unequivocal evidence that the hypertension that may develop early in gouty patients is of renal origin. Although renal disease due to gout is now a very uncommon development in patients whose hyperuricemia and hyperuricosuria is well controlled by medical treatment, it needs to be remembered that the potential to cause renal damage still exists as long as the potential for urate crystal deposition remains.

C. Pathology and Pathogenesis of the Renal Disease of Primary Gout

The evidence from observations over the years, and more recently using sophisticated techniques in selected populations, has suggested that the initial lesion causing renal disease in patients with gout is the formation of crystals either of urate (MSUM) or of uric acid (Figure 3). It suggests that urate deposited within the renal interstitium is in the form of monosodium urate monohydrate (MSUM), and this can induce an inflammatory response with the formation of interstitial microtophi (Figure 2); their formation will depend upon the local conditions involving urate concentration and pH at a particular site in the renal interstitial tissues. By contrast, the formation of uric acid crystals, which are usually amorphous, occurs within the lumen of the renal tubules and depends principally upon the concentration of uric acid within the tubular fluid and its tendency to precipitate at an acid pH (Figure 1). There is suggestive evidence that uric acid crystals can pass from an intraluminal site into an interstitial site and thereby form a nidus for epitaxial formation of further urate crystals. Either because of this or associated with it, the patient devel-

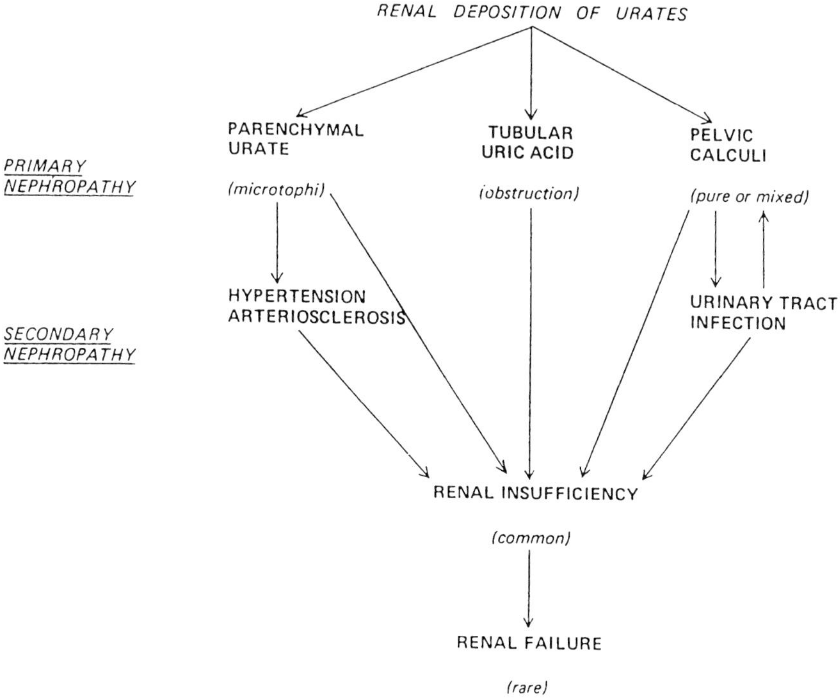

FIGURE 3 Mechanisms by which urate deposition within the kidney may produce renal disease. From Emmerson B. Gout, uric acid and renal disease. *MJA* 1976; I; 403–405. Copyright © 1976. *The Medical Journal of Australia*, reproduced with permission.

ops hypertension which, if it is not controlled, will promote the changes of a vascular and hypertensive nephropathy. Associated with this, renal calculi can occur and these may induce secondary renal injury of moderate degree related either to infection or obstruction. If the causes are effectively treated, this does not tend to progress. If severe hyperuricemia or hyperuricosuria, or hypertension and vascular disease, or urinary infection are allowed to persist, a critical degree of renal failure may develop. However, this is uncommon with effective treatment.

D. What Evidence Is There that Uric Acid can Cause an Acute Uric Acid Nephropathy (Hyperuricosuric Nephropathy)?

1. Evidence in Humans

The difficulty of documenting renal pathology secondary to gout is easier if there is clear evidence of a clinical situation where the urate abnormality is the primary phenomenon and any renal disease secondary. Urate overproduction is one primary state that can result in an acute deterioration of renal function (referred to as an acute uric acid nephropathy) (23). This condition is potentially reversible because it is due to the deposition of uric acid crystals in the collecting tubules, resulting in an obstructive nephropathy. Its development is always associated with a high uric acid concentration in the urine, often detected by a urinary uric acid/creatinine concentration ratio of greater than 1 (if expressed as in milligrams percent) or greater than 0.66 (if expressed in mmols per liter). If this type of nephropathy is not rapidly reversed by an alkaline diuresis, chronic renal damage can supervene. It is recognized in several clinical situations.

a. *Leukemias, Lymphomas, and Tumor Lysis from Chemotherapy*

In all of these conditions, there is greatly increased purine catabolism that results in severe overproduction of uric acid leading to a greatly increased excretion of urate in the urine (18,23). In these situations, there may be massive intrarenal and often ureteric deposits of urate and uric acid crystals, particularly in the collecting ducts of the kidney. This causes an obstructive nephropathy with superimposed acute tubular necrosis and inflammatory cell infiltration of the interstitium. It is usually prevented or reversed by the use of prophylactic allopurinol and the maintenance of an alkaline diuresis. Mannitol may be added if the diuresis is not adequate. If allopurinol is used, initial doses can be high (up to 600 mg a day), with a reduction as renal function stabilizes.

b. *Other Causes of a High Urinary Urate Concentration*

Potent uricosuric drugs, such as sulphinpyrazone, can cause a considerable increase in urate concentration in tubular fluid and urine during the phase of initiation of treatment. If the urine is concentrated or particularly acid at this time, the high urate concentration in tubular fluid can cause uric acid crystallization to occur and an episode of acute renal insufficiency. If recognized, this is readily reversible. Although rarely recognized by physicians, it has been reported that 20% of patients who present to a urologist with bilateral urinary tract obstruction have been receiving uricosuric therapy at the time.

In addition, some patients with renal hypouricemia due to failure of urate reabsorption in the tubules have a very high urate clearance and urinary urate excretion and have been reported to develop an acute uric acid nephropathy (24). This acute renal failure may be triggered by a transient decrease in fluid intake or increase in hydrogen ion excretion. This is a clear case where hyperuricosuria is present in the absence of hyperuricemia and illustrates the importance of the high uric acid concentration in the tubular fluid in inducing pathology. Similar nephropathies are also recognized with other types of crystals, most notably that caused by the even more insoluble 2,8 dihydroxyadenine, which is excreted in increased amounts in the severe deficiency of adenine phosphoribosyl transferase.

c. *Hypoxanthine Guanine Phosphoribosyltransferase (HGPRT) Deficiency*

Mutations of this purine reutilization enzyme result in severe urate overproduction from birth. Patients with these mutations initially have very high urine uric acid excretions and, while the kidney can excrete this large amount of produced urate, the patient may have a normal serum urate concentration (16). However, with time, some degree of renal insufficiency usually develops and the serum urate becomes elevated. In these patients it is clear that the urate abnormality is primary and any renal disease is secondary. Episodes of potentially reversible deterioration of renal function, often subclinical, may occur. Pathologically the crystals that are found are both uric acid and urate (MSUM). The development of renal insufficiency in such urate overproducers is not uniform or predictable and is consistent with an intermittent process promoting crystal formation within tubular fluid. With the development of renal disease, there is a steady rise in the serum urate concentration and a reduction in the excretion of urate in the urine. This is explicable pathologically by the intratubular deposits of uric acid crystals, its reversibility by an alkaline diuresis, by its prevention with allopurinol, and by the recognition of a crystal nephropathy on ultrasound where there may be an increase in echogenicity in the medullary pyramids and collecting ducts. Recognition that a primary abnormality of urate metabolism can lead to renal insufficiency has greatly strengthened our understanding of the role of uric acid crystals in the genesis of this nephropathy and has also placed emphasis upon the importance of the uric acid concentration in the tubular fluid and collecting ducts.

d. *Medullary Microtophi*

A number of autopsy reports have described the occasional presence of minute medullary microtophi in the renal medulla. These contain urate crystals and constitute a cellular reaction as in a classical microtophus. As well as in some patients with gout, they are also seen in patients with renal insufficiency, and sometimes in patients with no other disease who died from trauma (25). There is a suggestion that they occur less commonly in patients with diabetes who might have polyuria. Considerable more study needs to devoted to these to explain them fully. However, current observation suggests that uric acid can sometimes crystallize from any sufficiently concentrated or acid urine in the renal medulla and cause an inflammatory response. This emphasizes that there are still many aspects relating to uric acid and the kidney that are not yet fully elucidated.

2. Animal Studies of Renal Damage from Urate

Because they possess a functional uricase, most animals do not have a significant urate concentration in their tissues and are not useful models to study the effect of uric acid in inducing renal disease. However, two recent developments have provided us with useful animal models. The first involves the use of the uricase inhibitor oxonic acid that, when given with dietary supplements of uric acid, can induce renal disease with uric acid deposits (26). The other is the development of a mutation in the urate oxidase gene in rats that can lead to hyperuricemia and an obstructive nephropathy. In all cases, the renal pathology is reminiscent of that in the urate overproduction due to tumor lysis or HGPRT deficiency in humans. Macroscopically there are yellow accumulations within the medulla corresponding to the collecting ducts that contain negatively birefringent crystals. The intraluminal crystalline deposits produce an obstructive nephropathy and an increased urate concentration is found in renal tissues. Again, crystals cause damage to tubular lining cells, especially of the collecting ducts, which is followed by interstitial fibrosis, acute tubular necrosis, and abnormalities in the renal vasculature, thereby providing a useful model of the effect of excessive urate production upon renal structure and function. This model has confirmed two aspects relevant to the crystal hypothesis in that the lesions are prevented or reversed by a high urine flow rate and also that the administration of salicylate to the animals greatly lessens the inflammatory cellular response (26).

3. In Vitro Studies of the Reaction Between Urate Crystals and Cultured Renal Tubular Cells

Canine kidney cells in culture (MDCK) exhibit many of the characteristics of the epithelium of the collecting ducts and these cells react with MSUM crystals. The cell membrane reacts with the crystals and phagocytosis occurs with the formation of a phagolysosome and ultimately enzyme release from the cell (27). Crystals are found not only within the cells but also within the intercellular spaces. These in vitro studies support the hypothesis that some of the interstitial deposits of urate/uric acid in the kidney may originate in intratubular deposits that react with the tubular epithelium or pass into the interstitial tissues. They therefore provide in vitro support for the hypothesis of the importance of the urate concentration within the renal tubular lumen in causing crystal formation at that site, with the crystals then passing to the renal interstitium and inducing an inflammatory response in the process.

E. Synthesis

The important aspects of uric acid in causing renal disease, both acute and chronic, include a component of reversible obstruction of collecting ducts by urate/uric acid crystals, which lead to inflammation, transfer of crystals to the renal interstitium, and the development of chronic interstitial nephritis with microtophi. Secondary effects may cause glomerular scarring. The crystals may either originate within the renal tubule or the interstitium, or may migrate from the lumen to the interstitial site. To these must be added the adverse effects of uric acid calculi and the associated effects on the kidney of hypertension and vascular disease occurring independently or as a sequel to the renal damage (Figure 3).

IV. URIC ACID CALCULI

Uric acid calculi occur at some time in about 20% of patients with gout, sometimes antedating the first attack (28). However, only 25% of patients with uric acid calculi suffer from gout. This is because the risk of calculi depends upon conditions in the urine whereas the risk of gout depends upon the urate concentration in the serum and tissues. Pure urate stones are radiolucent and comprise up to 10% of all renal calculi. Bladder stones, which are rare in developed countries, often consist of ammonium urate and now occur principally in malnourished children in tropical countries. Calcium oxalate calculi may also be associated with a high urinary uric acid excretion, especially if hypercalciuria is also present. Such calculi are radio-opaque. Correction of the hyperuricosuria with allopurinol can prevent such calcium oxalate calculi (29).

A. Solubility of Urate and Uric Acid

Uric acid is least soluble in an acid urine and, as the pH falls, urine can become supersaturated. The solubility is greatly enhanced at pH values greater than 7.

B. Factors Contributing to Uric Acid Calculi

The factors determining uric acid calculus formation depend upon the urine becoming supersaturated with regard to uric acid and also upon the urine pH, so that any cause of a persistently acid urine will promote the formation of uric acid calculi. In addition, the presence of inhibitors of crystallization, including citrate and glycosaminoglycans, may have an important role in their prevention. Supersaturation of urine with urate will depend upon both the amount of urate being excreted and upon the urine volume (30).

1. Urate Excretion

In a balanced state, urinary urate excretion reflects urate production and this depends upon both intrinsic urate production and urate derived from the diet.

Intrinsic or genetic urate overproduction will occur in HGPRT deficiency or when there is an increase in nucleoprotein turnover as in a malignancy. Infants with primary urate overproduction due to HPRT deficiency may present with yellow/orange gravel on their diapers, consisting of pure uric acid. Conversely, a high urine urate derived from diet may occur from the consumption of moderate amounts of high purine foods (such as meat and yeast) or from the consumption of large amounts of moderate purine foods. Ethanol will also increase urate production. So important has dietary nucleoprotein consumption become in patients with calculi and high urinary urate excretions that some affected patients have been referred to as "purine gluttons" (29). A high urinary urate may be associated with a normal serum urate, so that the presence of a normal serum urate has no reflection upon whether a calculus is uric acid or not. Conversely, the presence of hyperuricemia does not necessarily suggest that an associated calculus consists of uric acid.

2. Urine Volume

The urine volume depends upon a number of factors including fluid intake and fluid loss from evaporation, which is increased by exercise, climate, or a raised temperature. In chronic diarrheal states such as post-ileostomy, dehydration can occur, which will give a more concentrated urine.

3. Urine pH

Some patients with gout and uric acid calculi are thought to have a reduction in ammonia production by the kidney that results in a persistently lower urine pH. It has not yet been definitely established whether this is a primary phenomenon or is secondary to renal damage. Systemic acidosis in chronic diarrhoeal states can lead to both a concentrated urine and lowered urinary pH, both predisposing to uric acid calculi.

C. Management

Examination of a 24-hr urine specimen is usually rewarding in elucidating the cause of a uric acid calculus in a particular patient. This can provide information about the urine flow rate, urinary urate concentration and excretion, and the urate and creatinine clearances on the patient's normal diet. The pH may need to be examined on each specimen of urine passed throughout the 24-hr period. A poor urine volume may be increased by sufficient fluid intake with the aim at excreting 2 l per day. A high urinary urate may be amenable to a reduction in dietary purines. A consistently acid urine may be corrected by the addition of potassium citrate. If the problem is persistent, the administration of regular allopurinol will correct hyperuricosuria (29,30) and would be of particular value if the 24-hr urinary urate excretion on the usual diet exceeds 5 mmols or 850 mg per day. This will reduce urate production and, if tolerated and acceptable, should prevent the formation of further uric acid calculi.

REFERENCES

1. R. E. Rieselbach and T. H. Steele. Intrinsic renal disease leading to abnormal urate excretion, *Nephron 14*:81 (1975).
2. B. T. Emmerson, P. J. Stride, and G. Williams. The clinical differentiation of primary gout from primary renal disease in patients with both gout and renal disease, *Adv Exp Med Biol 122A*:9 (1980).
3. B. T. Emmerson. Identification of the causes of persistent hyperuricemia, *Lancet 337*:1461 (1991).
4. L. B. Sorensen. Gout secondary to chronic renal disease: studies on urate metabolism, *Ann Rheum Dis 39*:424 (1980).
5. O. Ifudu, C. C. Tan, A. L. Dulin, B. G. Delano, and E. A. Friedman. Gouty arthritis in end-stage renal disease: Clinical course and rarity of new cases, *Am J Kidney Dis 23*:347 (1994).
6. B. T. Emmerson. Chronic lead nephropathy, *Kidney Int 4*:1 (1973).
7. D. A. Henderson. The aetiology of chronic nephritis in Queensland, *Med J Aust 1*:377 (1958).
8. G. V. Ball and L. B. Sorensen. Pathogenesis of hyperuricemia in saturnine gout, *New Engl J Med 280*:1199 (1968).
9. V. Batuman, J. K. Maesaka, B. Haddad, E. Tepper, E. Landy, and R. P. Wedeen. The role of lead in gout nephropathy, *New Engl J Med 304*:520 (1981).
10. J. R. Burke, J. A. Inglis, P. W. Craswell, K. R. Mitchell, and B. T. Emmerson. Juvenile nephronophthisis and medullary cystic disease—the same disease (report of a large family with medullary cystic disease associated with gout and epilepsy), *Clin Nephrol 18*:1 (1982).
11. E. Mejias, J. Navas, R. Lluberes, and M. Martinez-Maldonado. Hyperuricemia, gout and autosomal dominant polycystic kidney disease, *Am J Med Sci 297*:145 (1989).
12. W. D. Kaehny, D. J. Tangel, A. M. Johnson, W. J. Kimberling, R. W. Schrier, and P. A. Gabow. Uric acid handling in autosomal dominant polycystic kidney disease with normal filtration rates, *Am J Med 89*:49 (1990).
13. G. Calabrese, H. A. Simmonds, J. S. Cameron, and P. M. Davies. Precocious familial gout with reduced fractional urate clearance and normal purine enzymes, *Q J Med 277*:441 (1990).
14. J. H. Talbott and K. L. Terplan. The kidney in gout, *Medicine (Balt) 39*:405 (1960).
15. B. T. Emmerson, S. L. Nagel, D. L. Duffy, and N. G. Martin. Genetic control of the renal clearance of urate: A study of twins, *Ann Rheum Dis 51*:375 (1992).
16. B. T. Emmerson and P. G. Row. An evaluation of the pathogenesis of the gouty kidney, *Kidney Int 8*:65 (1975).

17. J. E. Seegmiller and P. D. Frazier. Biochemical considerations in the renal damage of gout, *Ann Rheum Dis 25*:668 (1966).
18. Y. S. Kanwar and J. R. Manaligod. Leukemic urate nephropathy, *Arch Pathol 99*:467 (1975).
19. R. Grahame and J. T. Scott. Clinical survey of 354 patients with gout, *Ann Rheum Dis 29*:461 (1970).
20. T. Yu and L. Berger. Impaired renal function in gout, *Am J Med 72*:95 (1982).
21. W. J. Fessel. Renal outcomes of gout and hyperuricemia, *Am J Med 67*:74 (1979).
22. D. Tarng, H. Lin, M. Shyong, J. Wang, W. Yang, and T. Huang. Renal function in gout patients, *Am J Nephrol 15*:31 (1995).
23. J. D. Conger. Acute uric acid nephropathy, *Med Clin North Am 74*:859 (1990).
24. C. M. M. Erley, R. R. Hirschberg, W. Hoefer, and K. Schaefer. Acute renal failure due to uric acid nephropathy in a patient with renal hypouricemia, *Klin Wochenschr 67*:308 (1989).
25. J. W. Linnane, A. F. Burry, and B. T. Emmerson. Urate deposits in the renal medulla—prevalence and associations, *Nephron 29*:216 (1981).
26. R. Bluestone, J. Waisman, and J. R. Klinenberg. The gouty kidney, *Semin Arth Rheum 7*:97 (1977).
27. B. T. Emmerson, M. Cross, J. M. Osborne, and R. A. Axelsen. Ultrastructural studies of the reaction of urate crystals with a cultured renal tubular cell line, *Nephron 59*:403 (1991).
28. T. Yu. Urolithiasis in hyperuricemia and gout, *J Urol 126*:424 (1981).
29. F. L. Coe. Uric acid and calcium oxalate nephrolithiasis, *Kidney Int 24*:392 (1983).
30. A. W. Williams-Larson. Urinary calculi associated with purine metabolism—uric acid nephrolithiasis, *Endocrinol Metab Clin North Am 19*:821 (1990).

18
Radiologic Manifestations of Gout

DANIEL S. URI
Mecklenburg Radiology Associates, Presbyterian Orthopedic Hospital, Charlotte, North Carolina

WILLIAM MARTEL
University of Michigan Hospital, Ann Arbor, Michigan

I. INTRODUCTION

The diagnosis of gout is frequently straightforward when typical clinical symptoms are present and characteristic crystals are recovered from affected tissues. Not infrequently, however, patients present with atypical signs and symptoms that may lead to difficulty in diagnosis. Patients in whom acute arthritic episodes were not present, or in whom they were subclinical and missed, may present with tophaceous deposits at the "onset" of the disease (1–4). Accelerated tophus formation may be found in some transplant recipients and, though uncommonly, tophaceous gout occurs in children (5,6). Radiologic examination can be helpful in the exclusion of those disorders that may be confused clinically with gout, and can be a valuable aid in the initial diagnosis. Furthermore, radiological studies provide a baseline for comparison during the course of the disease and can assist in the evaluation of the effectiveness of therapy.

II. ACUTE GOUT

The acute stage of gout is typically monoarticular with a predilection for the first metatarsophalangeal joint. However, the disease may first present with polyarticular manifestations and need not involve the first metatasophalangeal articulation at all; such "sparing" is more common in women (7). Radiographs are often "normal" in the acute arthropathy but commonly there is periarticular, nonspecific soft-tissue swelling and joint effusion (8). Hyperemia or disuse sometimes causes osteopenia. There are usually no bone erosions and the articular cartilage space is often normal. Symptoms usually last a few days, after which nonspecific soft-tissue swelling and effusion typically resolve. The initial episode of acute arthritis sometimes follows trauma or a major surgical procedure (9).

III. CHRONIC TOPHACEOUS GOUT

A. Distribution of Arthritis and Tophaceous Deposits

There is a distinct predilection for peripheral extremity involvement, particularly joints in the foot, hand, wrist, and elbow. A characteristic site of arthritis in the

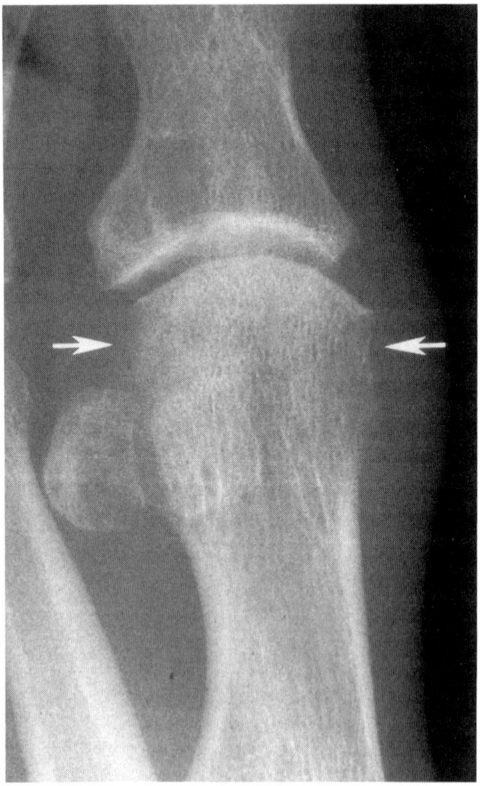

FIGURE 1 Two rarefactions, presumably secondary to subchondral tophi, are present in the lateral aspect of the proximal phalanx of the first metatarsophalangeal joint. Note marginal erosions of the metatarsal head (arrows). The thickness of the joint space is normal. (From Ref. 13.)

foot is the first digit, where soft-tissue swelling and bone erosion in the metatarsophalangeal joint is most common (1) (Figure 1). These erosions tend to affect the medial and dorsal margins of the first metatarsal head (10). Interphalangeal and tarsometatarsal involvement is not atypical; the ankle is often affected when widespread disease involves other joints of the foot.

In the hand virtually any joint may be affected, although there is a propensity for interphalangeal and carpal locations (Figure 2). Ulnar deviation of some digits and scapholunate diastasis may simulate rheumatoid arthritis, but the asymmetric distribution of involvement and the soft-tissue features allow for their distinction. Marginal (juxtachondral) erosions about the knee may occur in femorotibial and patellofemoral joint compartments. Inflammation of the prepatellar bursa and tophaceous deposits are common and patellar erosion may occur. Popliteal cyst formation and rupture of the quadriceps tendon have been described; however, their association with gout is somewhat tenuous. Olecranon bursal inflammation with associated soft-tissue swelling is common and adjacent osseous erosion is frequently present (11) (Figure 3). Tophaceous gout may be superimposed on osteoarthritis of the terminal interphalangeal

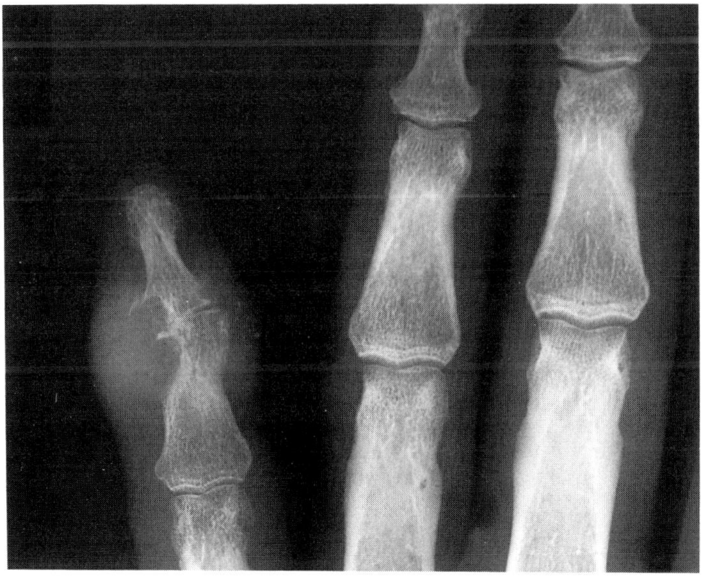

FIGURE 2 Eccentric soft-tissue swelling caused by tophus with contiguous bone erosions associated with an "overhanging edge." The increased density of the tophus suggests that it contains calcium.

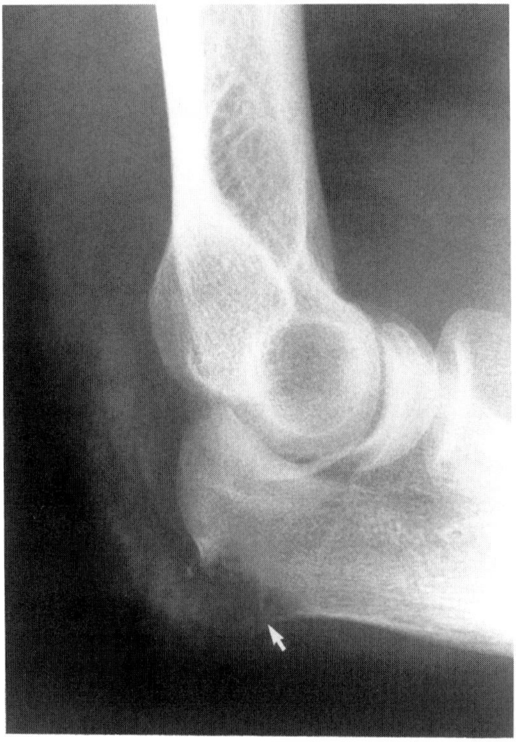

FIGURE 3 Amorphous calcification in tophus at the extensor aspect of the elbow associated with contiguous bone erosion of olecranon (arrow).

joints in keeping with a presumed predilection for previously "damaged" tissues (Figure 4).

Tophi are most frequently found within synovium, subchondral bone, tendon, and subcutaneous soft tissues. Tophaceous deposition, like articular involvement, tends to be appendicular with an asymmetric distribution. Deposits are typically nodular in appearance and radiographs frequently depict tophi as areas of increased density relative to adjacent soft tissues (Figure 2). This may be subtle if finely divided calcification is present or conspicuous if more coarse calcific deposits occur (Figure 5). The nature of the calcium salt accompanying monosodium urate in these cases is not definitely known though it could be calcium hydroxyapatite (H. Schumacher, personal communication). Periarticular soft-tissue swelling may also be due to bursal inflammation, which is most often

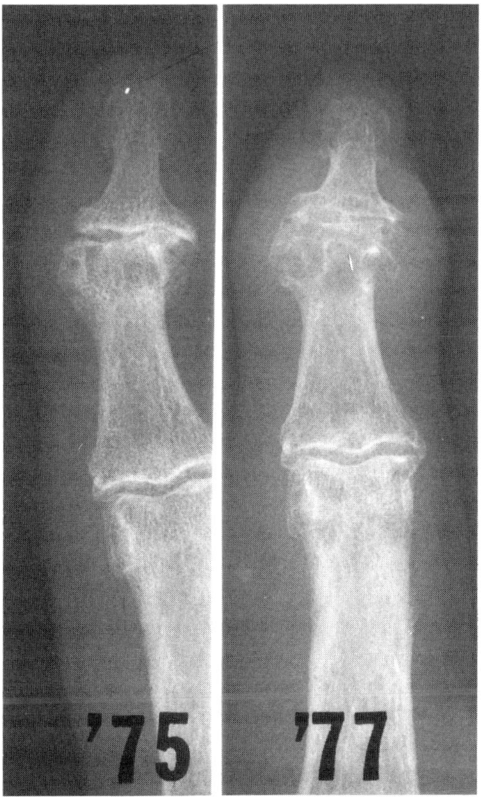

FIGURE 4 Tophaceous gout developing in a joint previously affected by erosive osteoarthritis.

prepatellar or near the olecranon; tophi are frequently nearby, as are bony erosions (Figure 3).

B. Articular Cartilage Spaces

Polyarticular involvement is common and typically asymmetric. The articular cartilage space is usually preserved until late in the disease, at which time uniform narrowing may develop, simulating an inflammatory arthritis (e.g., rheumatoid arthritis) (Figure 6a). In other cases, cartilage destruction may later be followed by secondary degenerative joint disease leading to nonuniform articular cartilage narrowing (12) (Figure 6b). A normal joint-space width in the presence of numer-

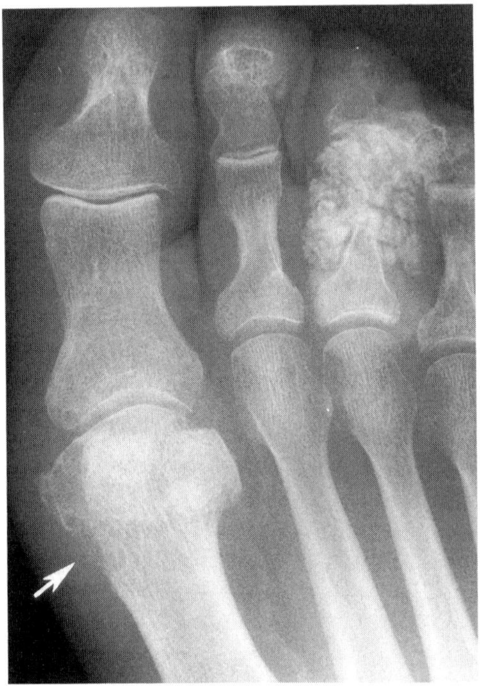

FIGURE 5 Floccular calcification in a tophus of the third toe, with severe erosion of the proximal phalanx. A smaller erosion is present on the medial surface of the first metatarsal head. (From Ref. 13.)

ous erosions is a characteristic feature of gout. The deposition of monosodium urate within subchondral locations may lead to structural weakening, microfracture, and ultimately osteochondral compression resulting in a "cupping" deformity (13). Late in the disease, destruction of cartilage and subchondral bone may be severe, leading to secondary degenerative changes, subluxation, or arthritis mutilans (Figure 7). Joint obliteration with ankylosis may occur but is rare (14).

The significance of chondrocalcinosis in gout is controversial and there are conflicting views regarding this finding. When present in gout, it tends to be restricted to fibrocartilagenous structures, especially in the knee and wrist. To the extent that such chondrocalcinosis is common in the elderly, it may be a coincidental finding and unrelated to gout. Widespread chondrocalcinosis or involvement of hyaline cartilage is distinctly unusual and probably indicates the coexistence of calcium pyrophophate–related arthropathy.

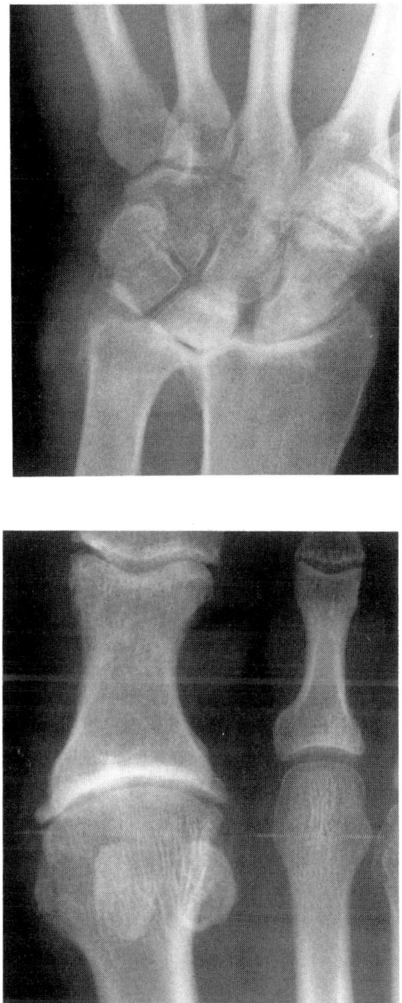

FIGURE 6 Gout in the foot and wrist. (a) Nonspecific uniform loss of cartilage space in the first metatarsal-phalangeal joint associated with marginal osteophytes secondary to longstanding gout and prior episodes of gouty inflammation in this joint. (b) Uniform loss of cartilage space and subchondral sclerosis in radiocarpal joint with scapholunate separation, secondary to tophaceous gout. Note dense tophus lateral to ulna and prominence ("mushrooming") of the ulnar styloid process.

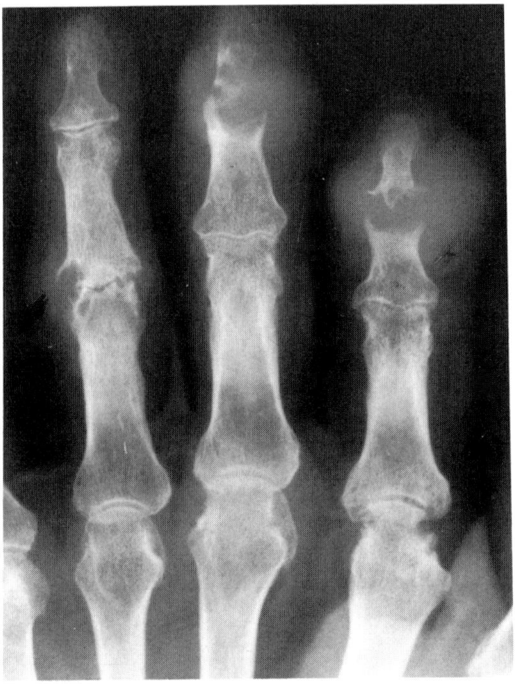

FIGURE 7 Chronic arthritis of multiple joints with a characteristic overhanging edge (arrow). There are massive intra-articular tophi in the terminal interphalangeal joints associated with extensive bone erosion. Note juxtachondral bone erosions in second metacarpophalangeal joint, similar to those seen in rheumatoid arthritis.

C. Osseous Erosions

The preservation of normal bone mineralization is common in the early phase of chronic gout. In advanced disease, osteopenia may develop following disuse. Bone erosions may be marginal ("bare areas") or juxtachondral and simulate the pattern of erosion found in inflammatory diseases such as rheumatoid arthritis (12) (Figure 7). This may be due to chronic synovitis associated with the urate arthropathy. Such erosions may have a somewhat sclerotic margin, giving them a well-defined appearance.

Intraosseous tophi formation and bone resorption may result in a subchondral cyst-like appearance (Figure 1). When prominent, intraosseous tophi may result in osteolytic lesions that have an aggressive appearance simulating neoplastic disease (15,16). These lesions predominate in lower extremity locations, particularly the patella, where they are typically superolateral and adjacent to a discernable soft-tissue tophus. Lesions are sharply marginated and often round or oval in shape. They may be oriented along the long axis of the bone and are frequently subchondral in location. Although intraosseous tophi, like their soft-tissue counterparts, may become calcified, this is uncommon. These calcified tophi predominate in the hands and feet, and may simulate osteonecrosis or enchondroma (17).

Osseous erosions may also be para-articular in location and are due to adjacent tophi. The erosions in tophaceous gout often have a characteristic configuration, with an "overhanging margin" of bone (18). This margin has a thin shell-like configuration that, while continuous with the adjacent bone, is displaced outward from its contour. The gradual enlargement of a subcortical tophus results in adjacent cortical resorption creating an erosion. This process also evokes periosteal new bone apposition that extends over the outer margin of the tophus creating the elevated and displaced "overhanging edge" (Figure 8). The inciting tophus usually appears as a relatively discrete soft-tissue nodule adjacent to such erosions. This resulting appearance may be compared to a small "blow-out" deformity and should not be confused with the "pocketed" erosions of rheumatoid arthritis. In the latter, the eroded cortex is not displaced away from the original bone contour and no expansion is present. The "overhanging margin" sign has been noted in 40% of gout patients who have bone erosions and

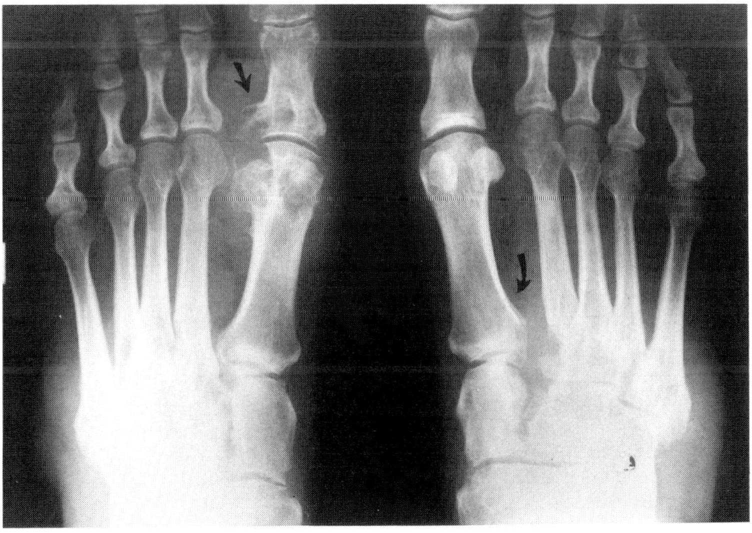

FIGURE 8 Marginal bone erosions with "overhanging edges" (straight arrow) with relative preservation of joint cartilage spaces and bone mineralization. Minimal linear periosteal bone apposition (curved arrow) adjacent to the tarsal tophus and bone destruction is present. Note the typical location of a tophus in the right tarsus.

typically occurs in the hands and feet. Although it is a very useful finding, it is not pathognomonic and may occasionally be simulated in other disorders, including psoriatic arthritis and sarcoidosis.

Isolated periosteal bone apposition may sometimes be observed adjacent to large tophi (11,12). This is usually minimal and almost always linear (Figure 8). It should not be confused with the irregular, frayed periosteal new bone apposition that occurs in psoriasis, for example. Incorporated proliferative changes along the metatarsal and metacarpal heads and ulnar styloid process may result in a club-shaped appearance that has been termed "mushrooming" by some authors (19,20) (Figure 6b).

D. Extra-Articular Tophi

Tophi may occur in virtually any location and have a propensity for areas exposed to repetitive mechanical stress or pressure. This is particularly the case along extensor surfaces at the elbow and prepatellar and dorsal foot locations (Figures 3 and 9). Tophi may also be deposited in tendons and ligaments leading to structural weakening and eventual rupture. Deposits within confined spaces such as the carpal tunnel may compress adjacent structures and result in entrapment neuropathy (21,22).

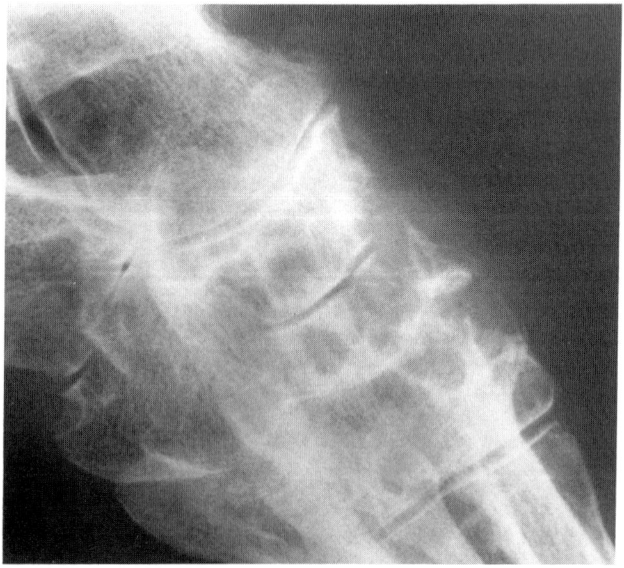

FIGURE 9 Extensive erosions of the extensor surface of the tarsal navicular and adjacent cuneiforms by overlying tophi. Note juxtachondral erosion of the cuboid. (From Ref. 13.)

E. Infrequent Sites of Involvement

Less frequent sites of involvement include the spine, sacroiliac joints, and hips; virtually any location may be affected. Gout of the spine is rare and may present with a variety of findings including disc-space narrowing and endplate erosion simulating discitis (23). Epidural soft-tissue tophi may also result in myelopathy or raduculopathy (24–26). The thoracic spine is least affected by gout; and involvement of more typical articular sites is usually present concurrently (24). Some reports emphasize the frequent coexistence of diffuse idiopathic skeletal hyperostosis and gout (27,28). However, similar to chondrocalcinosis, it is doubtful whether a true association between these entities exists, inasmuch as such hyperostosis is frequent in the general population. Prominent erosions or a cyst-like lesion with sclerotic margins may be present in sacroiliac joint involvement (29,30) (Figure 10). As with more characteristic sites involved in gout, the sacroiliac joint spaces are usually preserved and ankylosis is rare. Gout rarely involves the hip. The relationship between gout and osteonecrosis of the femoral head is unclear (31,32). Calcified intraosseous tophi may be mistaken for osteonecrosis, and deposition of monosodium urate in sites of prior osteonecrosis may occur due to biochemical factors; both lead to a false concept of an association between these disorders.

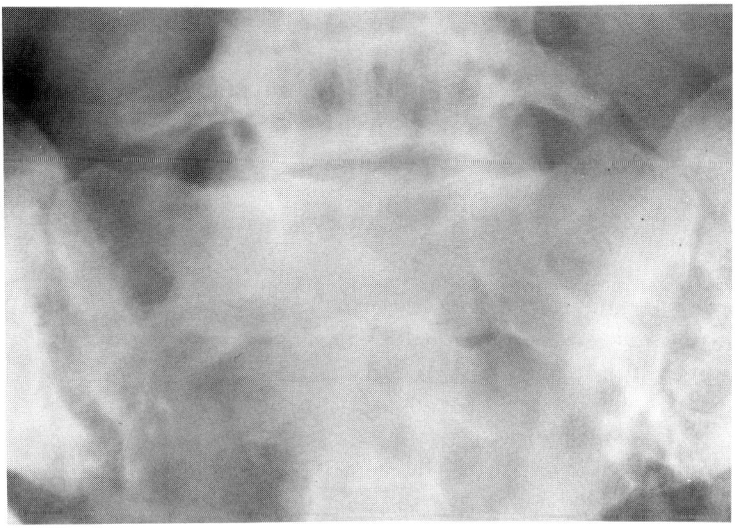

FIGURE 10 Tophaceous deposits in the sacroiliac joints associated with large bone erosions bilaterally. The left sacroiliac joint is obscured by superimposed bowel content. These lesions were verified at necropsy.

IV. OTHER IMAGING MODALITIES

Radionuclide studies are often abnormal in areas affected by gout; however, these are of limited clinical utility due to their low specificity. Although indium-111–labeled leukocyte imaging is a useful tool in the investigation of infection, false positive results in the setting of acute gout have been described (33). Abnormal uptake, especially when monoarticular, may be indistinguishable from septic arthritis. Nonspecific uptake patterns indistinguishable from Paget's disease, metastasis, and infection have been described with bone and gallium scintigraphy performed on patients with gout (34,35).

Magnetic resonance imaging (MRI) is not routinely utilized in the evaluation of gout and there are few reports of the imaging features. MRI studies may be obtained in patients presenting with unusual symptoms or with atypical radiographs. Tophi are typically of intermediate to low signal intensity on T1-weighted images regardless of location. More variability in signal intensity is present on T2-weighted sequences, with a tendency for low signal areas to be present (36). A low T2 signal has been attributed to calcification in tophi, but this is speculative. Intravenous gadolinium contrast administration usually demonstrates intense enhancement of tophi and adjacent synovial proliferation/pannus formation in those patients with articular involvement. These imaging features, while suggestive of gout, are nonspecific and overlap with those sometimes found in rheumatoid arthritis, pigmented villonodular synovitis, and fibromatous tumors (37,38).

V. DIFFERENTIAL DIAGNOSIS

Most patients with gout have a clinical diagnosis before chronic arthropathy develops. Nevertheless, the radiologic differential diagnosis is important to verify the clinical impression and exclude other entities that may manifest similar clinical findings.

Calcium pyrophosphate dihydrate (CPPD) crystal deposition disease may produce symptoms identical to those of gout. Chondrocalcinosis in CPPD is typically polyarticular, involving fibrocartilages and often hyaline cartilages, whereas in gout it is not widespread and generally occurs only in fibrocartilages (39,40). Pyrophosphate arthropathy may exhibit some features similar to gout, such as intraosseous cyst-like lesions, preservation of mineralization, and asymmetric joint involvement; however, the basic abnormality is a severe degenerative arthropathy without soft-tissue masses and the bone erosions are predominantly subchondral.

Psoriatic patients may exhibit hyperuricemia and similar radiologic features, including preservation of bone mineralization, asymmetric joint involvement, and marginal erosions (41). However, the distribution of affected extremity joints differs and vertebral and sacroiliac involvement is common in psoriasis but infrequent in gout. Asymmetric nodular soft-tissue swelling, characteristic of gout, is unusual in psoriasis. Both disorders may demonstrate periosteal bone apposition, but in gout this is usually linear and minimal whereas in psoriasis it is often irregular and may be extensive (Figure 11). Bony ankylosis is common in psoriasis but rare in gout. Subchondral cyst-like lesions are uncommon in psoriasis.

In typical rheumatoid arthritis there is a more or less symmetric arthritis, fusiform periarticular swelling, early joint-space narrowing, and osteopenia. Although erosions may develop at some "bare areas" in gout, this is not as conspicuous and widespread as in rheumatoid arthritis; "overhanging edges" are not a feature of rheumatoid arthritis (Figure 12). The robust or cyst-like form of rheumatoid arthritis may be a problem, especially in cases without osteopenia, but the pattern of bone lesions and absence of soft-tissue masses can be important clues (42). Furthermore, these cases with cyst-like lesions often exhibit subtle "bare area" erosions more typical of rheumatoid arthritis.

Amyloid deposition in bone, joint, and periarticular tissues may be mis-

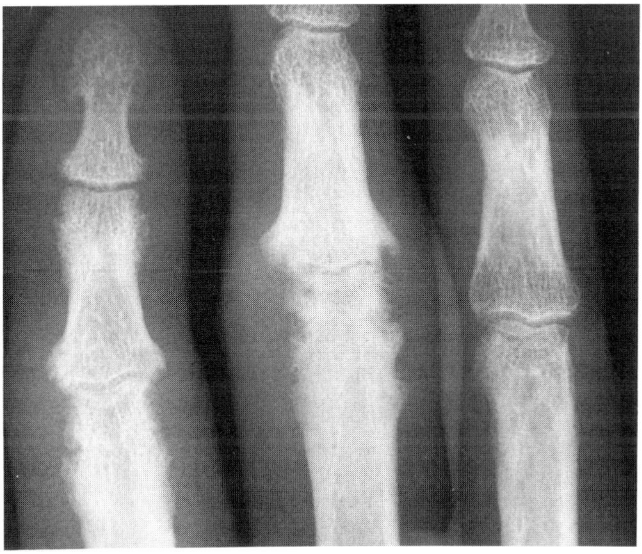

FIGURE 11 Psoriatic arthritis. Juxtachondral or "bare area" erosions in the distal interphalangeal joint of the index finger and the proximal interphalangeal joints of the index and middle fingers. This is associated with irregular proliferative periosteal bone production. In the middle finger the bone production simulates the "overhanging edge," but it is distinguished from gout in that the bone production in the latter is usually minimal and smooth and not irregular as in this case.

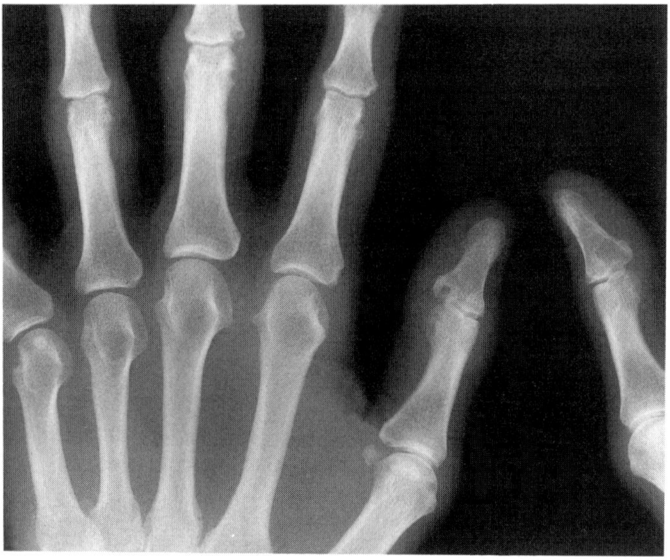

FIGURE 12 Rheumatoid arthritis. Pocketed erosions are present in characteristic locations. These are sharply demarcated but do not have an elevated margin. The contour of the eroded distal phalanx of the left thumb is not expanded. This erosion should not be confused with the "overhanging edge" sign in gout. The bone contour should be compared with that of the right thumb. (From Ref. 13.)

taken for tophi. This may be accompanied by articular bone erosion and cyst-like changes. These lesions usually develop in association with multiple myeloma or longstanding hemodialysis. In the latter condition the lesions may occur in a variety of sites but are most common in the wrist where they too may produce carpal tunnel syndrome.

Osseous sarcoidosis is most frequently found in the hands and may manifest soft-tissue swelling and bone erosion. The latter are frequently "lace-like" and are associated with osteopenia and occasionally marginal sclerosis. Phalangeal involvement is most frequent and articular involvement less common; the lesions are typically within bone near a joint and, except when large, do not affect the subchondral cortices.

REFERENCES

1. C. R. Barthelemy, D. A. Nakayama, G. F. Carrera, et al. Gouty arthritis: a prospective radiographic evaluation of sixty patients. Skeletal Radiol 11:1–8 (1985).

2. R. H. Smerling, S. H. Stern, E. M. Gravallese, et al. Tophaceous deposition in the finger pads without gouty arthritis. Arch Intern Med 148:1830–1832 (1988).
3. J. Varga, C. Giampaolo, and D. L. Goldenberg. Tophaceous gout of the spine in a patinet with no peripheral tophi: case report and review of the literature. Arth Rheum 28:1312–1315 (1985).
4. R. Wernick, C. Winkler, and S. Campbell. Tophi as the initial manifestation of gout. Arch Intern Med 152:873–876 (1992).
5. B. A. Baethge, J. Work, M. D. Landreneau, et al. Tophaceous gout in patients with renal transplants treated with cyclosporine. Am J Rheumatol 20:718–720 (1993).
6. D. M. Garagiola, S. A. Clark, R. A. Coyler, et al. Case report 536: Chronic tophaceous gout in a 17 year old male. Skeletal Radiol 18:377–379 (1989).
7. A. G. Fam, J. Stein, J. Rubenstein. Gouty arthritis in nodal osteoarthritis. J Rheumatol 23:684–689 (1996).
8. C. Bloch, G. Hermann, T. -F. Yu. A radiologic re-evaluation of gout: a study of 2,000 patients. Am J Rheumatol 134:781–787 (1980).
9. M. E. Ruiz, S. I. Erickson, G. F. Carrera, et al. Monoarticular gout following trauma: MR appearance. JCAT 17:151–153 (1993).
10. D. Resnick. The radiographic manifestations of gouty arthritis. CRC Crit Rev Diag Imaging 265–335 (1977).
11. J. T. Wright. Unusual manifestations of gout. Australas Radiol 10:365–374 (1966).
12. W. Martel. Differential diagnosis of the arthropathies. In: Radiology: Diagnosis-Imaging-Intrervention (J. M. Tavernas, ed.), Lippincott, Philadelphia, PA, chapter 33.
13. D. R. Pennes and W. Martel. Hyperuricemia and gout. Seminars Roentgenol 4:245–255 (1986).
14. G. R. Hughes, C. G. Barnes, R. M. Mason. Bony ankylosis in gout. Ann Rheum Dis 27:67–70 (1968).
15. R. Cope, R. Marsan, M. J. Castelli. Case report 732. Gout presenting as a large pseudotumor (tophus) in the proximal end of the tibia. Skeletal Radiol 21:269–270 (1992).
16. M. P. Recht, F. Seragini, J. Kramer, et al. Isolated or dominant lesions of the patella in gout: a report of seven patients. Skeletal Radiol 23:113–116 (1994).
17. D. Resnick and T. W. Broderick. Intraosseous calcifications in tophaceous gout. Am J Rheumatol 137:1157–1161 (1981).
18. W. Martel. The overhanging margin of bone: a roentgenologic manifestation of gout. Radiology 91:755–756 (1968).
19. W. Dihlmann and H. J. Fernholtz. Osteoplastiche reaktionen bei chronischer gicht. Fortschr Geb Roentgenst 120:216–217 (1974).
20. I. Watt and H. Middlemiss. The radiology of gout. Review article. Clin Radiol 26:27 (1975).
21. C. Ogilvie and N. R. Kay. Fulminating carpal tunnel syndrome due to gout. J Hand Surg 13:42–44 (1988).
22. C. H. Pai and C. H. Tseng. Acute carpal tunnel syndrome caused by tophaceous gout. J Hand Surg 18:667–669 (1993).
23. T. P. Duprez, J. Malghern, B. V. Berg, et al. Gout in the cervical spine: MR pattern mimicking diskovertebral infection. AJNR 17:151–153 (1996).

24. P. Fenton, S. Young, K. Prutis. Gout of the spine. JBJS 77:767–771 (1995).
25. J. Litvak and W. Briney. Extradural spinal deposition of urates producing paraplegia: a case report. J Neurosurg 39:656–658 (1973).
26. A. F. Reynolds, A. R. Wyler, H. T. Norris. Paraparesis secondary to sodium urate deposits into the ligamentum flavum. Arch Neurol 33:795 (1976).
27. I. Jajic. Gout in the spine and sacroiliac joints: radiological manifestations. Skeletal Radiol 8:209–212 (1982).
28. G. O. Littlejohn, S. Hall. Diffuse idiopathic skeletal hyperostosis and new bone formation in male gouty subjects. Rheumatol Int 2:83–86 (1982).
29. S. E. Malawista, J. E. Seegmiller, B. E. Hathaway, et al. Sacroiliac gout. JAMA 194:106–108 (1965).
30. R. Kerr. Sacroiliac joiny involvement by gout and hyperparathyroidism. Orthopedocs 11:187–190 (1988).
31. A. Cooper, R. Minutello, V. J. Vigorita, et al. Case report 763. Osteonecrosis and gout of femoral head. Skeletal Radiol 21:555–558 (1992).
32. L. De-Smet, D. Willemen, E. Kimpe, et al. Nontraumatic osteonecrosis of the capitate bone associated with gout. Ann Chir Main Memb Super 12:210–212 (1993).
33. C. J. Palestro, A. Vega, C. K. Kim, et al. Appearance of acute gouty arthritis on indium-111-labeled leukocyte scintigraphy. J Nuc Med 31:682–684 (1990).
34. D. Alarcon-Segouia, C. Lazo, J. Sepulveda, et al. Uptake of 99mTc-labeled phosphates by gouty tophi. J Rheumatol 1:314–318 (1974).
35. I. Boxen. Inability of bone and gallium imaging to differentiate acute gouty arthritis from septic arthritis. Clin Nuc Med 11:443–444 (1986).
36. J. S. Yu, C. Chung, M. Recht, et al. MR imaging of tophaceous gout. Am J Rheumatol 168:523–527 (1997).
37. H. Konig, J. Sieper, K. J. Wolf. Rhuematoid arthritis: evaluation of hypervascular and fibrous pannus with dynamic MR imaging enhanced with Gd-DTPA. Radiology 176:831–835 (1990).
38. S. F. Quinn, S. J. Erickson, P. M. Dee, et al. MR imaging in fibromatosis: results in 26 patients with pathological correlation. Am J Rheumatol 156:539–542 (1991).
39. W. Martel. Radiology of the rheumatic diseases. In: Arthritis and Allied Conditions, 6th ed. (J. L. Hollander and D. J. McCarty, eds.), Lea & Febiger, Philadelphia, PA, 1972, p. 115.
40. W. Martel, C. K. Champion, G. R. Thompson, et al. A roentegologically distinctive arthropathy in some patients with the pseudogout syndrome. Am J Rheumatol 109:587–605 (1970).
41. W. Martel, K. J. Stuck, A. M. Dorwin, et al. Erosive arthritis and psoriatic arthritis: a radiologic comparison in the hand, wrist and foot. Am J Rheumatol 134:125–135 (1980).
42. A. S. Rappoport, J. L. Sosman, B. N. Weissman. Lesions resembling gout in patients with rheumatoid arthritis. Am J Rheumatol 126:41–45 (1976).

19

Introduction to Other Crystalline Arthropathies

H. RALPH SCHUMACHER, JR.
University of Pennsylvania School of Medicine, Philadelphia, Pennsylvania

When Hollander and McCarty started their systematic examinations of synovial fluid in 1960, a new era began. The careful documentation of monosodium urate crystals in gout joint fluid was followed in 1962 by McCarty et al.'s (1) identification of a previously unrecognized crystal—the square, rod-like, or rhomboid calcium pyrophosphate dihydrate (CPPD). Those who continue to examine synovial fluids have also described a variety of other crystals that, as reviewed below, may be either important in causing less common arthropathies or sources of diagnostic confusion (2). Fortunately, the focus on the joint that was initially driven by the crystal diseases has continued, with many investigators now examining key mechanisms in a variety of diseases at the site of the local symptoms and tissue damage.

Genetic factors, which are becoming more commonly recognized in many diseases, are clearly important in some CPPD associated disease. Familial cases have now been reported from countries around the world. Genetic contributions to the deposition of the other common calcium crystal, hydroxyapatite, are less clear.

Chapter 20, by O'Duffy, reviews the evolution of the concept of CPPD deposition disease and provides his perspective. Acute attacks of "pseudogout" continue to be misdiagnosed by the unwary as caused by gout or infection. It is interesting how infrequently general physicians consider this diagnosis (3), and how often relatively subtle joint swelling is missed and patients are extensively evaluated for "fever of unknown origin" when the systemic reaction is clearly a response to the pseudogout (4).

When one meticulously examines all synovial fluids or articular tissue biopsies for crystals, CPPD crystals are noted in many older patients who are affected by otherwise typical osteoarthritis. (5, 6) In such patients there is a striking absence of the dramatic inflammation seen with acute attacks of pseudogout. The role of the CPPD crystals in such situations is not clear. Our recent observations have suggested that there are many such patients who, despite large numbers of crystals, never develop acute arthritis (7). In such settings, do these really represent a "disease"?

Although most CPPD crystals are found in the elderly, special attention needs to be paid to younger patients found to harbor CPPD. As reviewed by O'-Duffy, crystal identification may occasionally be the first clue to treatable underlying systemic diseases such as hemochromatosis, hyperparathyroidism, or hypomagnesemia. CPPD crystals also have been described in association with hyperalciuric hypercalcemia, ochronosis, Wilson's disease, acromegaly, and amyloidosis.

Treatment of routine CPPD disease is symptomatic, because no measures to alter crystal deposition or speed removal have yet been found. As one who is asked to see refractory cases, I have watched for clinical trials that might suggest some new, valuable treatments. One report suggested that magnesium decreased pain although it did not succeed in dissolving CPPD. I would consider use of some second line agents as used in rheumatoid arthritis (RA) for chronic inflammation associated with CPPD crystals. Hydroxychloroquine (8) and methotrexate are two that have been suggested on the basis of still-limited studies.

Lynne S. Steinbach and Donald Resnick, in Chapter 21, provide an additional review and describe their and others' uses of imaging in evaluating CPPD deposition disease. Although chrondrocalcinosis and synovial fluid crystals are often seen together, radiographic changes of typical chondrocalcinosis can be present for years in totally asymptomatic joints with no effusions; CPPD crystals can also be found in synovial fluids or tissues of patients without x-ray evidence of chondrocalcinosis. The prominence of early subchondral cysts emphasized by these authors needs explanation. Are there important parallel metabolic changes in subchondral bone? The synovial, tendon, and ligament calcifications noted radiographically have also interested us (9). The few synovial specimens we examined all appeared to have the calcification occurring in areas of chondrometaplasia.

Rapidly destructive osteoarthritis originally associated with apatite crystals has also been seen with CPPD crystal disease. We have found both CPPD and apatite crystals in a number of patients with rapid "noninflammatory" destruction of hips and shoulders ("Milwaukee shoulder"), knees, and other joints (10). Whether these crystals are a cause or result (or both) requires further study.

CPPD involvement of the spine is an area of increased recent interest. Destructive disc lesions can mimic infection or neuropathic joints. CPPD in the ligamentatun flavum and posterior longitudinal ligament can cause myelopathy and spinal stenosis.

Routine radiographic techniques remain the mainstay of imaging evaluation for CPPD. The few mentions of magnetic resonance (MR) imaging suggest that CPPD deposits show low signal intensity that may be difficult to distinguish from adjacent tissues. Inflammatory reaction around the crystals would be detected as increased signal on T2 weighted images. In the spine, MR imaging has been used to search for evidence and degree of cord compression. CT scanning has been used to demonstrate small calcifications in the carpal tunnel and spine.

A number of features of CPPD disease at various sites are reviewed. I would add the temporomandibular joint, from which escaping masses of CPPD crystals have mimicked parotid tumors (11). We earlier noted a distal phalanx mass of CPPD that was misdiagnosed as a tumor (12).

Chapter 23 by Masuda, Ryan, and McCarty reviews the approximately 20-year dogged pursuit by these investigators and their colleagues in Milwaukee to elucidate the details of pyrophosphate metabolism as related to the still incompletely understood formation of CPPD crystals in various settings.

Since CPPD crystals are so common in osteoarthritis, one hope is that reversal of these deposits might slow progression of OA. However, this is not certain as it has not been proved whether or exactly how the crystals cause tissue deterioration. Phagocytosis of crystals by synovial and inflammatory cells does lead to cell proliferation, release of a variety of destructive proteases and largely proinflammatory molecules. As noted in the review, inorganic pyrophosphate may have an important normal function as it inhibits apatite nucleation and growth, thus perhaps protecting cartilage and synovium from the mineralization that occurs in bone.

A few other fascinating puzzles also remain. Where do CPPD crystals primiarly deposit? One recent study even suggests the possibility of intracellular deposition. Why is the outer third of the knee meniscus apparently unable to elaborate inorganic pyrophosphate and develop crystal deposits? Why do CPPD crystals deposit only in articular structures?

Hydroxyapatite crystal disease, as reviewed by Dr. Adel G. Fam in Chapter 22, remains underappreciated and underrecognized compared to CPPD disease and especially compared to gout. There perhaps are several reasons for this:

1. Both CPPD and apatite deposition diseases lack the quick name recognition of gout. One solution suggested by Simkin was to call all these crystal associated diseases "gout," with the following qualification of what type of crystal caused the now less-specific "gout" (13). This approach has been adopted in the chapter by Reginato but not in the chapters on CPPD and apatite, further perpetuating the confusion for the unwary.

2. Although most reports and the earliest studies have called the disease(s) seen with apatite crystals either *apatite* or *hydroxyapatite crystal deposition disease*, there have also been proposals to call this *basic calcium phosphate disease*. When calcifications are analyzed with infrared spectroscopy their major compo-

nent is not pure hydroxyapatite but hydroxyapatite with varying amounts of carbonate substitution along with small amounts of octacalcium phosphate or tricalcium phosphate (14). McCarty et al. (15) and Schumacher et al. (16) have occasionally found patients with predominantly the octacalcium phosphate crystals. Very limited clinical-crystallographic correlations have not shown any clinical implications of the deposits with the different contents of apatite and other crystals, so most clinical descriptions tend to favor the term *apatite crystal deposition.* Prudhommeaux et al. (17) have shown some biologic differences among these crystals, so continued evaluations seen indicated. Chapter 22 by Fam is titled "Basic Calcium Phosphate (Calcium Apatite) Crystal Deposition Diseases," which confuses the matter more because apatite by definition contains calcium. *Asi es la vida.* Let me put in my vote for apatite crystal deposition disease and CPPD crystal deposition disease. As we will see, all these crystals can be asymptomatic or associated with a variety of features, so to be useful any classifications will probably need some modifiers to be truly clinically or pathophysiologically useful.

3. A distinct problem with the apatite crystals is that they are difficult to identify clinically since they do not produce nice birefringent particles for those now experienced in the clinical use of compensated polarized light microscopy. Individual apatite crystals are seen only by electron microscopy: Shiny 2–20μ nonbirefringent clumps of apatite crystals in SF can be suggestive and can be confirmed to contain calcium by stains such as alizarin red S (18). However, we could certainly use easier, more user-friendly ways to both screen and confirm the presence of apatite than by EM, elemental analysis, x-ray diffraction, and Fourier transform infrared spectroscopy. The most common syndrome of calcific periarthritis often can be recognized by the characteristic but not totally specific or sensitive calcific periarthritis deposits often seen on radiographs.

Attacks of acute calcific periarthritis are fairly well recognized at the shoulders but often misdiagnosed when occurring at less-common sites, such as the wrists, hands, and feet or even the retropharyngeal structures. Fam and Rubenstein (19) have provided some of the most dramatic descriptions of apatite crystal disease at (or adjacent to) the first MTP joints mimicking acute gout but occurring most often in young women. Despite dramatic symptoms and clinical signs, aspirations often yield pasty masses of crystals with very few leukocytes! There is a need for much more investigation into mechanisms of production of inflammation and of deposition of these common apatite deposits. What is available does suggest underlying connective tissue chondrometaplasia (20), as also seen with some CPPD. Other situations in which soft tissue apatite deposits occur might provide some clues to mechanisms, although the hyperphosphatemia seen in renal dialysis patients is not seen in idiopathic cases. The apatite calcifications in scleroderma and dermatomyositis or after local steroid injections seem more likely to be due to local connective tissue changes. I am not aware if these show any chondrometaplasia or have other local metabolic changes.

Dieppe et al. (21) and Schumacher et al. (22) almost simultaneously identified and called attention to apatite intraarticular disease in 1976 and 1977. At least in part because of difficulty in identifying the apatite in usual practice, we find that it is still underrecognized. It is not clear exactly how this relates to the rapidly destructive type of osteoarthritis of the elderly. This was first identified at the shoulders ("l'epaule senile hemorrhagigue"; "Milwaukee shoulder") but also occurs at other and probably smaller joints. Although invariably associated with apatite crystals, in many of these cases it is uncertain whether the apatite crystals are initiating factors or are released from the destroyed bone. Note that apatite and CPPD often occur together in such joints. The noninflammatory and often bloody effusions seen in these patients are important to identify, because clinical and radiographical concern may be raised about septic (or neurotrophic) joints. Apatite crystals have fascinating biologic effects, including mitogenic properties and the ability to stimulate proteolytic enzyme release, and continue to be studied by Cheung and co-workers (23).

The chapter by Fam reminds us that apatite crystals like CPPD are very common in osteoarthritis (OA) effusions. He asks whether they are a contributing factor or an epiphenomenon. Might we also consider whether they might not even play some physiological, ameliorative role? Louthrenoo et al.'s study on SF leukocyte counts in OA actually showed trends to lower counts in those effusions with apatite (24). We would agree that for now finding calcium crystals in classical OA joint effusions should not change treatment approaches. Further studies would be of interest.

Fads have come and gone in treating apatite calcinosis when serum Ca and P are normal. The calcium channel blocker diltiazem may have been useful in some scleroderma or other cases, although it seems to require many months for effect (25).

Antonio J. Reginato and Gerald Falasca take up the challenge of reviewing calcium oxalate and other miscellaneous arthropathies in Chapter 24. Anyone personally doing synovial fluid microscopic examinations on a regular basis must expect to be confronted by the less common but known crystals, by artifacts, and occasionally by something not previously described. These, as well as the other crystals, can occasionally be a first clue to an important, treatable, systemic disease. Finding unexpected or unexplained crystalline or other materials in SF can be one of the delights of medicine, leading one down fascinating trails of library and laboratory investigation (although I doubt anyone will have time to do this with the pressure of rapid visits that, hopefully temporarily, is resulting from managed care). One must really spend some time at the microscope. When Hoffman et al. first reported oxalate crystals in joint fluid in 1982 (26), for example, they had been passed off as CPPD because many rod and square forms were seen before we found the first telltale clump of envelope-like or bipyramidal crystals.

Primary oxalosis is reviewed; arthritis, in these cases as well as in acquired oxalosis, tends to occur as a result of renal failure and then the inability to keep up with the oxalate load. This leads to oxalate deposits in joints and bone as well as key viscera such as the heart and blood vessel walls.

I am fascinated by the fact that articular oxalate deposits have not yet been described in patients with bowel disease and increased oxalate absorption. Radiographic calcifications may be indistinguishable from CPPD or apatite, although bone changes reviewed here can help suggest oxalate disease.

A relatively recent development that makes it important to recognize primary oxalosis is the successful use of kidney and liver transplantation. Most other therapies, including renal dialysis, have failed. A new liver can provide enough enzyme to successfully lower oxalate production.

The authors of this chapter, although not attempting to be encyclopedic, also review the other crystals that can be seen in joints. One of the points worth emphasis is that some cholesterol crystals and other lipids can be needle-shaped and can be confused with urates. Maltese cross-like lipid liquid crystals in small numbers can be seen in many effusions, but large numbers can cause acute monoarthritis; cryoglobulin or paraprotein crystals in joints have occasionally been an important first clue to cryoglobulinemia. Cholesterol crystals have formed tophus-like deposits and cholesterol clefts can be seen in rheumatoid nodules. Crystalline depot corticosteroids continue to be seen in joint fluids or contaminate fluids after aspiration and can be confused with naturally occurring crystals.

Throughout this introduction, I have highlighted some of the many puzzles that remain in understanding pathogenesis of the calcium crystal diseases. This remains an exciting area for consideration by potential investigators.

REFERENCES

1. D. J. McCarty, N. N. Kohn, and J. S. Faires. The significance of calcium phosphate crystals in the synovial fluid of arthritic patients: the "pseudogout syndrome." I. Clinical aspects. *Ann Intern Med 56:*711 (1962).
2. H. R. Schumacher and A. J. Reginato, Atlas of synovial fluid and crystal identification, Lea and Febiger, Philadelphia, PA (1991).
3. R. S. Panush, K. Carias, N. Kramer, and E. D. Rosenstein. Acute arthritis in the hospital: Comparison of rheumatologic with nonrheumatologic care. *J Clin Rheum 1* (2):74 (1995).
4. M. U. Rahman, K. N. Shenberger, and H. R. Schumacher. Initially unrecognized calcium pyrophosphate dihydrate deposition disease as a cause of fever. *Am J Med 89:*115 (1990).
5. P. Gibilisco, H. R. Schumacher, J. Hollander, and K. Soper. Synovial fluid crystals in osteoarthritis. *Arth Rheum 28:*511 (1985).

6. P. A. Dieppe, D. V., Doyle, E. C. Huskisson, et al. Mixed crystal deposition disease and ostearthritis. *Brit Med J 1:*150 (1978).
7. N. Schlesinger, M. Sieck, G. Clayburne, and H. R. Schumacher. Does acute synovitis (pseudogout) occur in patients with chronic pyrophosphate arthropathy or are these separate syndromes? *Arth Rheum 40:*S49 (1997).
8. B. Rothschild and L. E. Yakubov. Evidence for an effect of hydroxychloroquine in chronic pyrophosphate in chronic pyrophosphate deposition disease. *J Clin Rheum 2* (3):170 (1996).
9. A. Beutler, S. Rothfuss, G. Clayburne, M. Sieck, and H. R. Schumacher. Calcium pyrophosphate dihydrate crystal deposition in synovium. Relationship to collagen fibers and chondrometaplasia. *Arth Rheum 36:*704 (1993).
10. L. Zakraoui, H. R. Schumacher, S. Rothfuss, M. Sieck, and G. Clayburne. Idiopathic destructive arthropathies: Clinical, light, electron microscopic studies. *J Clin Rheumatol 2:*9 (1996).
11. T. Ishida, H. D. Dorfman, and P. G. Bullough. Tophaceous pseudogout (tumoral calcium pyrophosphate dihydrate crystal deposition disease). *Human Pathol 26*(6):587 (1995).
12. H. R. Schumacher, H. Bonner, J. J. Thompson, W. L. Kester, and J. J. Benner. Tumor-like soft tissue swelling of the distal phalanx due to calcium pyrophosphate dihydrate crystal deposition. *Arth Rheum 27:*1428 (1984).
13. P. A. Simkin. Articular oxalate crystals and the taxonomy of gout. *JAMA 260:*128S, (1988).
14. D. J. McCarty, P. B. Halverson, G. F. Carrera, B. J. Brewer, and F. Kozin, "Milwaukee shoulder" association of microspheroids containing hydroxyapatite crystals, active collagenase, and neutral protease with rotator cuff defects. I. Clinical aspects. *Arth Rheum 24:*464 (1981).
15. D. J. McCarty, J. R. Lehr, and P. B. Halverson. Crystal populations in human synovial fluid. Identification of apatite, octacalcium phosphate, tricalcium phosphate. *Arth Rheum 26:*1220 (1983).
16. H. R. Schumacher, S. Rothfuss, J. R. Lehr, J. L. Miller, and A. Good. Octacalcium phosphate as sole or predominant calcium phosphate crystal in joint fluid. *Arth Rheum 31:*S19 (1988).
17. F. Prudhommeaux, C. Schiltz, F. Liote, A. Hina, et al. Variation in the inflammatory properties of basic calcium phosphate crystals according to crystal type. *Arth Rheum 39:*1319 (1996).
18. H. Paul, A. J. Reginato, and H. R. Schumacher. Alizarin red S staining as a screening test to detect calcium compounds in synovial fluid. *Arth Rheum 26:*191 (1983).
19. A. G. Fam and J. Rubenstein. Hydroxyapatite pseudopodagra: A syndrome of young women. *Arth Rheum 32:*741 (1989).
20. K. Sarkar and H. K. Uhthoff. Ultrastructural localization of calcium in calcifying tendinitis. *Arch Pathol Lab Med 102:*266 (1978).
21. P. A. Dieppe, E. C. Huskisson, P. Crocker, et al. Apatite deposition disease. *Lancet 1:*266 (1976).
22. H. R. Schumacher, A. P. Somlyo, R. L. Tse, and K. Maurer. Apatite crystal associated crystal arthritis. *Ann Int Med 87:*411 (1977).

23. G. M. McCarthy, P. G. Mitchell, and H. S. Cheung. The mitogenic response to stimulation with basic calcium phosphate crystals is accompanied by induction and secretion of collagenase in human fibroblasts. *Arth Rheum 34:*1021 (1991).
24. W. Louthrenoo, M. Sieck, G. Clayburne, S. Rothfuss, and H. R. Schumacher. Supravital staining of cells in noninflammatory synovial fluids: Analysis of the effect of crystals on cell populations. *J Rheum 18:*409 (1991).
25. G. M. A. Palmieri, J. I. Sebes, J. A. Aelion, and M. Moinuddin. Treatment of calcinosis with diltiazem. *Arth Rheum 38:*1646 (1995).
26. G. Hoffman, H. R. Schumacher, H. Paul, V. Cherian, R. Reed, A. Ramsay, and W. Franck. Calcium oxalate microcrystalline associated arthritis in end stage renal disease. *Ann Int Med 97:*36 (1982).

20

Calcium Pyrophosphate Deposition Disease

The Clinical Syndrome

J. Desmond O'Duffy
Mayo Clinic, Rochester, Minnesota

I. INTRODUCTION

Numerous reports of patients having radiologic and histologic evidence of diffuse calcifications in cartilage were made in the first half of this century (1). The first recognition of a distinct syndrome of episodic attacks of acute joint inflammation is credited to Zitnan and Sitaj in Czechoslovakia, who reported in 1957 calcifications in hyaline and fibrocartilage in a familial pattern of "chondrocalcinosis" (2). McCarty and colleagues in 1962 described 7 patients, all over 50 years of age, having nonurate crystals in symptomatic arthritic knee joint fluids (3). These crystals, unlike the needle-shaped crystals of monosodium urate in gout, had both rodlike and rhombic forms and had weakly positive birefringence when viewed in a polarizing microscope fitted with a red-plate compensator. Moreover, they identified the crystals using infrared spectrophotometry, emission spectroscopy, and X-ray diffraction studies as calcium pyrophosphate dihydrate (CPPD) (4). The Philadelphia workers deduced that their syndrome of joint "pseudogout" occurring in patients having radiologic chondrocalcinosis of joints was identical to that reported by Zitnan and Sitaj.

Since those seminal reports, interest in the syndrome of CPPD crystal deposition (1) has expanded in the following directions: recognition that CPPD arthropathy, like hypertension, may have discrete metabolic causes (5); careful anatomic and pathologic descriptions of crystal deposits; clinical syndromes of pseudogout and pyrophosphate arthropathy (6); mechanisms of the inflammation

TABLE 1 Diagnosis of CPPD Disease

Definite: 1	Demonstration of CPPD crystals in microscopic examination of synovial fluid, or pathologic examination of articular tissues, tendons, or bursae.
Probable: 2	Punctate and linear cartilage calcifications in two or more joints.

and joint damage (7); attempts to define the basis for CPPD in cartilage (8); and treatment.

Although diagnostic criteria for CPPD crystal disease have been proposed, it is practical to accept the diagnosis when the CPPD crystals are demonstrated in synovial fluid or articular tissues using compensated polarized light microscopy (Table 1). Although radiologic patterns, especially chondrocalcinosis, are suggestive, they are not of themselves diagnostic. In this chapter, CPPD crystal deposition disease will be considered primary when no metabolic disorder is present and secondary when another metabolic disorder known to associated with CPPD crystal deposition is present.

II. PATHOLOGY AND MECHANISMS

Direct inspection of the knee joint at autopsy or arthrotomy varies from near normal, as seen at diagnostic arthroscopy, to advanced osteoarthritis with chalky deposits on synovium resembling tophi when cadaver joints are carefully examined. CPPD deposits stain black with von Kossa's stain and are most dense in menisci and other fibrocartilages (9). Hematoxylin and eosin stains color CPPD purple. The earliest deposits in hyaline cartilage are in the midzone of cartilage (9,10) where some early loss of proteoglycan and cloning of chondrocytes is occurring. Tophi are typically <1 mm in diameter, are often in hypocellular synovial membrane, and are best studied in undecalcified sections. CPPD deposits resist water solubility much better than do sodium urate crystals, and may be sharply demarcated from the surrounding fibrocartilage. Although the initial reports suggested that CPPD deposits were exclusively an intra-articular phenomenon, it is now clear that they can be found in such extra-articular sites as the ligamentum flavum, fingers, ears, and para-articular tissues (2,11,12,13).

The pathogenesis of CPPD crystal deposition is still unknown except in the rare instance of hypophosphatasia. In that condition, pyrophosphatase deficiency allows the accumulation of its substrate pyrophosphate (PPi) (13). There are two proposed mechanisms for CPPD deposition in idiopathic disease: one in which CPPD is over produced in or has decreased removal from cartilage (14); and another in which it is proposed that an abnormality of cartilage collagen exists (10), and that synovial deposits are due to chondrometaplasia in synovial membrane (14). Whereas PPi is produced during synthesis of proteins, nucleic acids, lipids, and glycogen, among others, the serum and urinary levels are not elevated in CPPD disease (5,15). Since PPi is elevated in synovial fluid of degenerated and CPPD joints as compared to patients with gout and rheumatoid arthritis, it is reasonable to suspect local overproduction. At present, there is interest in an overactivity in cartilage chondrocytes of the enzyme adenosine pyrophosphohydrolase (ATP PPH) leading to local accumulation of PPi (5).

Proposed mechanisms of secondary CPPD deposition are the hypercalcemia in hyperparathyroidism and hypocalciuric hypercalcemia (5), inhibition of inorganic pyrophosphatase by ferrous ion in hemochromatosis, and loss of cofactor for pyrophosphatase in hypomagnesemia.

III. CLINICAL FEATURES

A. The Acute Attack

Because lavage of chondrocalcinotic joints with solubilizers of CPPD such as magnesium ions and disodium EDTA provoked attacks of pseudogout, it is assumed that acute attacks in general are due to release of preformed CPPD crystals from synovial membrane and joint cartilage. The alternative hypothesis, that CPPD crystals are crystallized in the synovial fluid, is considered unlikely. The thesis of "crystal shedding" from joint surfaces into synovial fluid is now favored by most experts in the field (6,7). The situation is analogous to gout wherein acute episodes are provoked by release of preformed crystals into the joint. In parallel with gout where sudden lowering of serum levels of urate provokes attacks, the provocation for pseudogout is often a sharp reduction in serum calcium level (16). The clinical setting is often seen in a patient who develops pseudogout within a few days of a major surgical operation or an acute vascular event. Parathyroidectomy for hyperparathyroidism is the most obvious scenario for this event but hypocalcemia is a feature of other major surgical operations and is also a transient sequel to major vascular illnesses, such as stroke, and myocardial infractions.

Hospital cases of acute pseudogout probably represent a more severe spectrum of inflammation than community acquired attacks but provide more accurate observations. In hospital patients, more than one joint is affected 50% of the time and the most frequent joints affected are knees (26–88%), wrists (20–33%), and ankles (3–14%), with shoulders and small joints of the hands and feet inflamed in a minority of cases (17,18). Acute or subacute attacks develop over a day or two, and are associated with pain, swelling, and some erythema and local warmth. Errors in diagnosis in hospitalized patients are frequent, as leukocytosis, fever, and even disorientation often lead to extensive testing for infectious causes (19). A swollen knee joint often is associated with a popliteal synovial cyst that can mimic venous occlusion (Figure 1). Inexperience of the house staff

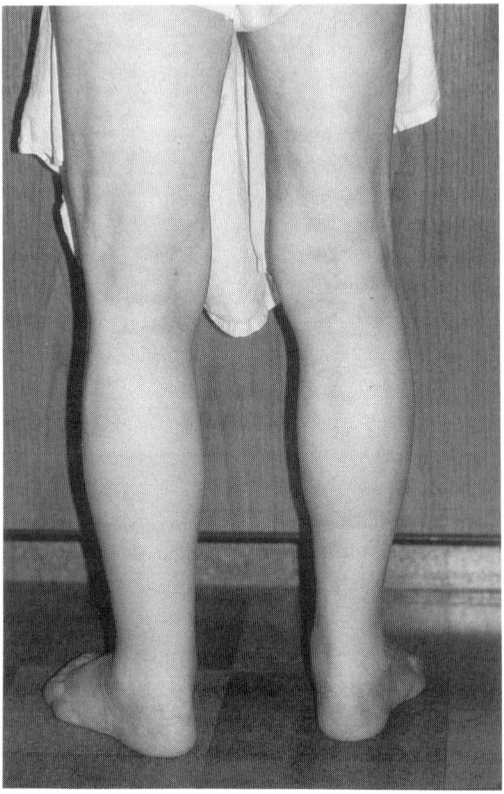

FIGURE 1 Acute pseudogout in the left knee presenting as "pseudophlebitis." Popliteal vein is compressed by associated popliteal cyst in an 80-year-old man.

in joint aspiration techniques adds to diagnostic delay. Because elevated erythrocyte sedimentation rate, leukocytosis, and fever are present in some combination in most patients, it is common to see referred patients already taking antibiotics. Elderly patients having polyarticular attacks may present with delirium and "fever of unknown origin" due to polyarticular pseudogout (19).

Synovial fluid examination in nearly all instances of acute pseudogout shows phagocytosed CPPD crystals (Figure 2). The crystals are usually smaller in diameter than the cell ingesting them, i.e., <10 microns, but range in length from 1 to 15 microns. In the polarized microscope fitted with a red-plate compensator, the sign of birefringence for CPPD crystals is weakly positive, whereas in gout the sign of birefringence is strongly negative (3,20). Some crystals are nonrefractile. The crystals' shape varies from triclinic (rhombic) to monoclinic

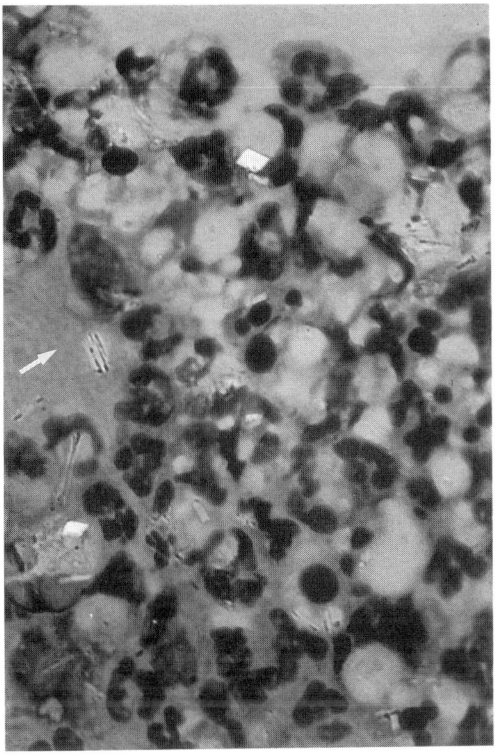

FIGURE 2 Wright's stain shows intracellular and extracellular positivity birefringent crystals. Arrow shows direction of slow vibration of light.

(needle) (Figure 2) and experience with the polarized light microscope is needed for accurate identification (20). Wet preps of synovial fluid are the most convenient for a quick diagnosis, but crystals tolerate cytospin preparations that are Wright stained. The fluid is usually mildly turbid but can be hemorrhagic or occasionally opaque resembling sepsis (3,21). The synovial fluid has low viscosity, and the leukocyte count in it varies from 4,000 to 60,000 mm^3. The count in serially aspirated joints declines sharply with time such that after a week of onset counts decline to a mean of <10,000. The predominant cell is a polymorphonuclear leukocyte, typically >90% of the total (5), and the usual shape of crystals in acute attacks is monoclinic (22). Fluids aspirated between acute episodes show mostly extracellular crystals and have low cell counts. Occasionally a bursa such as the olecranon may be found to contain CPPD crystals. Other crystals may be encountered along with CPPD crystals in joint or bursal episodes, e.g., sodium urate or basic calcium phosphate (5). Crystals degrade in unstained slides and tend to disappear over several days.

When fluid is aspirated from any acute joint, it is mandatory that bacterial culture be obtained. One to two percent of crystal-containing acute joints are in fact septic joints (23). We proposed that crystals in these cases of septic joint were "innocent bystanders" that were lysed by the inflammatory process from the surfaces of infected joints. While it is not mandatory to X-ray all newly inflamed joints, it is desirable to do so and also reassuring to note that in nearly all of the pseudogout joints the X-ray shows chondrocalcinosis (24).

Alizarin red staining for calcium-containing crystals is unnecessary in dealing with acute joints as it is both insensitive and nonspecific (25).

B. Other Clinical Syndromes

Several neurological syndromes can be associated with deposits of CPPD crystals. Patients may present with extensive cervical spondylosis and a gait disorder, having the syndrome of cervical myelopathy (6). The ligamentum flavum deposits of CPPD can also produce compression of the cauda equina at the lumbar level, resulting in a syndrome of neurogenic claudication due to lumbar stenosis (26,27). An acute meningitis-like syndrome is suspected when a patient having polyarticular pseudogout presents with nuchal rigidity and fever, i.e., pseudomeningitis (6,28). It has been claimed that carpal tunnel syndrome can result from a local tenosynovitis caused by CPPD, but close inspection of these reports leaves me unconvinced that the crystals found were in fact CPPD.

Charcot joints have clearly been shown to contain CPPD (5,29) but the causality is unclear. Tophaceous deposits of CPPD suggested radiologically by McCarty et al. in the ear of a patient in their first report (3) have also been found in several other nonarticular sites, i.e., digits, tendons, and muscle. Isolated joints, especially knees that have been subjected to previous meniscectomy or trauma (30), can have such localized deposits. The olecranon bursa has been reported to contain CPPD crystals.

When we consider that patients having newly discovered crystals in their joints cluster in the age range of 60–85 (3,6,18), it is clear that most patients having deposits in their joints have been, for most of their lives, either asymptomatic or only mildly affected by an arthropathy. In most respects, this arthropathy resembles idiopathic osteoarthritis (2). Whether this "pyrophosphate arthropathy" is equivalent to or more severe than idiopathic osteoarthritis is not an answerable question because longitudinal cohort comparisons have not been done. Radiologists viewing chondrocalcinotic joints from their perspective have not agreed whether pyrophosphate arthropathy is more severe than or roughly equivalent in severity to idiopathic osteoarthritis (30,31).

In my experience, the most difficult cases to diagnose accurately are patients seen during an emerging phase of a polyarthritis, especially polymyalgia rheumatica and rheumatoid arthritis, whose synovial fluid is found to contain intracellular CPPD crystals. These patients have been called "pseudorheumatoid" (5), but in many cases the clinical course favors one of these two conditions. Although CPPD crystals are present along with radiologic chondrocalcinosis, the new event that draws them to our attention is the appearance of another provoking synovitis. I have seen CPPD crystals disappear after rheumatoid arthritis becomes established. The average duration of troublesome symptoms in polymyalgia rheumatiza (PMR) is 2–3 years and the course may be more severe in patients having "innocent bystander" crystals being liberated from previously symptomless CPPD deposits. Nevertheless, there are well-described instances (32) and even kindreds (33) of patients having chronic smoldering arthropathy due to CPPD deposits in joints. Familial CPPD deposition is well described in at least 10 countries with a pattern of autosomal dominant transmission (5). A slow evolution to diffuse degenerative joint disease has been suggested in French and Slovakian series of patients.

IV. RADIOLOGY AND NATURAL HISTORY

The natural history of CPPD disease is not well understood. While it has been questioned that there is an accelerated degeneration of joints in CPPD disease (31), the evolution to advanced degenerative changes in the peripheral joints of some patients has been well described (34–37). Severe disease, with stiffening of the spine and peripheral joints, seems unique to certain Chilean patients, whose disease mimics ankylosing spondylitis (36). Radiologic reports have highlighted the increasing prevalence of chondrocalcinosis in aging individuals along with very gradual degeneration of joints (35). Genant championed the use of Type M industrial film in detecting the subtle calcific deposits in thin body parts such as hands and feet (38). Linear and punctate calcification of fibrocartilage and hyaline cartilage in multiple sites, bilaterally and symmetrically, is characteristic (Figures 3 and 4). Synovial calcification, best seen in lateral views of the knees, can resemble synovial chondromatosis (30). The fibrocartilages of the knee menisci, symphysis pubis, and triangular ligament of the wrist are especially prone to show linear calcium, but hyaline cartilage at all bone ends is involved, as is the fibrocartilage of the intervertebral discs (35,38). The changes of degenerative joint disease overlap with those of primary osteoarthritis (OA). A few clues to CPPD disease are cysts in carpal bones; patellofemoral

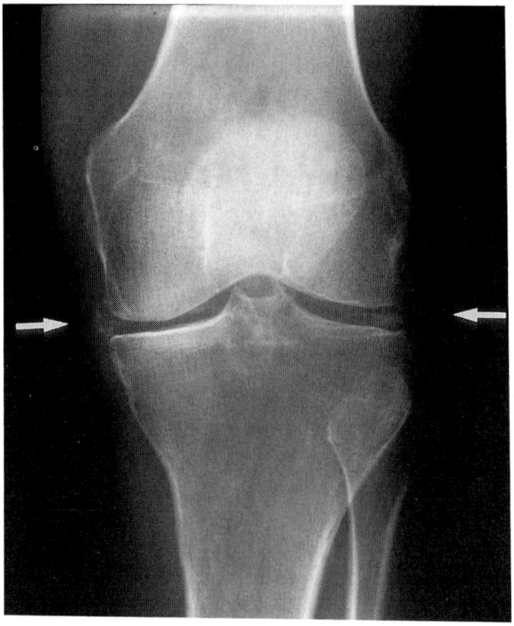

FIGURE 3 Chondrocalcinosis of knee menisci and hyaline cartilage with associated degenerative change.

OA; as well as wrist, carpus, and shoulder degeneration. Extra-articular calcific deposits in tendons and capsular calcification in small joints are common but less specific (17).

Riestra and colleagues (31) attempted to compare the arthropathy in CPPD crystal deposition disease with an age-matched group of patients with primary osteoarthritis. They found no tendency to more severe joint damage in CPPD disease and only minor differences between groups (31). Workers in Britain and in Slovakia have recently revisited the question of how the polyarthropathy progresses (39,40). We may conclude that over decades there is a slow deterioration in peripheral and axial joints. When scanning X-rays for calcific deposits, the viewer may see "cloud-like" masses of fine calcific flecks, which denote synovial membrane deposits (30). Bright-light examination of X-rays and underpenetrated technics enhance detection of calcific deposits. Occasionally, CPPD crystals are detected in synovial effusions of osteoarthritic joints that reveal no radiologic calcification. Locations that are neglected radiologically include the sternoclavicular, temporomandibular, and acromioclavicular joint articular discs (41) as well as the cervical and lumbar spine (5).

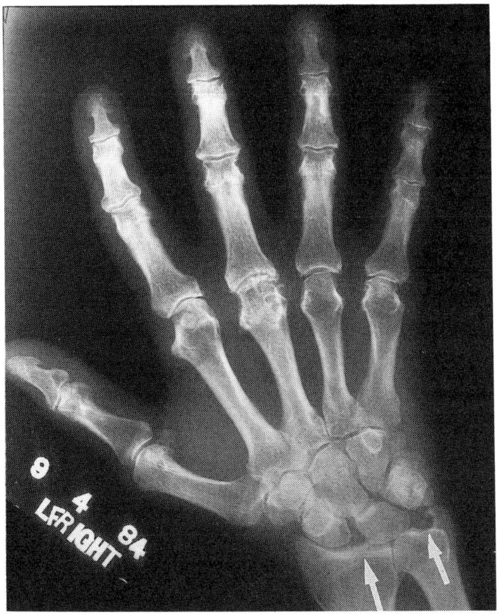

FIGURE 4 Faint chondrocalcinosis of triangular ligament of the wrist and intercarpal joints (arrows). Degenerative change at second and third metacarpophalangeal joints. Not hemochromatosis.

V. ASSOCIATED DISORDERS

Table 2 lists states that predispose to deposition of CPPD. The strongest evidence links CPPD to hyperparathyroidism (6,42), a disorder that may be declining in prevalence. Since chondrocalcinosis is radiologically evident in 5–30% of individuals older than 60 (5), a cause-and-effect relationship with coexistent

TABLE 2 Associated Conditions

Definite	Hyperparathyroidism
	Hemochromatosis
	Hypomagnesemia
	Hypophosphatasia
Possible	Hypothyroidism
	Hypocalciuric hypercalcemia
	Neuropathic joints
	Gout

metabolic disorders of old people is often difficult to prove (5). In my view, it is more appropriate to seek causes in young people (<50) than in the elderly, who are not likely to benefit from discovery of comorbidity. A practical approach would be to assess the following after finding CPPD or chondrocalcinosis in a select population: serum calcium, iron and/or ferritin, and magnesium. This roughly agrees with the opinion of Doberty and Dieppe (6).

In three series of consecutively studied patients with CPPD deposition, metabolic associations were sought. Hyperparathyroidism was present in 3–6% and hemochromatosis in 0–2% (17,42,43) while hypomagnesemia was found in only 1 of 115 total patients studied. The question of hypothyroidism being linked to CPPD has proponents (44,45) and at least one doubter (46). Hypophosphatasia is detected by finding a very low serum alkaline phosphatase and elevated urinary ethanolamine in a patient having metabolic bone disease. These patients may present in early adulthood with dense chondrocalcinosis in joints as well as fractures of the long bones (13). Because alkaline phosphatase activity includes that of pyrophosphatase, it follows that homozygous expression of the enzyme deficiency results in heavy accumulation of CPPD (13,47). Despite the association of treatable metabolic disease with CPPD, an exhaustive search in the "frail elderly" is not indicated (6,43).

Hemochromatosis should always be considered when CPPD disease is found (48), because iron removal can prevent hepatic cirrhosis. The recent discovery of a gene HLA-H, related to the MHC class I family, will further stimulate the discovery of new patients and kindreds of patients with hereditary hemochromatosis (49). At present, hemochromatosis is suspected in the following clinical setting of joint disease: involvement of metacarpophalangeal and wrist joints, chondrocalcinosis, a confusing overlap of "osteoarthritis with rheumatoid distribution," as well as mild hyperglycemia and elevated aspartate transaminase (50). Table 3 is a list, with references, of the most common diseases confused with CPPD disease. Interestingly, most of these may coexist with CPPD. The occurrence of attacks of pseudogout during pregnancy is recently described, but is unexplained (46,56).

TABLE 3 Differential Diagnosis

Disorder	Reference	Method of diagnosis
Gout	5	Monosodium urate crystals
Calcium apatite	52	Extra-articular crystals and attacks
Septic arthritis	51,23,53	Positive bacterial culture
Osteoarthritis	6,35	X-ray
Synovial chondromatosis	54	X-ray, arthrotomy
Stress fracture	55	X-ray

VI. TREATMENT

The acute attack of pseudogout responds best to aspiration of the joint with intra-articular injection of a potent corticosteroid (16,18), such as betamethasone (Celestone) or depomethylprednisolone (Depo-Medrol). In the knee, the injected volume is 1–2 ml. Joint rest combined with a nonsteroidal anti-inflammatory drug, e.g., sulindac 200 mg, twice daily for 4–7 days, are also effective. Intravenous colchicine has less appeal, due to potential toxicity, but is also effective: if used, the total dose should not exceed 2–3 mg and no more colchicine should be given for one week. Oral prednisone 30 mg daily for a week is a preferable alternative in the frail elderly with renal, hepatic, or bone marrow impairment and in patients with polyarticular pseudogout.

Prevention of attacks with daily oral colchicine may be considered in those few patients who have three or more attacks per year. Several neutrophil responses to CPPD crystals liberated into joints, including chemotaxis and response to cytokines such as leukokine B4, are lessened (57). The dosage range is 0.6–1.2 mg daily. Myopathy, neuropathy, and bone marrow toxicity are possible side effects. There is no satisfactory medical treatment for the calcific deposits and polyarticular degenerative changes that can progress in elderly patients with CPPD deposition disease. Even successful treatment of associated and causative conditions such as hyperparathyroidism and hemochromatosis does not reverse chondrocalcinosis and its associated degenerative arthritis (58). Intra-articular yttrium-90 caused some improvement in one study (59), and the same workers also tried oral treatment with magnesium carbonate in a six-month controlled trial (60). Magnesium treated patients had less symptoms while on treatment. Arthroscopic lavage of the knee in some patients with degenerative changes in knees said to harbor crystals has been tried. Total joint replacement is frequently carried out in knees, hips, and shoulders for the degenerative changes of CPPD deposition. Cervical and lumbar laminectomies are also carried out for myelopathy and lumbar stenosis, respectively, in the uncommon instances that these are caused by deposition of this material.

REFERENCES

1. W. D. Bundens, Jr., C. T. Brighton, and G. Weitzman. Primary articular-cartilage calcification with arthritis (pseudogout syndrome), *Bone Joint Surg 47-A(1)*:111–122 (1965).
2. D. Zitnan and S. Sitaj. Calcifications multiples du cartilage articulaire, *9th International Congress sur les Maladies Rheumatismales* 2:291 (1957).
3. D. J. McCarty, Jr., N. N. Kohn, and J. S. Faires. The significance of calcium

phosphate crystals in the synovial fliud of arthritic patients: The "pseudogout syndrome." I. Clinical aspects, *Ann Intern Med 56(5)*:711–737 (1962).

4. N. N. Kohn, R. E. Hughes, D. J. McCarty, Jr., et al. The significance of calcium phosphate crystals in the synovial fluid of arthritic patients: The "pseudogout syndrome." II. identification of crystals, *Ann Int Med 56(5)*:738–745 (1962).
5. L. M. Ryan and D. J. McCarty, Jr. Calcium pyrophosphate crystal deposition disease, pseudogout, and articular chondrocalcinosis, In: Arthritis and Allied Conditions: Textbook of Rheumatology, 13th Edition (Koopman, ed.), Williams and Wilkins, Baltimore, MD, 1997, pp. 2103–2125.
6. M. Doherty and P. Dieppe. Clinical aspects of calcium pyrophosphate dihydrate crystal deposition, *Rheum Dis Clin North Am 14(2)*:395–414 (1988).
7. P. A. Dieppe and M. Doherty. The role of particles in the pathogenesis of joint disease, *Curr Top Pathol 71*:199–233 (1982).
8. J. W. Rachow and L. M. Ryan. Adenosine triphosphate pyrophosphohydrolase and neutral inorganic pyrophosphatase in pathologic joint fluids: Elevated pyrophosphohydrolase in calcium pyrophosphate dihydrate crystal deposition disease, *Arth Rheum 28(11)*:1283–1288 (1985).
9. H. R. Schumacher, Jr. Pathology of crystal deposition diseases, *Rheum Dis Clin North Am 14(2)*:269–288 (1988).
10. A. O. Bjelle. Morphological study of articular cartilage in pyrophosphate arthropathy, *Ann Rheum Dis 31*:449–456 (1972).
11. H. A. Sissons, G. C. Steiner, F. Bonar, et al. Tumoral calcium pyrophosphate deposition disease, *Skeletal Radiol 18*:79–87 (1989).
12. T. Ishida, H. D. Dorfman, and P. G. Bullough. Tophaceous pseudogout (tumoral calcium pyrophosphate dihydrate crystal deposition disease), *Human Pathol 26(6)*:587–593 (1995).
13. J. D. O'Duffy. Hypophosphatasia associated with calcium pyrophosphate dihydrate deposits in cartilage, *Arth Rheum 13(4)*:381–388 (1970).
14. A. Beutler, S. Rothfuss, G. Clayburne, et al. Calcium pyrophosphate dihydrate crystal deposition in synovium, *Arth Rheum 36(5)*:704–715 (1993).
15. A. Caswell, D. F. Guilland-Cumming, P. R. Hearn, et al. Pathogenesis of chondrocalcinosis and pseudogout. Metabolism of inorganic pyrophosphate and production of calcium pyrophosphate dihydrate crystals, *Ann Rheum Dis 42*:suppl 27–37 (1983).
16. J. D. O'Duffy. Pseudogout syndrome in hospital patients, *JAMA 226(1)*:42–44, (1973).
17. A. G. Fam, J. R. Topp, H. B. Stein, et al. Clinical and roentgenographic aspects of pseudogout: A study of 50 cases and a review, *CMA J 124*:545–551 (1981).
18. G. Ho Jr. and M. DeNuccio. Gout and pseudogout in hospitalized patients, *Arch Intern Med 153*:2787–2790 (1993).
19. D. Bong and R. Bennett. Pseudogout mimicking systemic disease, *JAMA 246(13)*:1438–1440 (1981).
20. P. Phelps, A. D. Steele, and D. J. McCarty, Jr. Compensated polarized light microscopy: identification of crystals in synovial fluids from gout and pseudogout, *JAMA 203(7)*:166–170 (1968).
21. L. W. Stevens and H. Spiera. Hemarthrosis in chondrocalcinosis (pseudogout), *Arth Rheum 15(6)*:651–653 (1972).

22. A. Swan, B. Heywood, B. Chapman, et al. Evidence for a causal relationship between the structure, size, and load of calcium pyrophosphate dihydrate crystals, and attacks of pseudogout, *Ann Rheum Dis 54*:825–830 (1995).
23. L. P. Zyskowski, J. C. Silverfield, and J. D. O'Duffy. Pseudogout masking other arthritides, *J Rheum 10*:449–453 (1983).
24. M. Skinner and A. S. Cohen. Calcium pyrophosphate dihydrate crystal deposition disease, *Arch Intern Med 123*:636–644 (1969).
25. E. Hamilton, M. Pattrick, J. Hornby, et al. Synovial fluid calcium pyrophosphate dihydrate crystals and alizarin red positivity: analysis of 3000 samples, *Brit J Rheum 29*:101–104 (1990).
26. R. B. Delamarter, J. E. Sherman, and J. Carr. Lumbar spinal stenosis secondary to calcium pyrophosphate crystal deposition (pseudogout), *Clin Ortho Rel Res 289*:127–130 (1993).
27. T. Sadique, J. G. Bradley, and A. M. Jackson. Central spinal stenosis due to pseudogout: a case report, *J Bone Joint Surg 76-B(4)*:672–673 (1994).
28. M. Hammoudeh and A. R. Siam. Pseudogout mimicking meningitis, *Brit J Rheum 32(4)*:351–352 (1993).
29. S. Jacobelli, D. J. McCarty, D. C. Silcox, et al. Calcium pyrophosphate dihydrate crystal deposition in neuropathic joints, *Ann Int Med 79*:340–347 (1973).
30. C. S. Resnik and D. Resnick. Calcium pyrophosphate dihydrate crystal deposition disease, In: Current Problems in Diagnostic Radiology (Keats, ed.), Year Book Medical Publishers, Inc., Chicago, IL, 1982, pp. 2–40.
31. J. L. Riestra, A. Sanchez, V. Rodriques-Valverde, et al. Roentgenographic features of the arthropathy associated with CPPD crystal deposition disease. A comparative study with primary osteoarthritis, *J Rheum 12(6)*:1154–1158 (1985).
32. R. W. Moskowitz, B. K. Harris, A. Schwartz, et al. Chronic synovitis as a manifestation of calcium crystal deposition disease, *Arth Rheum 14(1)*:109–116 (1971).
33. A. J. Reginato. Calcium pyrophosphate dihydrate gout and other crystal deposition diseases, *Curr Opin Rheum 3*:676–683 (1991).
34. C. J. Menkes, F. Simon, F. Delrien, et al. Destructive arthropathy in chondrocalcinosis articularis, *Arth Rheum 19*:329–348 (1976).
35. D. Zitnan and S. Sitaj. Natural course of articular chondrocalcinosis, *Arth Rheum 19*:363–370 (1976).
36. A. J. Reginato. Articular chondrocalcinosis in the Chiloe islanders, *Arth Rheum 19*:395–404 (1976).
37. E. B. D. Hamilton. Residual joint damage due to calcium pyrophosphate dihydrate (CPPD) deposition, *Eur J Rheum Inflam 1(2)*:102–104 (1978).
38. H. K. Genant. Roentgenographic aspects: calcium pyrophosphate dihydrate crystal deposition disease (pseudogout), *Arth Rheum 19*:307–328 (1976).
39. M. Doherty, P. Dieppe, and I. Watt. Pyrophosphate arthropathy: a prospective study, *Brit J Rheum 32*:189–196 (1993).
40. D. Zitnan, J. Lukac, E. Rovenska, et al. What is the fate of families with occurrence of primary articular chondrocalcinosis observed in Slovakia since 1955, *Acta Rheum Balenol Pistiniana 11*:41–48 (1993).
41. G. Huang, D. Bachmann, J. A. M. Taylor, et al. Calcium pyrophosphate dihydrate

crystal deposition disease and pseudogout of the acromioclavicular joint: radiographic and pathologic features, *J Rheum 20(12)*:2077–2082 (1993).

42. D. J. McCarty, D. C. Silcox, F. Coe, et al. Diseases associated with calcium pyrophosphate dihydrate crystal deposition, *Am J Med 56*:704–714 (1974).
43. M. H. Ellman, N. L. Brown, and A. P. Porat. Laboratory investigations in pseudogout patients and controls, *J Rheum 7(1)*:77–81 (1980).
44. B. B. Dorwart and H. R. Schumacher. Joint effusions, chondrocalcinosis and other rheumatic manifestations in hypothyroidism, *Am J Med 59*:780–790 (1975).
45. R. M. McLean and D. N. Podell. Bone and joint manifestations of hypothyroidism, *Sem Arth Rheum 24(4)*:282–290 (1995).
46. D. J. McCarty. Calcium pyrophosphate dihydrate crystal deposition disease, *Brit Soc Rheum 32*:177–180 (1993).
47. T. Shinozaki and K. P. H. Pritzker. Regulation of alkaline phosphatase: implications for calcium pyrophosphate dihydrate crystal dissolution and other alkaline phosphatase functions, *J Rheum 23(4)*:677–683 (1996).
48. A. C. Jones, A. J. Chuck, E. A. Arie, et al. Diseases associated with calcium pyrophosphate deposition disease, *Sem Arth Rheum 22(3)*:188–202 (1992).
49. J. N. Feder, A. Gnirke, W. Thomas, et al. A novel MHC class I-like gene is mutated in patients with hereditary haemochromatosis, *Nat Gene 13*:399–408 (1996).
50. R. Faraawi, M. Harth, A. Kertesz, et al. Arthritis in hemochromatosis, *J Rheum 20(3)*:448–452 (1993).
51. N. J. Doll and F. N. Jackson. Acute pseudogout simulating septic arthritis, *JAMA 242(16)*:1768 (1979).
52. A. G. Fam and J. Rubenstein. Hydroxyapatite pseudopodagra: a syndrome of young women, *Arth Rheum 32(6)*:741–747 (1989).
53. M. E. Mavrikakis, I. V. Athanassiades, L. G. Antoniades, et al. Pseudogout presenting as sepsis in an elderly man, *Am J Med 91*:559 (1991).
54. M. H. Ellman, M. I. Krieger, and N. Brown. Pseudogout mimicking synovial chondromatosis, *J Bone Joint Surg 57-A(6)*:863–865 (1975).
55. D. J. Ross, P. A. Dieppe, I. Watt, et al. Tibial stress fracture in pyrophosphate arthropathy, *J Bone Joint Surg 65-B(4)*:474–477 (1983).
56. M. Regan, A. K. Clarke, and M. Doherty. Case reports: pseudogout provoked by pregnancy, *Brit Soc Rheum 32*:245–247 (1993).
57. R. A. Terkeltaub. Pathogenesis and treatment of crystal-induced inflammation, In: Arthritis and Allied Conditions: Textbook of Rheumatology, 13th Edition (Koopman, ed.), Williams and Wilkins, Baltimore, MD, 1997, pp. 2085–2102.
58. E. B. D. Hamilton, A. B. Bomford, J. W. Laws, et al. The natural history of arthritis in idiopathic hemochromatosis: progression of the clinical and radiologic features over ten years, *Quart J Med 199*:3321–3329 (1981).
59. M. Doherty and P. A. Dieppe. Effect of intra-articular yttrium-90 on chronic pyrophosphate arthropathy of the knee, *Lancet 1*:1243–1246 (1981).
60. M. Doherty and P. A. Dieppe. Double-blind placebo-controlled trial of magnesium carbonate in chronic pyrophosphate arthropathy, *Ann Rheum Dis 42*:106–107 (1983).

21

Imaging of Calcium Pyrophosphate Dihydrate (CPPD) Crystal Deposition Disease

LYNNE S. STEINBACH
University of California—San Francisco, San Francisco, California

DONALD RESNICK
University of California—San Diego and Veterans Affairs Medical Center, San Diego, California

Calcium pyrophosphate dihydrate (CPPD) crystal deposition disease, the subject of this manuscript, is induced by CPPD crystals. It is characterized by acute, subacute, or chronic joint inflammation and deposition of CPPD crystals in hyaline cartilage, fibrocartilage, and other soft tissue structures. In 1958, Zitnan and Sitaj were the first to recognize the condition subsequently termed CPPD crystal deposition disease (1). Three years later, Revault et al. discussed 41 cases of this disorder (2), and the following year McCarty emphasized the significance of CPPD crystals in synovial fluid and stressed the importance of chondrocalcinosis in this disorder. Martel subsequently described the first characteristic radiographic features in a prospective study in 1970 (3). We have learned a great deal about imaging findings of CPPD crystal deposition disease (4). New facts about the disorder and clues to radiological diagnosis continue to be revealed. This article will provide a review of imaging characteristics of this disease, with emphasis upon some recent findings.

I. NOMENCLATURE

One of the more confusing aspects of this arthropathy is the associated nomenclature. A variety of terms have been used. We utilize the following guidelines, realizing that not everyone agrees with them. *Chondrocalcinosis* is a more general term that is reserved for pathologically or radiologically evident cartilage calcification. It can include CPPD, dicalcium phosphate dihydrate, or calcium hydroxyapatite crystals, or combinations of the three. *Calcium pyrophosphate dihydrate (CPPD) crystal deposition disease* is a specific term for a disorder characterized by the exclusive presence of CPPD crystals in or around joints. The term *pseudogout* is not a radiological diagnosis; rather, it is reserved for a gout-like clinical syndrome produced by CPPD crystal deposition disease that is characterized by intermittent acute attacks of arthritis. *Pyrophosphate arthropathy* is a term that describes a particular pattern of structural joint damage that occurs in CPPD crystal deposition disease. This arthropathy is similar to osteoarthritis but has some separate distinct features. Cartilage calcification may be absent on radiographs in patients with pyrophosphate arthropathy (5). *Articular and periarticular calcification* may occur with CPPD crystal deposition disease; however, calcium deposits other than CPPD crystal accumulation also can produce this type of calcification.

II. CLASSIFICATION

CPPD crystal deposition disease can be classified as sporadic, hereditary, or secondary (6). The sporadic, or idiopathic, form tends to occur in middle-aged and elderly patients without a sexual predominance (7–9). Different hereditary types have been described in families all over the world. The hereditary forms usually have a female predominance, appear at a relatively early age, and are accompanied by more severe arthropathy. CPPD crystal deposition may be seen in association with other diseases (i.e., the secondary form of the disease). Association with the four H's—primary hyperparathyroidism, hemochromatosis, hypomagnesemia, and hypophosphatasia—is well documented (10).

III. PATHOPHYSIOLOGY

CPPD crystal deposition disease occurs with a frequency of 1 in 1,000 persons, approaching 45% in patients aged 85 years or older (11,12). The etiology of CPPD crystal deposition in cartilage is unknown. Several factors may influence this deposition; however, the importance of age changes in normal cartilage or local tissue damage related to preexisting joint disease as a cause of crystal deposition has been reported in recent years and is part of the "amplification loop hypothesis" (13). It has been proposed that cartilage damage that occurs with increasing age predisposes to crystal deposition by changing the concentration of proteoglycan and inhibitory factors and increasing inorganic phosphate turnover (14,15).

Secondary chondrocalcinosis of the knee meniscus also results from surgical intervention (16). This is attributed to liberation of intracellular pyrophosphates from chondrocytes into the extracellular space during surgery.

Histologic, biochemical, and electron microscopic studies of a familial form of CPPD crystal deposition disease suggest that affected patients have a primary abnormality of the cartilaginous matrix with secondary crystal deposition (17).

Other mechanisms for CPPD crystal deposition in cartilage have been postulated. A defect in the metabolism or production of inorganic pyrophosphate (PPi) may be present because synovial fluid PPi concentration is elevated, especially following a pseudogout attack (18). Elevated levels of PPi in the joint is not specific for this arthropathy, having been demonstrated also in osteoarthritis. Elevated levels of extra-articular calcium and pyrophosphatase inhibition by divalent ions such as iron, calcium, and copper have also been implicated. It is postulated that divalent ions may accelerate cartilage damage, producing structural joint changes in association with CPPD crystal deposition (19).

Synovitis results when polymorphonuclear leukocytes phagocytize the CPPD crystals, releasing chemotactic factors (20). The acute exacerbations of the disease associated with synovitis may be related to shedding of the crystal within the joint. Such shedding is seen with joint lavage using crystal solubilizers, in patients with decreased blood calcium concentration, and when there is significant cartilage destruction (as in neuropathic osteoarthropathy and infection). This is further substantiated by the observation that radiologically evident chondrocalcinosis sometimes disappears during pseudogout attacks.

CPPD crystals occasionally coexist in the same articular or periarticular site with other crystalline deposits, including calcium hydroxyapatite and monosodium urate. Multiple types of crystals are frequently present in asymptomatic joints. Urate, hydroxyapatite, and CPPD crystals can produce calcifications in gouty tophi. The significance of the coexistence of multiple crystal types in one location needs further investigation.

VI. CLINICAL MANIFESTATIONS

The clinical presentations of CPPD crystal deposition disease are highly variable, ranging from asymptomatic disease to severe pain associated with a destructive arthropathy. Indeed, this disease has been called a "great mimicker" of other arthritides (3). Ryan and McCarty described six patterns of joint involvement (21). Furthermore, occasionally, several of these clinical patterns present at different times during the course of the arthritis.

The *asymptomatic* form of this arthropathy is probably the most common; however, it is difficult to document this because many asymptomatic patients are never seen by a physician. Absence of symptoms occurs in at least 10–20% of documented cases of CPPD crystal deposition disease.

A large percentage of patients with CPPD crystal deposition disease present with an arthritis that simulates *osteoarthritis*. An occasional acute inflammatory component is seen in 35–60% of such patients. This osteoarthritic form is a chronic and progressive arthritis that is frequently bilateral and symmetric, presenting in the knee, hip, metacarpophalangeal, elbow, ankle, wrist, and glenohumeral joints. Flexion contractures are common, especially in the knee and elbow.

Patients with CPPD crystal deposition disease also may be symptomatic. For example, attacks of pseudogout occur in 10–20% of symptomatic patients. The pseudogout syndrome is caused by shedding of pyrophosphate crystals into the joint fluid. The attacks are self-limited and can last from one day to several weeks. They generally are less painful than those of gout and are most common in the knee, but other sites including the hip, glenohumeral, elbow, ankle, wrist, acromioclavicular, talocalcaneal, and metatarsophalangeal joints also are affected. Fever and elevation of the erythrocyte sedimentation rate may accompany pseudogout attacks.

Two to six percent of patients with CPPD crystal deposition disease present with an arthritis that simulates *rheumatoid arthritis*. These attacks are characterized by morning stiffness, fatigue, synovial thickening, restricted joint motion, and an elevated erythrocyte sedimentation rate, and they persist from four weeks to several months.

CPPD crystal deposition disease also can have a *pseudoneuropathic* presentation in as many as 2% of patients (22–26). Indeed, CPPD crystalline arthropathy should be considered in the differential diagnosis of rapidly progressive destruction of large joints.

Other miscellaneous uncommon clinical presentations of CPPD crystal deposition disease include symptoms suggestive of rheumatic fever, psychogenic disease, trauma, and ankylosing spondylitis (27–30).

Treatment of CPPD crystal deposition disease includes aspiration of large effusions, nonsteroidal anti-inflammatory medication, corticosteroids, and low doses of colchicine, which are helpful if the patient has recurrent episodes of pseudogout. Patients with pseudoneuropathic joints often do well with joint replacement.

V. RADIOLOGIC MANIFESTATIONS

CPPD crystal deposition disease is characterized by calcification in and around joints and structural joint changes termed *pyrophosphate arthropathy*. This arthropathy resembles osteoarthritis; however, it occurs in articulations not usually affected by osteoarthritis, often affecting nonweight-bearing regions such as the radiocarpal, metacarpophalangeal, elbow, and glenohumeral joints, followed in frequency by the hip, and glenohumeral joint. It usually is bilateral and symmetric and is most common in the knee, wrist, and metacarpophalangeal joints. Furthermore, CPPD crystal deposition disease has an unusual intra-articular distribution in certain joints such as the knee and wrist, where patellofemoral and radiocarpal joint space narrowing may be seen.

Radiographically, chondrocalcinosis usually is apparent in CPPD crystal deposition disease, but the arthropathy can also precede radiographically detectable cartilage calcification, the calcification may not always be dense enough to be visualized on conventional radiographs, or it may be difficult to identify such calcification if the joint is severely deranged (31, 32).

The joints are mineralized normally with narrowing of various articulations and subchondral sclerosis. Osteophytes are common, but occur not always with the frequency seen in osteoarthritis. Subchondral cysts are one of the hallmarks of this arthropathy (Figure 1). The cysts usually are larger and

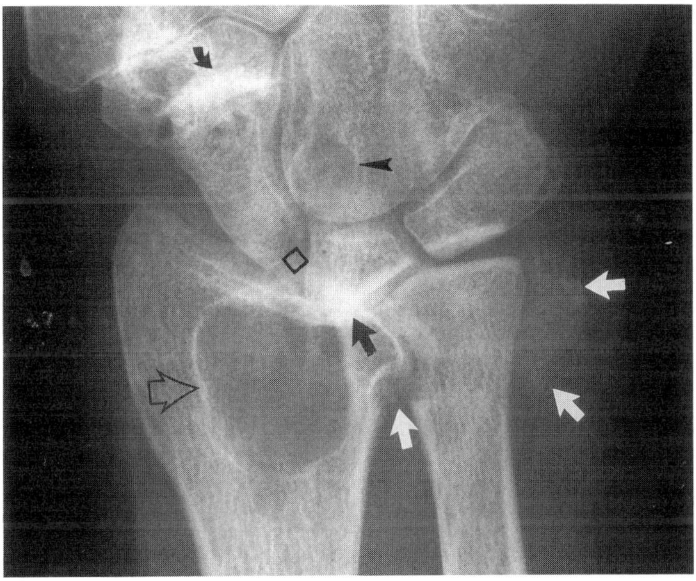

FIGURE 1 Multiple wrist abnormalities in CPPD arthropathy. This PA wrist study demonstrates several features of pyrophosphate arthropathy: (1) a large well-circumscribed lytic lesion in the distal radius, which represents a subchondral cyst (hollow black arrow); (2) a similar but smaller cyst is seen in the capitate (arrowhead); (3) radiocarpal joint narrowing, particularly at the lunate articulation (solid black arrow); (4) narrowing of the triscaphe joint (curved arrow); (5) scapholunate dissociation (diamond); and (6) tumoral deposit of CPPD crystals in the soft tissues around the distal ulna at the distal radioulnar joint, producing erosion along the radial aspect of the ulna (white arrows). (Published with permission from Ref. 4.)

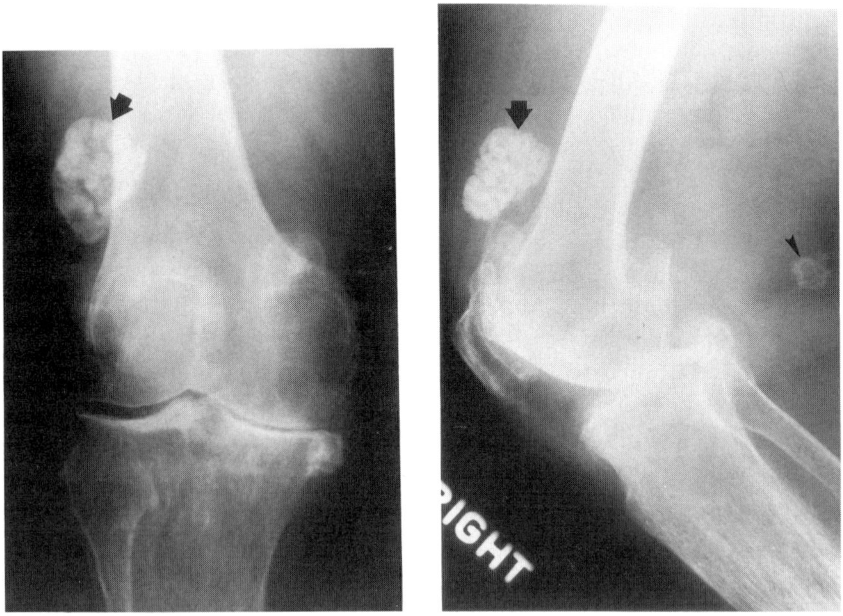

(a) (b)

FIGURE 2 (a) AP and (b) lateral radiographs of the knee show synovial osteochondromatosis associated with CPPD arthropathy. A large loose body lies in the suprapatellar bursa (arrow). There is a smaller one in a popliteal cyst (arrowhead). There are degenerative changes in the patellofemoral joint. [Part (b) published with permission from Ref. 4].

more numerous and widespread than in osteoarthritis, and they frequently are multiple. Cysts may form before cartilage loss is evident. Osseous fragmentation and collapse may be related to fracture of these cystic lesions. Intra-articular osteochondral bodies commonly are associated with CPPD crystal deposition disease (33) (Figure 2). These may be loose in the joint cavity or embedded in cartilage or synovium.

A. Cartilage

Chondrocalcinosis is usually caused by CPPD crystal deposition. In 5% of cases, however, it can be related to other crystals such as dicalcium phosphate dihydrate and hydroxyapatite (5). Both hyaline and fibrocartilage can contain CPPD crystals. The CPPD crystal tends to be deposited in the middle layer of degenerated hyaline cartilage. These deposits are thin, linear, and parallel the subjacent subchondral bone (Figure 3). CPPD crystals are deposited on the sur-

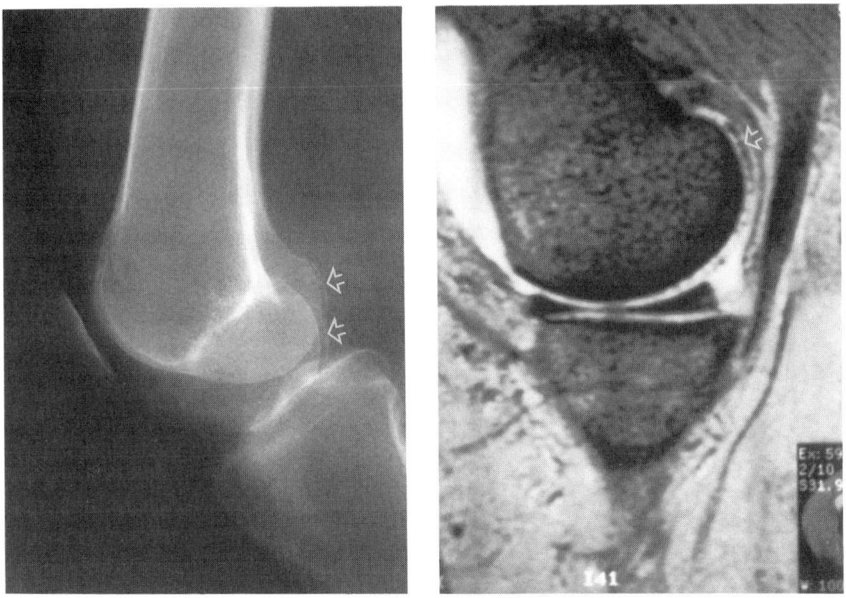

(a) (b)

FIGURE 3 (a) Hyaline cartilage calcification is demonstrated paralleling the posterior femoral condyles (arrows) on an off-lateral radiograph of the knee. (b) A corresponding gradient echo T2* sagittal magnetic resonance image (MRI) through the medial compartment of the knee shows the calcification as a region of low signal intensity within the hyaline cartilage (arrow).

face of the hyaline cartilage, when there is superficial chondral erosion (34,35). Hyaline cartilage calcification is most common in the wrist, knee, elbow, and hip.

CPPD crystal deposition in fibrocartilage is most commonly observed in the menisci of the knee (Figure 4), triangular fibrocartilage of the wrist, labra of the acetabulum, symphysis pubis, and anulus fibrosus of the intervertebral disc (25). Other less common sites of CPPD crystal deposition in cartilage include the articular discs of the sternoclavicular and acromioclavicular joints and glenoid labra (36,37).

B. Synovium and Capsule

Synovial calcification is common in CPPD crystal deposition disease (33). Synovial deposits are more common in the wrist, knee (Figure 5), and metacarpophalangeal and metatarsophalangeal joints. These deposits are cloud-like and

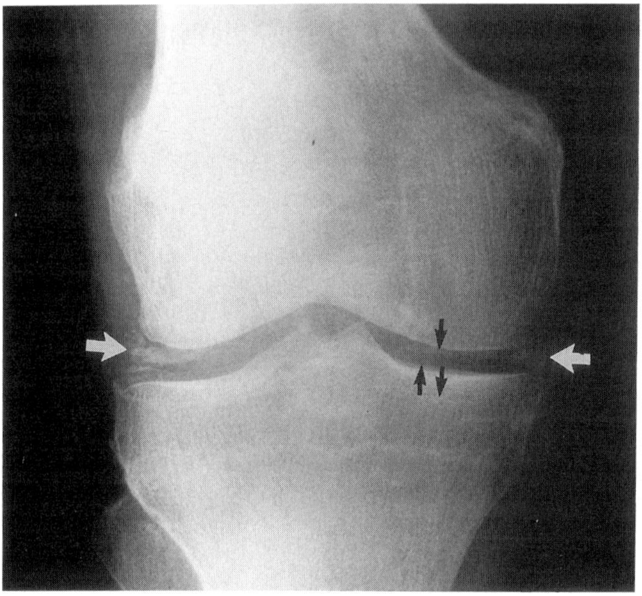

FIGURE 4 This AP knee radiograph demonstrates both meniscal and hyaline cartilage calcification. Meniscal calcification is characterized by triangles of high density (white arrow), whereas the hyaline cartilage calcification parallels the articular surface (black arrow). The medial and lateral joint compartments are of normal height, a feature commonly seen with CPPD crystal deposition disease.

can simulate calcifications in idiopathic synovial osteochondromatosis. Calcium hydroxyapatite crystals also deposit in the synovium, particularly if there are associated severe degenerative changes. The synovial membrane may demonstrate acute and chronic inflammatory changes in association with CPPD crystal deposition disease. It is not known if the crystals migrate into the synovium from the adjacent cartilage or are deposited directly within the synovium. Capsular calcification may appear as a linear peripheral density and may be difficult to distinguish from early synovial calcification. It is most commonly observed in the elbow, glenohumeral, metatarsophalangeal, and metacarpophalangeal joints.

C. Tendons, Ligaments, and Bursae

Tendon calcifications are observed with high frequency in patients with CPPD crystal deposition disease (32,38,39). An incidence of 13.5% was reported in

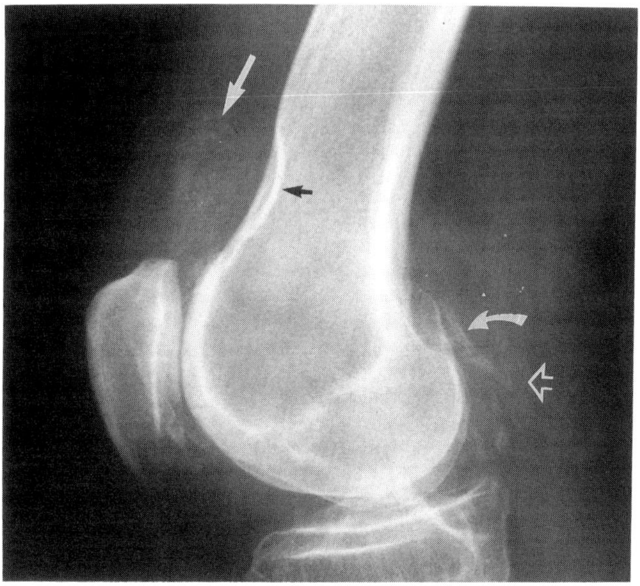

FIGURE 5 This lateral knee radiograph demonstrates several findings characteristic of CPPD crystal deposition disease. There is calcification of the synovium that lines the suprapatellar bursa (arrow) as well as the posterior capsule (open arrow). The gastrocnemius tendon is also calcified (curved arrow). Smooth erosion is present along the anterior aspect of the distal femur above the patella (black arrow). This is related to abutment of the patella against the femur, a common finding in this disorder.

such patients in one study (39). Those tendons more frequently involved include the supraspinatus, triceps, quadriceps (Figure 6), gastrocnemius, and Achilles (Figure 7) tendons. Hip adductor and rectus femoris tendon calcification may also be seen. Tendon calcifications commonly are linear or punctate and usually can be distinguished from the more homogeneous, discrete, and nodular calcifications of calcium hydroxyapatite crystal deposition (25). Calcification often extends far from the tendon attachment. There is a high correlation between the existence of these tendon calcifications and the extent and intensity of calcific deposits in other joints (38). Direct translocation of CPPD crystals from the articular or bursal surfaces may be reponsible for some of the tendinous calcification (40).

Ligaments can also calcify. Sometimes, the calcification is not dense enough to be visualized on conventional radiographs. We have recently seen cruciate ligament involvement in a cadaveric case with CPPD crystal deposition disease (Figure 8). The ligamentum flavum (Figure 9) and dura mater can con-

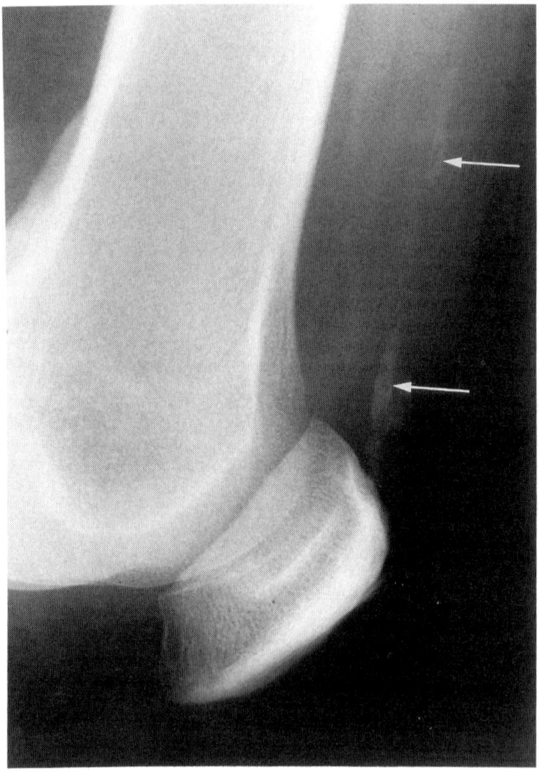

FIGURE 6 The quadriceps tendon is calcified in a linear pattern typical of CPPD crystal deposition disease (arrows).

tain calcific deposits. Bursal calcification is most common in the olecranon and subacromial bursae.

D. Other Extra-Articular Soft Tissues

Soft tissue and vascular calcification may be seen in CPPD crystal deposition disease (32,41–44). In particular, tumor-like masses of CPPD crystals can be seen in the extra-articular soft tissues (Figure 1). This manifestation of CPPD crystal deposition disease, known as "tophaceous pseudogout," is rare. In one study, seven cases of massive focal CPPD crystal deposition disease were identified in atypical locations (45). The patients ranged in age from 31 to 86

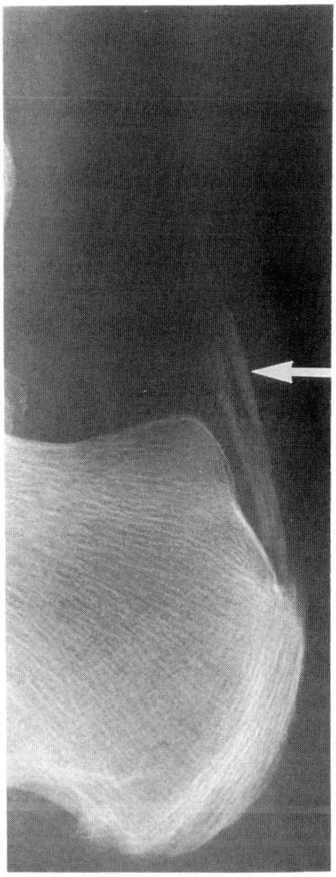

FIGURE 7 Tendon calcification in CPPD arthropathy. Extensive linear calcification of the Achilles tendon (arrow). There was also hyaline cartilage calcification in the ankle joint (not shown). (Published with permission from Ref. 4.)

years and six of them were women. Although the mechanism for development of these masses is not known, it has been postulated that hypertrophic metaplastic chondrocytes accumulating proteoglycans intracellularly provide a seeding site for crystal formation. These calcified masses may initially be mistaken for benign and malignant chondroid or other soft-tissue tumors (46). Misdiagnosis sometimes leads to unnecessary surgery. They usually can be differentiated from the lobular pattern of calcification in tumoral calcinosis by their granular and more delicate appearance (47,48). Calcified soft tissue masses related to CPPD crystal deposition are of intermediate to low signal intensity on magnetic resonance (MR) imaging examinations (49). They can

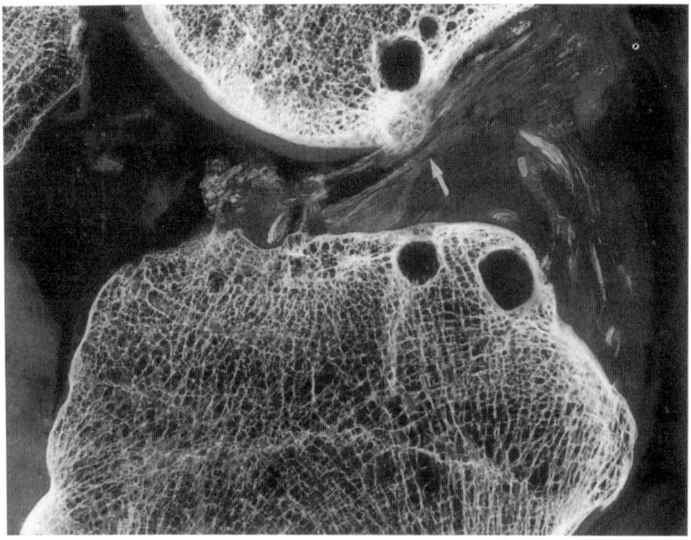

(a)

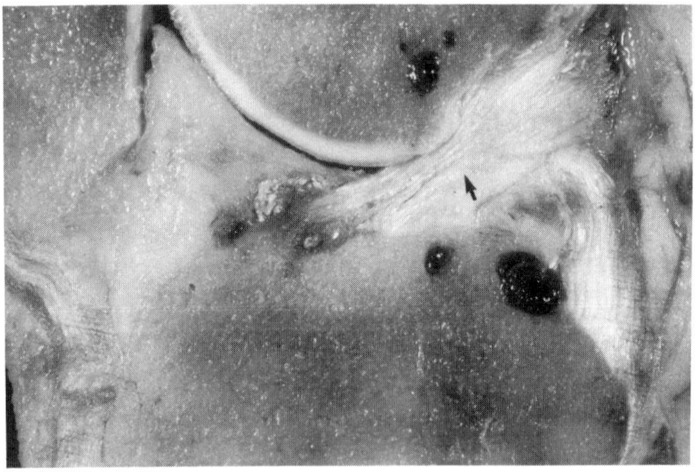

(b)

FIGURE 8 Anterior and posterior cruciate ligament calcification in CPPD arthropathy. (a) CPPD crystal deposition is demonstrated on a sectional lateral radiograph of a cadaver knee (white arrow). (b) The linear CPPD crystalline deposits are confirmed on a photograph of the specimen (black arrow). Note the subchondral cysts on both sides of the joint. Courtesy of Joachim Brossmann, M.D. (Published with permission from Ref. 4.)

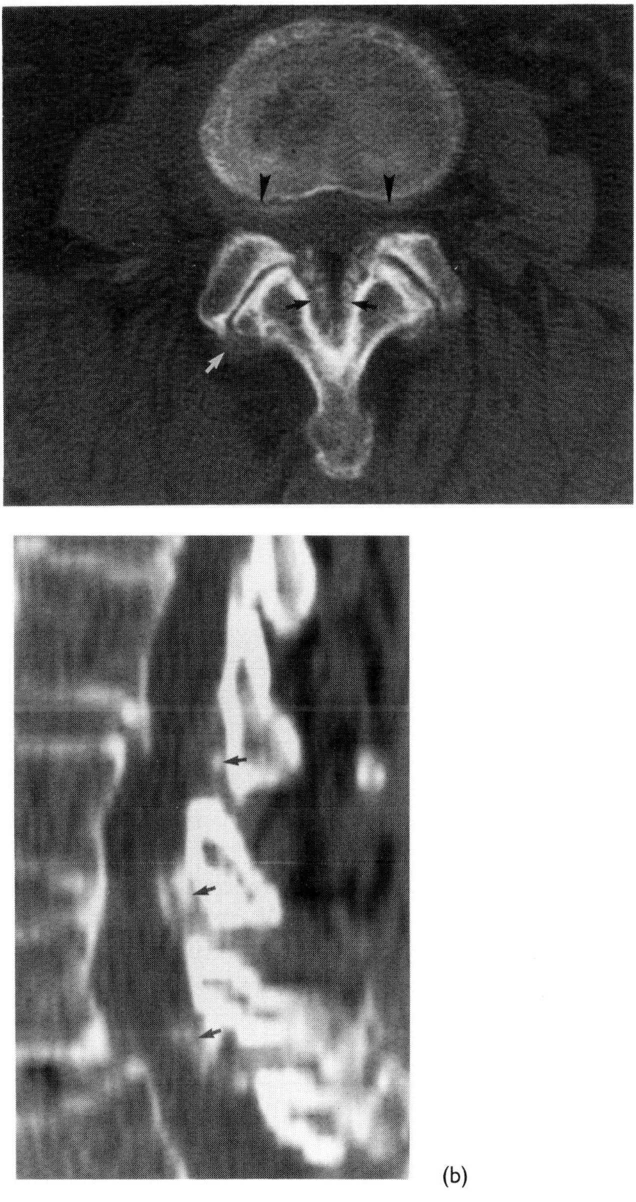

(a)

(b)

FIGURE 9 (a) The ligamentum flavum is calcified (black arrows) on this axial CT image obtained in the upper lumbar region with bone windows and (b) on a sagittal CT reformation of the lumbar spine in the same patient. Notice that the annulus fibrosus is also calcified (arrowheads), a feature often seen in CPPD crystal deposition disease. In addition, there is some calcification of the capsule surrounding a degenerated facet joint (white arrow).

present as the only manifestation of CPPD crystal deposition disease (45). Pressure erosion of adjacent osseous structures may be seen. It is important to identify the CPPD crystals, as these masses have also been mistaken for malignant cartilaginous tumors on histologic evaluation because of the presence of chondroid metaplasia (45,50).

E. Common Sites of Involvement

The joints most frequently involved are the knee, wrist, symphysis pubis, elbow, and hip. Unlike osteoarthritis, the glenohumeral joint and elbow often are involved. An ideal screening series for detecting chondrocalcinosis includes anteroposterior radiographs of each knee, posteroanterior radiographs of each wrist, and an anteroposterior radiograph of the pelvis.

1. Knee

The knee is the most commonly involved joint in CPPD crystal deposition disease. Disproportionate narrowing of the patellofemoral joint is a characteristic finding that is seen occasionally (Figure 10). The medial and lateral compartments frequently are of normal width (Figure 4); however, these compartments may become narrowed. In fact, pyrophosphate arthropathy more commonly involves the medial femorotibial than the patellofemoral compartment (25). Isolated patellofemoral narrowing is a finding that should suggest underlying CPPD crystal deposition disease in the older patient, however, even in the absence of joint calcification. Anterior femoral scalloping is occasionally seen proximal to the patella, related to abutment of the patella against the femur (Figure 5). Similar patellofemoral changes may appear in patients with primary hyperparathyroidism or renal osteodystrophy without CPPD crystal deposition disease.

Wedge-shaped meniscal calcification is more frequent than linear hyaline calcification (43), and the lateral meniscus is more commonly calcified than the medial meniscus. Chondrocalcinosis is thought to be secondary to post-traumatic or degenerative meniscal changes, or both types of changes (16). Posterior hyaline cartilage calcification is more common than anterior hyaline cartilage calcification (40). The synovium, capsule, ligaments, and tendons (Figures 5–11) also may be calcified, and these findings may be of aid in diagnosing CPPD crystal deposition disease in those joints with advanced cartilage loss where visualization of chondrocalcinosis is difficult. Medial or lateral gastrocnemius tendon calcification was seen in 15 of 37 patients with CPPD crystal deposition disease in a recent study (40) and was exclusive to this disorder. The quadriceps tendon can also calcify (Figures 6 and 11), although less commonly than the gastrocnemius (Figures 5 and 11). Intra-articular bodies occasionally are seen in association with degenerative changes of the cartilaginous and subchondral regions.

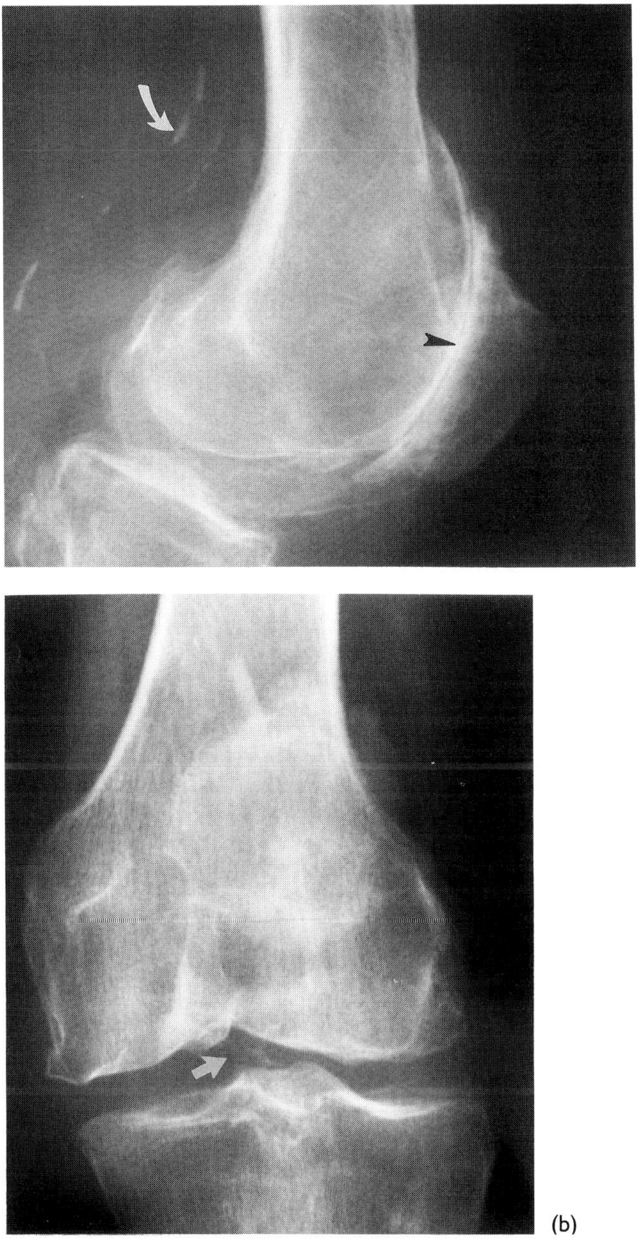

(a)

(b)

FIGURE 10 Isolated patellofemoral joint narrowing and cruciate ligament calcification in CPPD arthropathy. (a) Marked patellofemoral joint narrowing and degenerative changes (arrowhead) contrast with (b) the spared medial and lateral joint compartments. This finding alone raises the question of underlying pyrophosphate arthropathy. The anterior and posterior cruciate ligaments are calcified (arrow), confirming the diagnosis. The popliteal artery is calcified (curved arrow). (Published with permission from Ref. 4.)

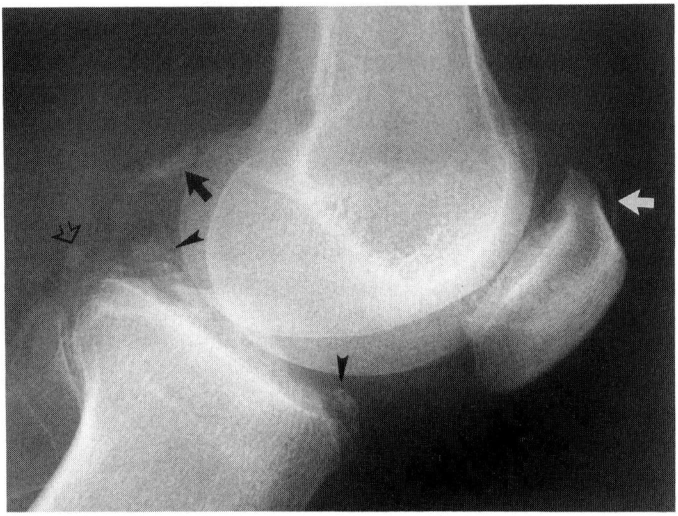

FIGURE 11 This lateral knee radiograph demonstrates many features of CPPD crystal deposition disease. There is calcification of the quadriceps (white arrow) and medial head of the gastrocnemius (black arrow) tendons on this lateral knee radiograph. Notice the meniscal calcification (arrowheads) and ossified loose body (open arrow) as well. There are characteristic subchondral lucencies in the superior aspect of the patella posteriorly adjacent to a region of hyaline cartilage calcification of the anterior femur. The popliteal artery is also calcified.

2. Wrist and Hand

In the wrist, the lunotriquetral ligament has been recently shown to be the a more common site of calcification than the triangular fibrocartilage (TFC), although the TFC is frequently calcified (51) (Figure 12). Degenerative tears of the TFC and degeneration of the articular cartilage of the lunate have been associated with CPPD crystal deposits (52). Hyaline cartilage calcification is most frequent between the scaphoid and lunate (Figure 13).

There is often associated radiocarpal joint space narrowing (Figure 14). A scapholunate advanced collapse (SLAC) pattern of arthritis, sometimes seen after wrist trauma, is the most common form of structural joint damage in the wrist in patients with CPPD crystal deposition disease (3,52,53). Compromised scapholunate and volar radioscapholunate ligaments subsequently lead to rotary subluxation of the scaphoid and scapholunate dissociation in the SLAC wrist. The capitate then migrates proximally and dorsally into the abnormally large space that exists between the capitate and lunate with eventual degenerative change in the radiocarpal joint. The scaphoid moves proximally and may appear

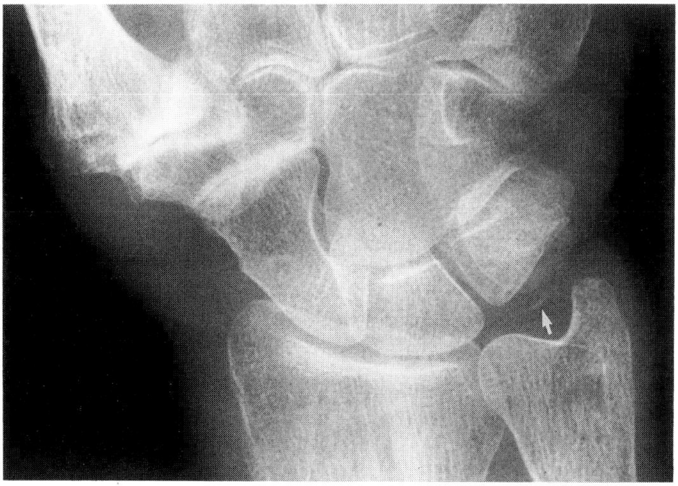

FIGURE 12 CPPD crystal deposition disease produces calcification in the region of the triangular fibrocartilage (arrow) on this PA wrist radiograph. There is also sclerosis and narrowing of the triscaphe and first carpometacarpal joints.

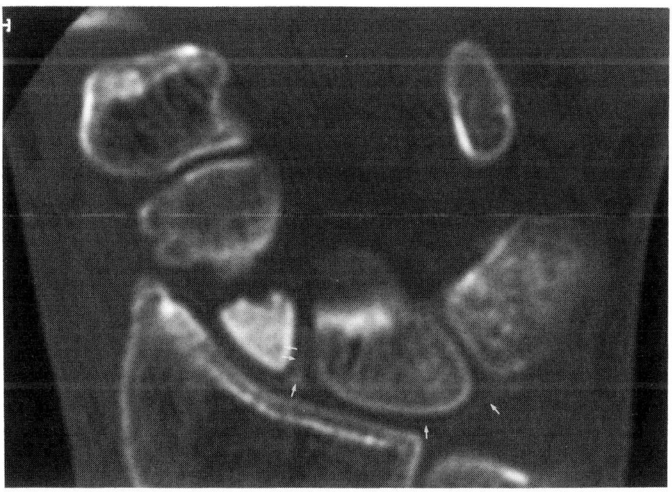

FIGURE 13 A coronal CT of the wrist in an older patient with avascular necrosis of the proximal scaphoid following a nonunion fracture of the waist also shows calcification of the hyaline cartilage of the proximal scaphoid and lunate and along the proximal lunate and triquetrum (arrows).

deformed or compressed by the adjacent radius (Figure 14). This results in the "stepladder" appearance. There is often narrowing of the radioscaphoid and capitolunate joint spaces. The radiolunate space generally is spared (54–56). A dorsal intercalated segment instability pattern commonly ensues. The triscaphe joint (located between the scaphoid, trapezium, and trapezoid) also is commonly affected in CPPD crystal deposition disease (Figures 1, 12, and 14).

Narrowing of the metacarpophalangeal joints (especially the second and third) also is frequent in CPPD crystal deposition disease (Figure 15), with spar-

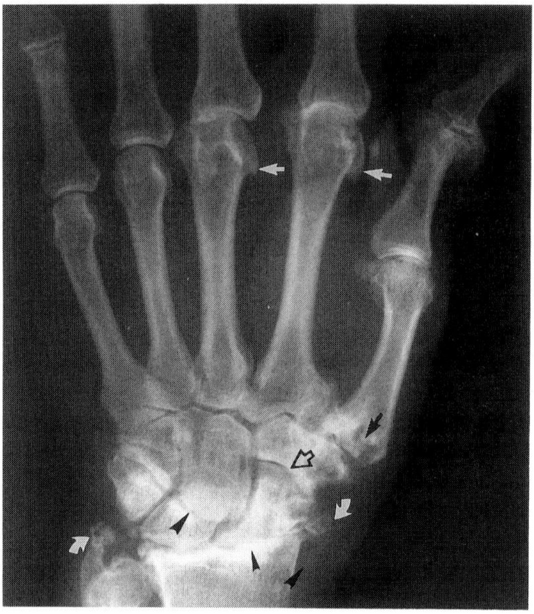

FIGURE 14 SLAC wrist, metacarpophalangeal, and other carpal joint involvement associated with CPPD arthropathy. The radioscaphoid and capitolunate joints are narrowed with subchondral sclerosis, typical of scapholunate advanced collapse (arrowheads). There is also involvement of the triscaphe joint (hollow arrow). The degenerative changes of the first carpometacarpal joints are frequent in osteoarthritis; however, the presence of large subchondral lucencies, which probably represent cysts, favor underlying pyrophophate arthropathy in this joint as well (solid black arrow). Such cysts are also seen adjacent to the second and third metacarpophalangeal joints, which are narrowed with drooping osteophytes, typical for this arthropathy (white arrows). There is a loose body in the radiocarpal joint and the prestyloid recess is calcified (curved white arrows). Cartilage and ligament calcification is present at the ulnocarpal articulation. (Published with permission from Ref. 4.)

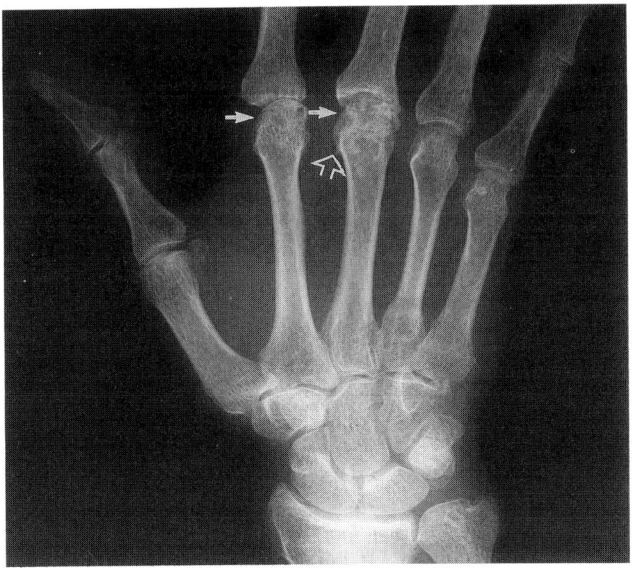

FIGURE 15 Pyrophosphate arthropathy without cartilage calcification. This arthropathy manifests as asymmetric narrowing of the second and third metacarpophalangeal joints (arrows). There is a drooping osteophyte along the radial aspect of the third metacarpal head (open arrow). This is a characteristic finding. There is no evidence of chondrocalcinosis in the joints or in the region of the triangular fibrocartilage. (Published with permission from Ref. 4.)

ing or only mild changes in the interphalangeal joints. This region may also reveal sclerosis, cyst formation, and subchondral collapse, particularly of the metacarpal head. Another finding in this disease are the so-called drooping osteophytes, which are seen along the radial aspects of the metacarpal heads. This feature is more characteristic of hemochromatosis, however. Patients with hemochromatosis often have CPPD crystal deposition disease with specific involvement of the second and third metacarpophalangeal joints. The fourth and fifth metacarpophalangeal joints are involved more frequently in patients with hemochromatosis than in those with idiopathic CPPD crystal deposition disease (57). It must be remembered that persons engaged in manual labor may develop similar changes in the metacarpophalangeal joints, termed the "Missouri metacarpal syndrome" (58).

Capsular calcification is occasionally identified in CPPD crystal deposition disease, especially about the metacarpophalangeal joints (Figure 16). Carpal tunnel syndrome is seen in association with synovitis related to CPPD crystal depo-

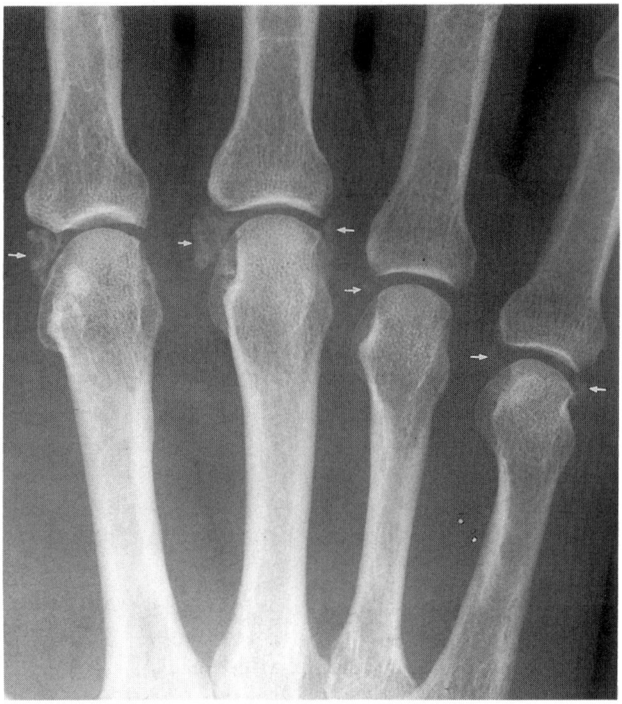

FIGURE 16 Synovial and capsular involvement in CPPD arthropathy. There is calcification of the capsule and synovium around the second through fifth metacarpophalangeal joints (arrows). (Published with permission from Ref. 4.)

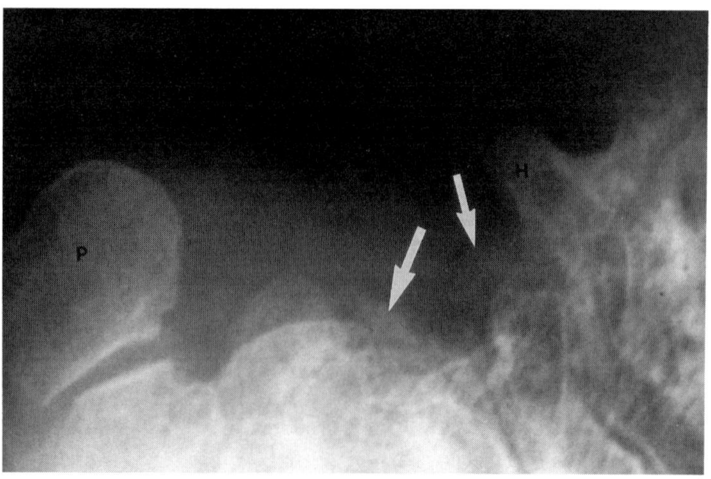

FIGURE 17 Calcification is present within the carpal tunnel (arrows) on this carpal tunnel view obtained in a patient with CPPD crystal deposition disease and acute symptoms of carpal tunnel syndrome. P = pisiform; H = hook of the hamate.

sition disease (52,59). A carpal tunnel view or cross sectional imaging using CT scanning can demonstrate the calcifications in the carpal tunnel (Figure 17).

3. Symphysis Pubis

This fibrocartilaginous joint frequently demonstrates calcification and occasional severe erosive changes (25) (Figure 18). Considerable bone fragmentation is occasionally seen in this region in patients with CPPD crystal deposition disease.

4. Elbow

Hyaline cartilage, capsular, and synovial calcification is occasionally visualized in this joint (Figure 19). The biceps and triceps tendons may calcify. CPPD crystal deposition disease is accompanied by joint space narrowing, resorption of the proximal portion of the ulna and radius, subchondral sclerosis and cyst formation, and bone fragmentation. Elbow contractures also develop in association with CPPD crystal deposition disease.

5. Hip

As in the knee, calcification is seen in both fibrocartilage and hyaline cartilage (Figures 18 and 20). The calcified acetabular labrum presents as a small radio-

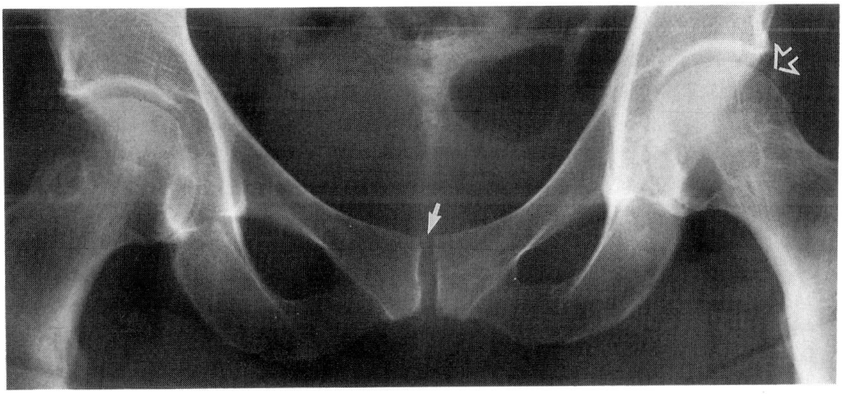

FIGURE 18 Linear calcification parallels the borders of the symphysis pubis of this patient (arrow), who also has hyaline cartilage calcification of both hips (open arrow). The well circumscribed lytic lesions in the femoral necks are also probably related to CPPD crystal deposition disease, but could just represent incidental herniation pits from friction of overlying capsule and tendons anterior to the hip.

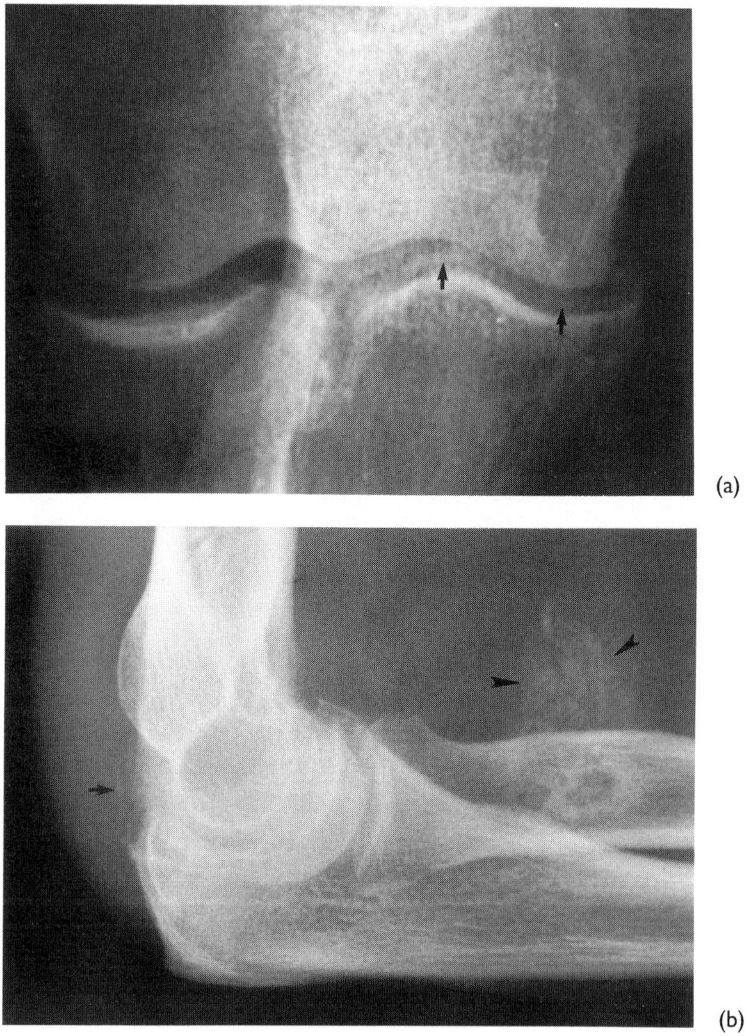

FIGURE 19 This man had acute elbow pain clinically diagnosed as a septic arthritis, but found to represent a pseudogout attack once (a) AP and (b) lateral radiographs of the elbow were reviewed. They reveal calcification of the hyaline cartilage (arrows) and of the bursa surrounding the insertion of the biceps tendon at the radial tuberosity (arrowheads). Weakly positive birefringent crystals were found on analysis of the elbow joint effusion and there was no evidence of infection.

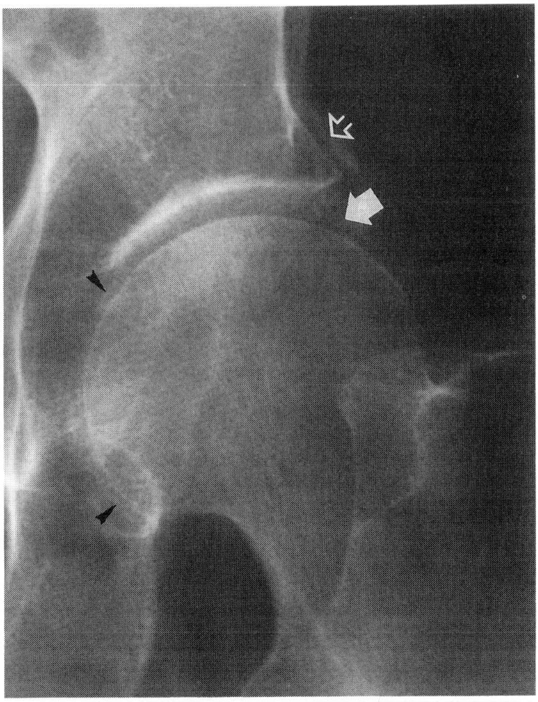

FIGURE 20 Hyaline and fibrocartilage calcification in the hip. The fibrocartilaginous acetabular labrum is associated with a typical triangular calcification superolateral to the femoral head (arrow). There is also an extra-articular linear calcification lateral to the acetabulum at the site of the rectus femoris tendon (open arrow). Curvilinear hyaline cartilage calcification parallels the medial femoral head (arrowheads). (Published with permission from Ref. 4.)

dense triangle along the peripheral aspect of the acetabulum superolaterally (Figure 20). Chondrocalcinosis is often apparent in the hyaline cartilage leading to a radiodense curvilinear line that parallels the femoral head (Figures 18 and 21). Surrounding tendons, including the rectus femoris (Figure 20), hamstrings, and adductor insertion (Figure 21) may also calcify. Narrowing of the hip joint is commonly superolateral, in a pattern similar to osteoarthritis. Alternatively, the hip joint may reveal concentric narrowing with axial migration, simulating the appearance of an inflammatory arthropathy. A rapidly destructive pattern of osteoarthritis in the hip has been described (60). The cause is not known, but some cases may be related to CPPD crystal deposition disease.

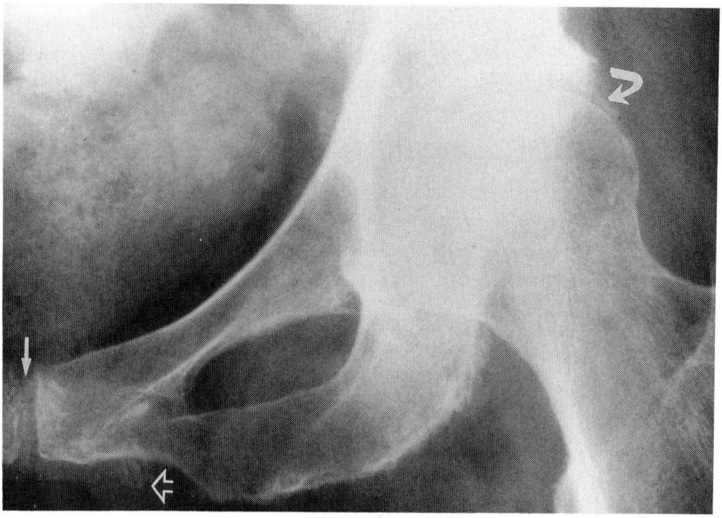

FIGURE 21 This patient has CPPD crystal deposition in the symphysis pubis (arrow), adductor tendon insertion (open arrow), and hyaline cartilage of the hip (curved arrow).

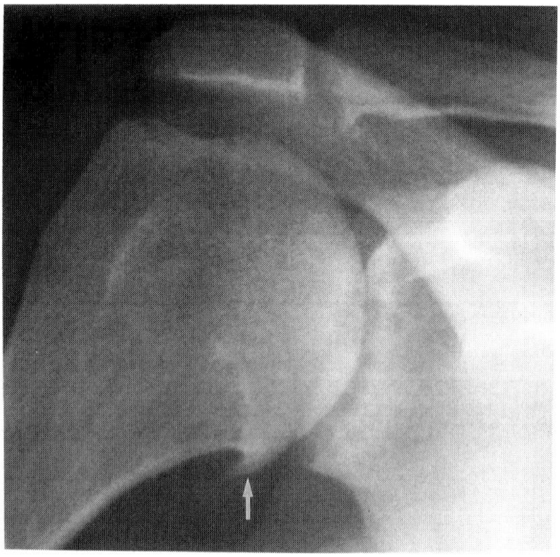

FIGURE 22 The glenohumeral joint is narrowed with small subchondral lucencies compatable with cysts and sclerosis and there is an inferomedial osteophyte (arrow) related to CPPD crystal deposition disease, which is a common cause of degenerative changes in the shoulder. There was no calcification in the shoulder joint, but the knees of this patient showed chondrocalcinosis.

6. Glenohumeral Joint

In the glenohumeral joint, CPPD crystal deposition disease resembles osteoarthritis with subchondral bone formation and cysts and osteophytes (Figure 22). Tendinous, capsular, and bursal deposits are occasionally seen (Figure 23). Rotator cuff tears are common in patients with CPPD crystal deposition disease. The Milwaukee shoulder syndrome is a rapidly progressive, destructive arthritis characterized by recurrent large effusions, rotator cuff tear, and destruction of cartilage and subchondral bone (61–63). It is most common in older women who often relate a history of trauma to the affected shoulder. It probably represents a severe form of mixed CPPD and hydroxyapatite crystal deposition disease (61), although some believe that it is purely a manifestation of hydroxyapatite crystal deposition disease.

7. Acromioclavicular Joint

CPPD crystal deposition disease also occurs in the acromioclavicular (AC) joint (36, 37, 64). This is a relatively infrequent but clinically important site of involvement. A calcified and/or cystic mass can present in the region of the AC joint, often just above the articulation (Figure 24). Calcification is most common in the articular disc. In one series, 65% of the AC joints had soft-tissue

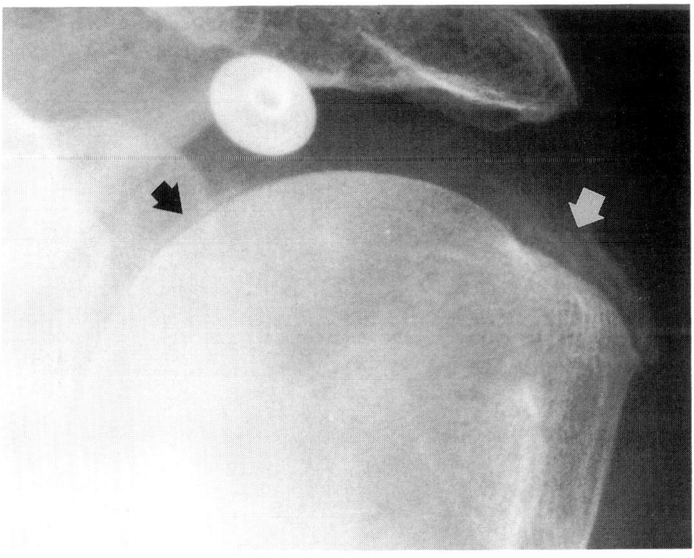

FIGURE 23 The supraspinatus tendon contains characteristic linear calcification of CPPD crystal deposition disease (white arrow). There is also calcification of the hyaline cartilage that parallels the superomedial humeral head (black arrow).

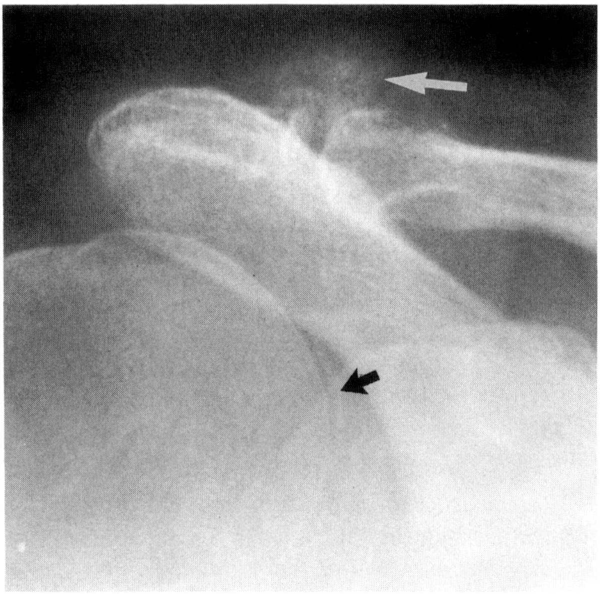

FIGURE 24 Acromioclavicular involvement with CPPD arthopathy. A calcified mass of CPPD crystals lies above the acromioclavicular joint (white arrow). There is sparing of the joint surfaces with no evidence of narrowing. The hyaline cartilage of the glenohumeral joint is also calcified (black arrow). (Published with permission from Ref. 4.)

swelling and calcified deposits above the joint (36). It may be difficult to identify the fibrocartilaginous calcification on conventional radiographs due to the obliquity of the joint. Careful evaluation of radiographs of this joint with a bright light is recommended, especially in elderly patients with acute shoulder pain and no history of trauma, in order to exclude CPPD crystal deposition disease. Cooper and coworkers discussed the importance of recognizing the presence of underlying CPPD crystal deposition disease when a calcified mass is seen around the acromioclavicular joint, in order to avoid misdiagnosis and inappropriate surgery (37).

8. Ankle and Foot

Calcification is not common in the ankle joint in patients with CPPD crystal deposition disease, and arthropathy in this site is unusual. The anterior talocalcaneonavicular joint is selectively affected when CPPD involves the ankle and hindfoot (25). In this location, joint space narrowing, subchondral sclerosis, fragmentation, and dorsal soft tissue swelling are seen, resembling the appearance of a neuropathic joint. The adjacent Achilles tendon and plantar fascia may be calcified (39) (Figure 7). Capsular calcification may be seen in the forefoot, especially about the metatarsophalangeal joints (Figure 25). Soft-tissue swelling and periarticular calcification medial to the first metatarsophalangeal joint can simulate radiographic findings of gout.

9. Spine

CPPD crystal deposition disease of the spine usually is asymptomatic. Many of the patients with CPPD crystal deposition disease are elderly and have unrelated degenerative disease of the spine. CPPD crystal deposition disease can produce severe degenerative disc disease often involving multiple levels. The spine may be the only site affected by CPPD crystal deposition disease (65). Acute and chronic CPPD crystal deposition disease can produce destructive lesions of vertebral bodies and disc spaces that can be confused with infectious discitis. Severe

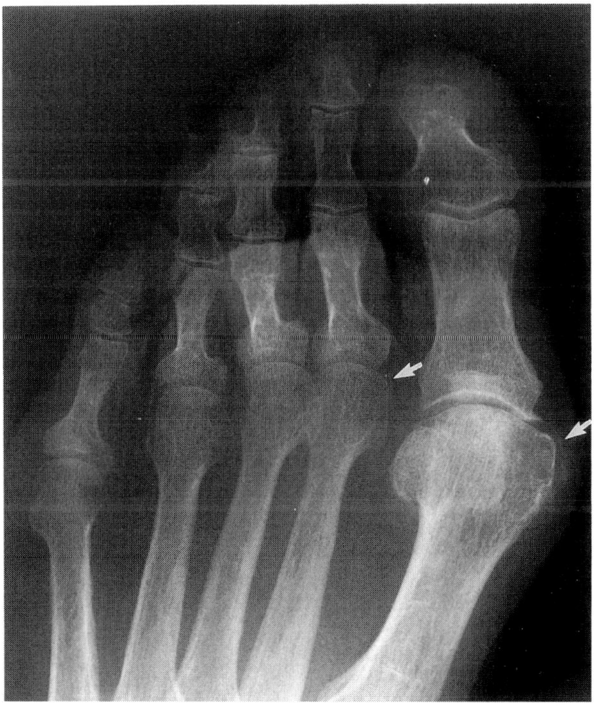

FIGURE 25 Capsular calcification is seen medial to the first and second metatarsophalangeal joints (arrows). In addition, there is mild degenerative change of the first MTP joint associated with hallux valgus, unrelated to the CPPD crystal deposition disease.

bone sclerosis, intervertebral disc space narrowing, and osteophyte formation in CPPD crystal deposition disease can simulate a neuropathic disorder. A destructive arthropathy that can lead to spondylolisthesis also may be noted in the facet joints. CPPD crystals can deposit in either the annulus fibrosus or nucleus pulposus of the disc, or in both structures (Figure 9). Calcification usually begins in the outer fibers of the annulus fibrosus. Thin, vertical annular calcification can simulate the syndesmophytes of ankylosing spondylitis. The nucleus pulposus is less commonly calcified in CPPD crystal deposition disease (41), but calcification of this structure may be seen in patients with a genetic predisposition to CPPD crystal deposition disease (29). Previous disc surgery may predispose to subsequent CPPD crystal deposition (65).

CPPD crystals may be deposited in the ligamentum flavum and posterior longitudinal ligament, leading to myelopathy, cord compression, and spinal stenosis (65–67) (Figure 9). The thoracic and lumbar regions are often affected, especially at the L2–3 disc level (68). MR imaging has demonstrated low-signal-intensity CPPD crystal deposits in the ligamentum flavum (69). These deposits may be difficult to distinguish from the low signal intensity of the ligamentum flavum itself. Discrete subchondral lucencies may be seen in the apophyseal joints, similar to those seen in the appendicular joints.

CPPD crystals may accumulate about the odontoid process in the area of the transverse ligament, producing cord compression, bone erosion (12), and even atlantoaxial subluxation. CPPD crystal deposition disease should be considered in elderly patients with gradual onset of cervical myelopathy and severe degenerative changes of the upper cervical spine. CT can aid in the identification of calcification and the degree of cord compression. MR imaging is preferred in this situation, however, because it allows for a more complete evaluation of the spinal cord.

10. Sacroiliac Joints

Sacroiliac joint abnormalities have been identified in approximately 50% of patients with CPPD crystal deposition disease (32). Abnormalities include subchondral erosions, reactive sclerosis and cyst formation, vacuum phenomena, and articular cartilage calcification. Calcification of the interosseous sacroiliac ligament also has been observed (70).

VI. DIFFERENTIAL DIAGNOSIS

Conditions that can simulate CPPD crystal deposition disease radiographically include osteoarthritis, neuropathic osteoarthropathy, synovial osteochondromatosis, hydroxyapatite crystal deposition disease, septic arthritis, gout, osteonecrosis, ochronosis, and spondyloarthropathies. It is helpful to analyze clinical and laboratory data and to examine the radiographs for the presence of distinctive characteristics of CPPD crystal deposition disease.

Radiographic features such as local calcification and chondrocalcinosis, large subchondral cyst-like lucencies, extensive subchondral sclerosis, collapse and fragmentation of joint surfaces, involvement of joints or components of joints that are not commonly affected by osteoarthritis, variable osteophyte formation, and osseous debris aid in distinction of this disorder from *primary osteoarthritis*.

Calcifications in hydroxyapatite crystal deposition disease (HADD) are more homogeneous or cloud-like and chondrocalcinosis is rare. Tendinous calcification in HADD disease differs from the elongated calcification seen in CPPD crystal deposition disease. In the setting of severe structural joint abnormality, osseous density is usually preserved in *neuropathic joint disease*, whereas this may not be true in CPPD crystal deposition disease. Pain is usually mild or absent in the presence of neuropathic joint disease, unlike the neuropathic form of CPPD crystal deposition disease. Lack of osteopenia and erosion usually allow differentiation of this arthropathy from inflammatory arthritides such as *rheumatoid arthritis* and *septic arthritis*. In chronic cases, joint erosion may be severe, simulating rheumatoid arthritis. Radiologic findings of joint or periarticular calcification and distribution of the arthropathy in CPPD crystal deposition disease usually allow differentiation from these arthritides. Distinguishing between CPPD crystal deposition disease and *gout* may be complicated by the occasional coexistence of these two arthropathies in the same joint or person. The presence of "punched out" or juxta-articular osseous erosion is useful for diagnosing gouty arthropathy. Lack of chondrocalcinosis in association with periarticular calcification may suggest other causes such as dystrophic calcification, metastatic calcification, or tumoral calcinosis.

VII. CONCLUSION

CPPD crystal deposition disease is widespread in elderly persons and has various clinical presentations that can be confounding to clinicians. Underlying knowledge of the various imaging presentations of CPPD crystal deposition disease aids in a more accurate diagnosis. Further studies that focus on pathophysiology, epidemiology, and the relation of this disease to aging should improve our understanding of the cause of this arthropathy.

REFERENCES

1. D. Zitnan and S. Sitaj. Mnoh opocetna familiarha kalcifikaaz artikularynch chrupiek, *Bratislouske Lakarske Listy 38*:217 (1958).

2. P. P. Revault, G. Vignon, E. Lejeune, et al. Diffuse articular chondrocalcinosis (apropos of six personal cases), *J Med Lyon 42*:65 (1961).
3. W. Martel, C. K. Champion, G. R. Thompson, and T. L. Carter. A roentgenologically distinctive arthropathy in some patients with the pseudogout syndrome, *Am J Roentgenol 109*:587 (1970).
4. L. S. Steinbach and D. Resnick. Calcium pyrophosphate dihydrate crystal deposition disease revisted, *Radiology 200*:1 (1996).
5. D. J. McCarty, J. M. Hogan, R. A. Gatter, et al. Studies on pathological calcifications in human cartilage. I. Prevalence and types of crystal deposits in the menisci of two hundred-fifteen cadavers. *J Bone Joint Surg 48A*:309 (1966).
6. R. W. Moskowitz. Diseases associated with the deposition of calcium pyrophosphate or hydroxyapatite, In: Textbook of Rheumatology, (W. N. Kelley and E. D. Harris, eds.), W. B. Saunders Company, Philadelphia, PA, 1983, pp. 1337–1354.
7. D. R. Mitrovic, A. Stankovic, O. Iriarte-Borda, et al. The prevalence of chondrocalcinosis in the human knee joint: An autopsy survey, *J Rheumatol 15*:633 (1988).
8. D. T. Felson, J. J. Anderson, A. Naimark, et al. The prevalence of chondrocalcinosis in the elderly and its association with knee osteoarthritis: The Framingham study, *J Rheumatol 16*:1241 (1989).
9. R. Sanmarti, D. Panella, M. A. Brancos, et al. Prevalence of articular chondrocalcinosis in elderly subjects in a rural area of Catalonia. *Ann Rheum Dis 52*:418 (1993).
10. A. C. Jones, A. J. Chuck, E. A. Arie, D. J. Green, and M. Doherty. Diseases associated with calcium pyrophosphate deposition disease, *Sem Arth Rheum 22*:188 (1992).
11. D. J. McCarty. Crystals and arthritis, *Dis Mon 40*:253 (1994).
12. G. Rivera-Sanfeliz, D. Resnick, P. Haghighi, W. Wong, and T. Lanier. Tophaceous pseudogout, *Skeletal Radiol 25*:699 (1996).
13. P. A. Dieppe. Crystal deposition and inflammations, *O J Med 53*:309 (1984).
14. K. Ishikawa, I. Masuda, T. Ohira, et al. A histological study of calcium pyrophosphate dihydrate crystal-deposition disease, *J Bone Joint Surg [Am] 71*:875 (1989).
15. M. Doherty. Pyrophosphate arthropathy-recent clinical advances, *Ann Rheum Dis 42(Suppl)*:38 (1983).
16. A. Fisseler-Eckhoff and K. M. Muller. Arthroscopy and chondrocalcinosis, *Arthroscopy 8*:98 (1992).
17. A. Bjelle. Cartilage matrix in hereditary pyrophosphate arthopathy, *J Rheumatol 8*:959 (1981).
18. R. D. Altman, O. E. Muniz, J. C. Pita, et al. Articular chondrocalcinosis. Microanalysis of pyrophosphate (PPi) in synovial fluid and plasma, *Arth Rheum 16*:171 (1973).
19. P. S. Jensen and C. E. Putman. Current concept with respect to chondrocalcinosis and the pseudogout syndrome, *Am J Roentgenol 123*:531 (1975).
20. R. L. Tse and P. Phelps. Polymorphonuclear leukocyte motility in vitro. V. Release of chemotactic activity following phagocytosis of calcium pyrophosphate crustals, diamond dust and urate crystals, *J Lab Clin Med 76*:403 (1970).
21. L. M. Ryan and D. J. McCarty. Calcium pyrophosphate crystal deposition disease: pseudogout; articular chondrocalcinosis. In: Arthritis and Allied Conditions (D. J. McCarty, ed.), Lea & Febiger, Philadelphia, PA, 1985, pp. 1515–1546.

22. C. J. Menkes, F. Simon, M. Chouraki, et al. Les arthropathies destructices de la chondrocalcinose, *Rev Thum Mal Osteoartic 40*:115 (1973).
23. A. J. Richards and E. B. D. Hamilton. Destructive arthropathy in chondrocalcinosis articularis, *Ann Rheum Dis 33*:196 (1973).
24. J. Villiaumey, B. Larget-Piet, C. DiMenza, et al. Caracteres symptomatiques et evolutifs des destructions articulaires observees au cours de la chondrocalcinose, *Rev Thum Mal Osteoartic 42*:263 (1975).
25. D. Resnick, G. Niwayama, T. G. Georgen, et al. Clinical, radiographic and pathologic abnormalities in calcium pyrophosphate dihydrate deposition disease (CPPD): Pseudogout, *Radiology 122*:1 (1977).
26. S. Jacobelli, D. J. McCarty, D. C. Silcox, et al. Calcium pyrophosphate dihydrate crystal deposition in neuropathic joints. Four cases of polyarticular involvement, *Ann Intern Med 79*:340 (1973).
27. D. J. McCarty. Calcium pyrophosphate dihydrate crystal deposition disease—1975, *Arth Rheum 19(Suppl)*:275 (1976).
28. J. K. Van der Korst, J. Geerards, and F. C. M. Driessens. A hereditary type of idiopathic articular chondrocalcinosis. Survey of a pedigree, *Am J Med 56*:307 (1974).
29. A. M. Reginato, E. R. Valanzuela, V. C. Martinez VC, et al. Polyarticular and familial chondrocalcinosis, *Arth Rheum 13*:197 (1970).
30. A. J. Reginato, V. Schiapachasse, C. M. Zmijewski, et al. HLA antigens in chondrocalcinosis and ankylosing chondrocalcinosis, *Arth Rheum 22*:928 (1979).
31. D. Resnick and P. D. Utsinger. The wrist arthropathy of "pseudogout" occurring with and without chondrocalcinosis, *Radiology 113*:633 (1974).
32. W. Martel, D. K. McCarter, M. A. Solsky, et al. Further observation of the arthropathy of calcium pyrophosphate dihydrate crystal deposition disease, *Radiology 141*:1 (1981).
33. M. H. Ellman, M. I. Krieger, and N. Brown. Pseudogout mimicking synovial chondromatosis, *J Bone Joint Surg 57*:863 (1975).
34. H. R. Shumacher. Ultrastructural findings in chondrocalcinosis and pseudogout, *Arth Rheum 19(Suppl)*.413 (1976).
35. A. Fondimare, J.-P. Talon, P. Deshayes, et al. Etude anatomophathologique de la chondrocalcinose articulare a propos de II observations, *Presse Med 79*:707 (1971).
36. G. S. Huang, D. Bachmann, J. A. M. Taylor, et al. Calcium pyrophosphate dihydrate crystal deposition disease and pseudogout of the acromioclavicular joint: radiographic and pathologic features, *J Rheumatol 20*:2077 (1993).
37. A. M. Cooper, C. Hayward, and B. D. Williams. Calcium pyrophosphate deposition disease-involvement of the acromioclavicular joint with pseudocyst formation, *Br J Rheumatol 32*:248 (1993).
38. E. Kanterewicz, R. Sanmarti, D. Panella, and J. Brugues. Tendon calcifications of the hip adductors in chondrocalcinosis: A radiological study of 75 patients, *Br J Rheumatol 32*:790 (1993).
39. J. C. Gerster, C. A. Baud, R. Lagier, I. Boussina, and G. H. Fallet. Tendon calcifications in chondrocalcinosis. A clinical, radiologic, histologic and crystallographic study, *Arth Rheum 20*:717 (1977).
40. K. Foldes, L. Lenchik, S. Jaovisidha, P. Clopton, D. J. Sartoris, and D. Resnick. As-

sociation of gastrocnemius tendon calcification with chondrocalcinosis of the knee, *Skeletal Radiol 25*:621 (1996).
41. D. J. McCarty and M. E. Haskin. The roentgenographic aspects of pseudogout (articular chondrocalcinosis): an analysis of 20 cases, *Am J Roentgenol 90*:1248 (1963).
42. R. W. Moskowitz and D. Katz. Chondrocalcinosis and chondrocalsynovitis (pseudogout syndrome): analysis of twenty-four cases, *Am J Med 43*:322 (1967).
43. H. K. Genant. Roentgenographic aspects of calcium pyrophosphate dihydrate crystal deposition disease (pseudogout), *Arth Rheum 19(suppl)*:307 (1976).
44. C. S. Resnick and D. Resnick. Crystal deposition disease, *Semin Arth Rheum 12*:390 (1983).
45. T. Ishida, H. D. Dorfman, and P. G. Bullough. Tophaceous pseudogout (tumoral calcium pyrophosphate dihydrate crystal deposition disease, *Human Pathol 26*:587 (1995).
46. S. Yu, R. Li, and Z. Bian. Tumoral calcium pyrophosphate dihydrate deposition disease, *Chinese Med J 105*:780 (1992).
47. L. S. Steinbach, J. O. Johnston, E. F. Tepper, G. Honda, and W. Martel. Tumoral calcinosis: Radiologic-Pathologic Correlation, *Skeletal Rad 24*:573 (1995).
48. I. Ohshio, T. Ogino, S. Satoh, M. Konari, and K. Nagashima. Tumourous deposition of calcium pyrophosphate dihydrate crystals in the wrist, *J Hand Surg 16B*:219 (1991).
49. J. Blechman, P. Sminkin, and R. Kier. MRI of pseudogout in atypical locations, *Soc Magnetic Resonance (abs)*:1526 (1995).
50. H. A. Sissons, G. C. Steiner, F. Bonar, et al. Tumoral calcium pyrophosphate deposition disease, *Skeletal Radiol 18*:79 (1989).
51. B. Y. Yang, D. J. Sartoris, S. Djukic, D. Resnick, and P. Clopton. Distribution of calcification in the triangular fibrocartilage region in 181 patients with calcium pyrophosphate dihydrate crystal deposition disease, *Radiology 196*:547 (1995).
52. W. Doherty and J. L. Lovallo. Scapholunate advanced collapse pattern of arthritis in calcium pyrophosphate deposition disease of the wrist, *J Hand Surg 18A*:1095 (1993).
53. C. Chen, V. P. Chandnani, H. S. Kang, D. Resnick, D. J. Sartoris, and J. Haller. Scapholunate advanced collapse: A common wrist abnormality in calcium pyrophosphate dihydrate crystal deposition disease, *Radiology 177*:459 (1990).
54. H. K. Watson and F. L. Ballet. The SLAC wrist: scapholunate advanced collapse pattern of degenerative arthritis, *J Hand Surg 1984*:358 (1984).
55. H. K. Watson and L. H. Brenner. Degenerative disorders of the wrist, *J Hand Surg 10A*:1002 (1985).
56. D. Resnick and G. Niwayama. Carpal instability in rheumatoid arthritis and calcium pyrophosphate deposition disease. Pathogenesis and roentgen appearance, *Ann Rheum Dis 36*:311 (1977).
57. T. C. Adamson III, C. S. Resnik, J. Guerra Jr, et al. Hand and wrist arthropathies of hemochromatosis and calcium pyrophosphate deposition disease: Distinct radiographic features, *Radiology 147*:377 (1983).
58. W. Williams, R. Cope, W. Gant W, et al. Metacarpophalangeal arthropathy associ-

ated with manual labor (Missouri metacarpal syndrome), *Arth Rheum 30*:1362 (1987).

59. A. J. Rate, R. W. Parkinson, T. H. Meadows, and W. J. Freemont. Acute carpal tunnel syndrome due to pseudogout, *J Hand Surg 17B*:217 (1992).
60. Z. S. Rosenberg, S. Shankman, G. C. Steiner, et al. Rapid destructive osteoarthritis: Clinical, radiographic, and pathologic features, *Radiology 182*:213 (1992).
61. D. J. McCarty, P. B. Halverson, G. F. Carrera, et al. "Milwaukee shoulder"–association of microspheroids containing hydroxyapatite crystals, active collagenase, and neutral protease with rotator cuff defects, *Arth Rheum 24*:464 (1981).
62. P. B. Halverson, D. J. McCarty, H. S. Cheung, et al. Milwaukee shoulder syndrome: Eleven additional cases with involvement of the knee in seven (basic calcium phophate crystal deposition disease), *Semin Arth Rheum 14*:36 (1984).
63. P. A. Dieppe, M. Doherty, D. G. MacFarlane, et al. Apatite associated destructive arthritis, *Br J Rheumatol 23*:84 (1984).
64. R. C. Marcove, S. W. Wolfe, J. H. Healey, et al. Massive solitary tophus containing calcium pyrophosphate dihydrate crystals at the acromioclavicular joint, *Clin Orthop Rel Res 227*:305 (1988).
65. M. Salcman, A. Khan, and D. A. Symonds. Calcium pyrophosphate arthropathy of the spine: Case report and review of the literature, *Neurosurgery 34*:915 (1994).
66. C. R. Wells, S. Morgello, and E. DiCarlo. Cervical myelopathy due to calcium pyrophosphate dihydrate deposition disease, *J Neurol Neurosurg Psych 54*:658 (1991).
67. R. B. Delmarter, J. E. Sherman, and J. Carr. Lumbar spinal stenosis secondary to calcium pyrophosphate crystal deposition (pseudogout), *Clin Orth Rel Res 289*:127 (1993).
68. A. J. Richards and E. B. D. Hamilton. Spinal changes in idiopathic chondrocalcinosis articularis, *Rheumatol Rehabil 15*:138 (1976).
69. T. R. Brown, S. F. Quinn, and A. N. D'Agostino. Deposition of calcium pyrophosphate dihydrate crystals in the ligamentum flavum: Evaluation with MR imaging and CT, *Radiology 178*:871 (1991).
70. D. Resnick and C. Pineda. Vertebral involvement in calcium pyrophosphate dihydrate crystal deposition disease. Radiographic-pathologic correlation, *Radiology 153*:55 (1984).

22

Basic Calcium Phosphate (Calcium Apatite) Crystal Deposition Diseases

ADEL G. FAM
Sunnybrook Health Science Centre, University of Toronto, Toronto, Ontario, Canada

Hydroxyapatite (HA) is the main mineral constituent of bone. Pathologic calcifications, such as shoulder calcific tendinitis and subcutaneous calcinosis in scleroderma, often contain a mixture of basic calcium phosphate (BCP) crystals, including partially carbonate-substituted HA (CHA), octacalcium phosphate (OCP), and occasionally tricalcium phosphate (TCP) (1,2).

Deposition of HA and other related BCP crystals in and around the joints is associated with three main articular syndromes (Table 1): acute calcific periarthritis; acute hydroxyapatite arthritis; and apatite-associated destructive arthropathy, including "Milwaukee shoulder-knee syndrome" (1–3). Of these, acute calcific periarthritis is the most clearly defined and most widely recognized clinical entity.

I. PERIARTICULAR BCP CRYSTAL DEPOSITION

A. Asymptomatic Periarticular BCP Calcific Deposits

Asymptomatic, inert radiographic periarticular calcifications in one or both shoulders occur in about 2.7–7.5% of adults (1,3). Only a minority of patients, particularly those with large periarticular deposits, may develop symptoms.

TABLE 1 Basic Calcium Phosphate (Calcium Apatite) Crystal Deposition Diseases

Periarticular BCP crystal deposition
- Asymptomatic periarticular deposits
- Acute calcific periarthritis
  - Idiopathic
    - Unifocal, including hydroxyapatite pseudopodagra
    - Multifocal
  - Secondary
    - Chronic renal failure
    - Scleroderma
    - Following local corticosteroid injections
  - Familial
- Chronic calcific tendinitis
- Calcific tendinitis with cortical erosions

Intraarticular BCP crystal deposition
- Acute hydroxyapatite arthritis
- Apatite-associated destructive arthritis (AADA) including Milwaukee shoulder-knee syndrome
- IA BCP crystal deposits in osteoarthritis, and CPPD crystal deposition disease

Subcutaneous and soft tissue BCP crystal deposition:
- Metastatic, e.g., renal failure, hyperparathyroidism
- Dystrophic, e.g., scleroderma, dermatomyositis
- Idiopathic, e.g., tumoral calcinosis
- Calciphylaxis, e.g., renal failure

B. Acute Calcific Periarthritis

Acute calcific periarthritis (ACP), acute calcific tendinitis, idiopathic calcifying tenosynovitis, peritendinitis calcarea, or acute calcific bursitis is characterized by painful, self-limited episodes of acute periarticular inflammation, associated with transient juxta-articular radiologic calcific deposits (1–5). The deposits are often heterogeneous with partially carbonate-substituted HA, small amounts of OCP, and occasionally TCP crystals.

1. Clinical and Laboratory Findings

ACP affects both sexes equally, most commonly between the ages of 40 and 70 years (4,5). An acute onset with intense joint pain is frequent. An antecedent history of trauma is sometimes obtained. Within hours, the affected joint becomes exquisitely tender, swollen, and warm; there is painful restriction of movements, and sometimes erythema and local edema (1–5). A low-grade fever may occur, and the intense local inflammation may resemble acute cellulitis or acute gouty arthritis (3).

The shoulder (supraspinatus > infraspinatus > teres minor > subscapularis > bicipital tendons > subacromial bursa) is the most common site (Table 2). This is followed by the hip (near greater trochanter or acetabulum) (6), knee (tendon attachments at the medial and lateral aspects), elbow (near epicondyles or triceps tendon) (Figure 1a), wrist (flexor carpi ulnaris tendon), and ankle joints. Involvement of the joints of the hands, feet, and cervical spine (particularly at C1/C2 with calcification within the longus colli muscle: acute calcific retropharyngeal tendinitis) (7) (Figure 1B), is rare. Most patients experience a single episode of ACP affecting one joint. Recurrent calcific periarthritis, affecting multiple sites, is rare (3,8,9).

ACP of the first metatarsophalangeal (MTP) joint, or "hydroxyapatite pseudopodagra," occurs predominantly in young, premenopausal women (Figure 1C) (10,11). This is in contrast to an almost equal sex distribution in patients with ACP in general (4,5). The role of womens' footwear in this striking gender difference is not clear. It is also unclear whether the increased frequency of hydroxyapatite pseudopodagra in women is a true finding, or simply due to underdiagnosis of the disorder in men. Since gout predominantly affects adult men, a presumptive diagnosis of gouty podagra is often made in male patients without foot radiographs or a diagnostic arthrocentesis (10,11). ACP of the finger joints also occurs more commonly in women (12).

The most revealing radiographic finding during an attack of ACP is the presence of calcific deposit(s) in the vicinity of the affected joint (1–12). The deposits are often regular in outline, round or linear in shape, and homogeneous in appearance. Clinical resolution of the acute inflammatory attack is often associated with gradual resorption of the periarticular deposit within 2–4 weeks (range is a few days to a few months) (3).

ACP is sometimes associated with a noninflammatory "sympathetic" joint effusions (total synovial leukocyte count $<2000/mm^3$), presumably secondary to the juxta-articular acute inflammation (3). "Inflammatory" (total synovial leukocyte count $>2000/mm^3$) joint effusions are rare, and may result from rupture of a large periarticular BCP crystal mass into an adjacent joint space. A toothpaste-like

Table 2 Sites of Acute Calcific Periarthritis

Shoulder	60%
Hip	15%
Less common areas	25%
knee, ankle, elbow, wrist	
MCP, PIP, DIP	
First MTP (hydroxyapatite pseudopodagra)	
C1/C2 (acute calcific retropharyngeal tendinitis)	

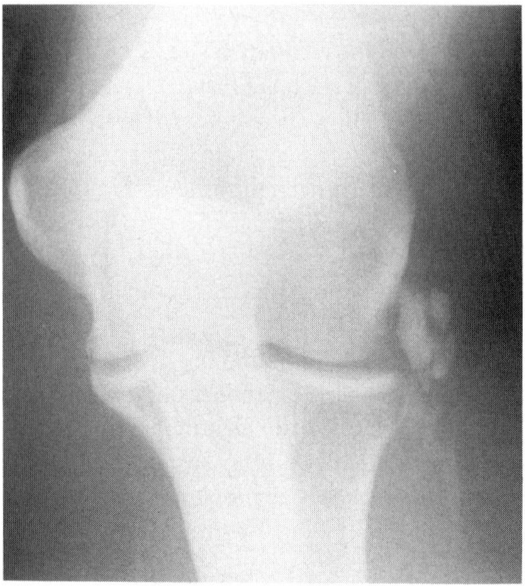

(A)

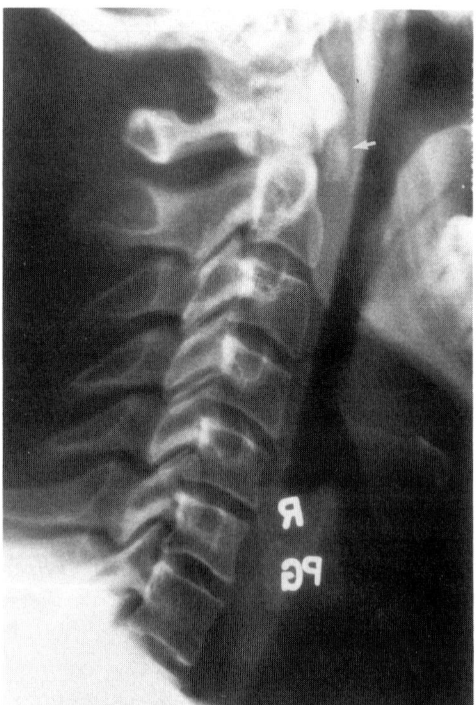

(B)

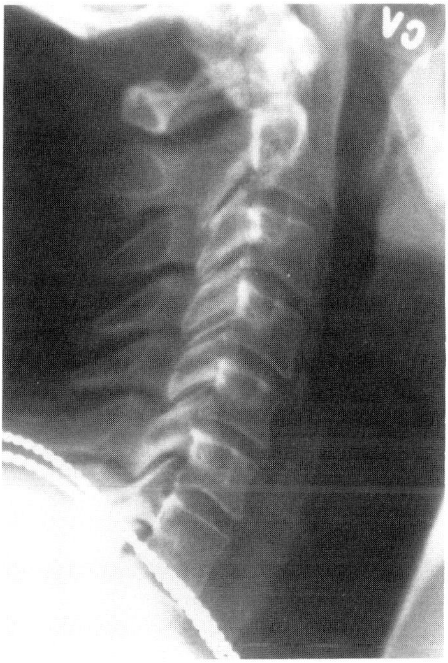

(C)

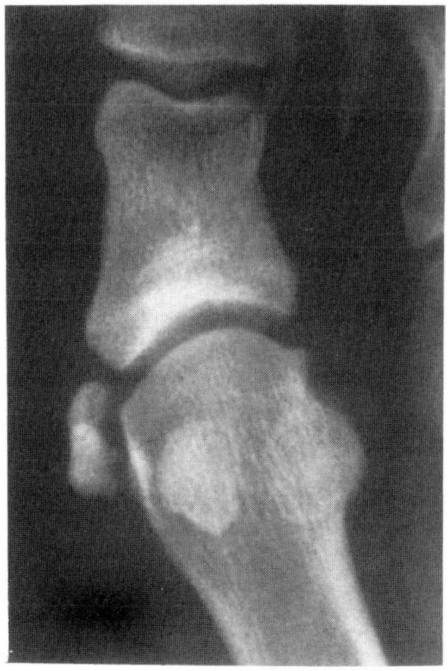

(D)

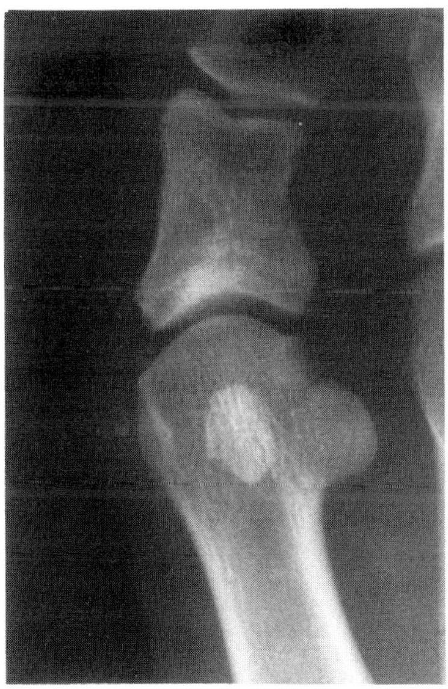

(E)

FIGURE 1 Acute calcific periarthritis. (A) Left elbow: calcific deposits near the lateral epicondyle. (B) Acute calcific retropharyngeal tendinitis: i, calcific deposit anterior to the atlantoaxial joint (arrow); ii, followup radiograph showing disappearance of the calcific deposit. (C) Hydroxyapatite pseudopodagra: i, calcific deposit medial to the first MTP joints; ii, followup radiograph showing almost complete disappearance of calcific density.

calcific material, containing masses of BCP crystals, can sometimes be aspirated from the periarticular calcification (8).

a. Treatment and Outcome

Most attacks of ACP respond to treatment with high-dose nonsteroidal anti-inflammatory drugs (NSAIDs), including indomethacin and naproxen (3,6–12). Local corticosteroid injections and oral or parenteral corticosteroids are useful treatment alternatives in patients with comorbid conditions contraindicating the use of NSAIDs, such as renal insufficiency, congestive heart failure, or peptic ulcer disease.

Needle aspiration of the periarticular calcific deposit, with or without saline irrigation, may be beneficial in some patients with ACP of the shoulder (2,13). However, this is rarely necessary given that most episodes of ACP resolve within two weeks.

b. Pathogenesis

ACP is a sporadic and idiopathic disorder in the majority of patients, and there are no known local or metabolic abnormalities.

Familial ACP is rare (9,14,15). No HLA specificity or other genetic marker has been identified. A familial form, associated with hand arthritis, shoulder periarthritis, intervertebral disc calcifications, HA-containing costal cartilage calcific deposits (apatite chondrocalcinosis), and multiple periarticular calcifications, has been reported (15).

Pathologically, calcific deposits in ACP are located in the vicinity of joints in tendons (often near insertion sites in poorly vascularized segments), peritendinous tissues, bursae, or ligaments. Original studies have suggested that the deposits represent a "dystrophic" calcification occurring at sites of tendon trauma. However, there is evidence to indicate that calcifying tendinitis is an active, cell-mediated process in which relative hypoxia and mechanical changes result in focal metaplasia of tendinous tissues into fibrocartilage (16). This is followed by local deposition of HA crystals within chondrocyte-derived extracellular matrix vesicle-like structures (16).

An attack of ACP is thought to result from rupture of a calcific deposit into an adjacent, soft-tissue space or bursa, setting off an acute, self-limited, BCP crystal-induced inflammatory reaction (1–3,6,8,10). The radiographic evidence of dispersal of the calcification after resolution of an acute ACP episode indirectly supports "crystal shedding" as the pathogenetic mechanism in ACP. Phagocytosis of HA crystals by neutrophil and synovial macrophages results in the release of lysosomal enzymes and other inflammatory mediators (17,18). The mechanisms of degradation of HA crystals are unclear, but dissolution of the crystals probably occurs within the acidic environment of phagolysosomes of fibroblasts, monocytes, and giant cells (19).

2. Secondary Forms of ACP

a. ACP in Renal Dialysis Patients

Periarticular calcifications occur frequently in patients with end-stage renal disease undergoing long-term dialysis. Common sites include shoulders, finger joints, hips, and ankles. The deposits, which consist of BCP crystals, are often asymptomatic but can sometimes cause attacks of ACP (20–22). Occasionally, large "tumoral" calcific masses may develop in the vicinity of joints (21,22) (Figure 2A).

Episodes of dialysis-associated ACP can often be prevented through normalization of serum phosphate levels by low-phosphate diet, use of calcium supplements to bind phosphate in the gastrointestinal tract, increasing the frequency and efficiency of dialysis, or renal transplantation (20–22).

b. ACP in Scleroderma

Although subcutaneous and periarticular calcifications are frequent in patients with systemic sclerosis, ACP is rare (23) (Figure 2B). A recent study of scleroderma-associated ACP indicates: (1) ACP appears to be more common in patients with limited cutaneous scleroderma (CREST syndrome) than in those with diffuse cutaneous scleroderma; (2) resorption of periarticular calcific deposits following resolution of acute attacks occurs both less frequently and incompletely in scleroderma-associated ACP compared to the idiopathic form; and (3) recurrent attacks of ACP in scleroderma tend to affect the same site (23).

c. Periarticular Calcifications and ACP Following Intra-Articular Corticosteroid Injections

Hydroxyapatite-containing periarticular and subcutaneous calcifications may rarely develop following single or multiple intra-articular (IA) corticosteroid injections, particularly of hand joints (24,25) (Figure 2C). The calcific deposits are thought to result from leakage of the drug into the periarticular tissues, causing tissue necrosis and secondary calcification. They are often symptomless, but may rarely cause inflammatory episodes of ACP (25).

C. Chronic Calcific Periarthritis

Intratendinous calcific deposits, particularly in the rotator cuff tendons of the shoulder, are sometimes associated with chronic aching and local tenderness (chronic calcific tendinitis) (2,5). A previous history of recurrent episodes of ACP is common. It is difficult to ascertain whether the pain is due to the tendinitis or to the calcific deposits themselves.

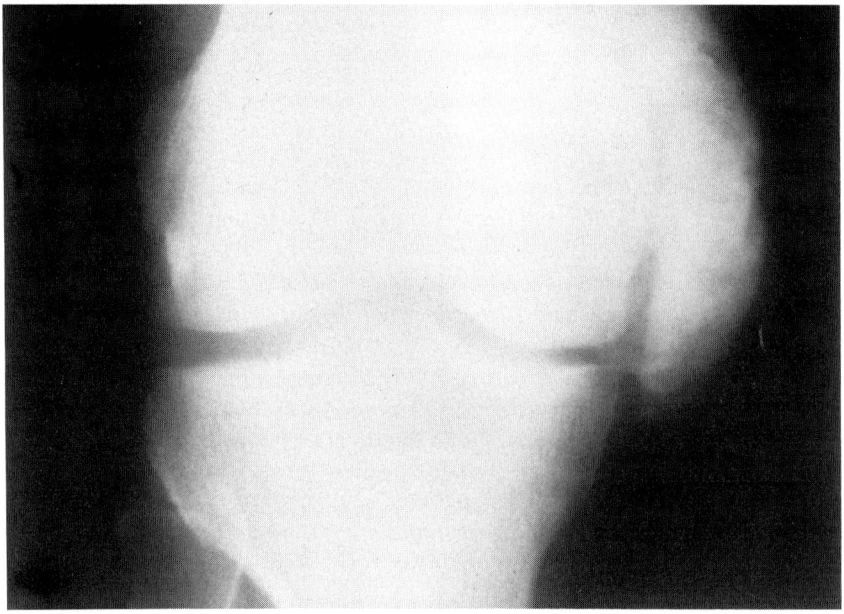

(A)

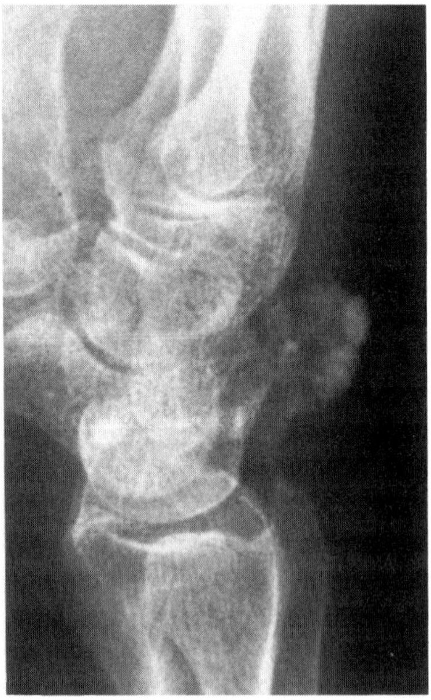

(B)

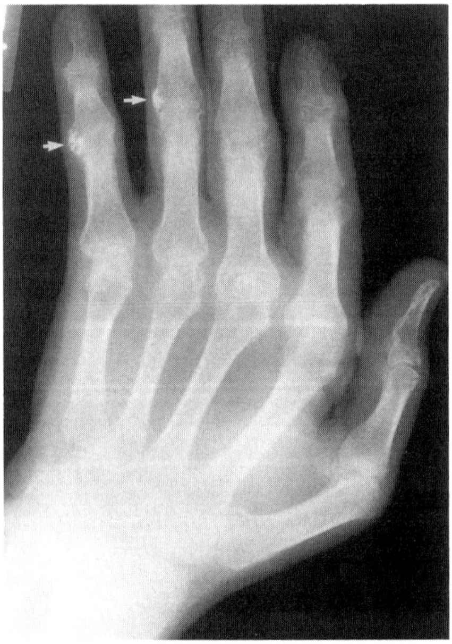

(C)

FIGURE 2 Secondary acute calcific periarthritis. (A) A large "tumoral" calcific deposit medial to the right knee in a patient with renal failure. (B) A periarticular calcific mass over the dorsum of right wrist in a patient with scleroderma. (C) Periarticular calcifications (arrows) following intraarticular corticosteroid injections of the left 4th and 5th proximal interphalangeal (PIP) joints, in a patient with rheumatoid arthritis.

Treatment is similar to that of noncalcific shoulder tendinitis: use of NSAIDs and physical modalities including heat application and range of movement exercises. Early mobilization of the shoulder is important in minimizing disability and reducing the risk of adhesive capsulitis. Needle aspiration of the calcific deposit is difficult, and its therapeutic value remains unproven. Local corticosteroid injections are often beneficial. Surgical or arthroscopic excision of large periarticular calcific deposits is indicated in refractory cases.

D. Calcific Periarthritis (Tendinitis) Associated with Cortical Bone Erosions

This is an uncommon manifestation of BCP crystal deposition disease (26,27). Common sites include the tendon insertions of the gluteus maximus, adductor magnus, pectoralis major, and deltoid muscles. The onset is often acute with severe local pain and tenderness. Subacute and chronic symptoms are less frequent. Radiologic features include fluffy calcification near the tendon insertion, associated with cortical erosions or cysts of the adjacent bone (Figure 3A). The calcification often conforms to the shape of the tendon insertion, and appears to taper away from the site of bone erosion like a "comet tail." Computed tomography allows better definition of the tendinous calcific deposits and of the cortical erosive lesions (Figure 3B). Radionuclide bone scans often demonstrate increased uptake at the site of cortical erosions. The erosions, and abnormalities on T_2-weighted magnetic resonance imaging, are thought to represent inflammatory changes and increased vascularity associated with acute calcific tendinitis. Pathologically, foci of paste-like, chalky calcific material are present within the tendon insertion. These consist of masses of HA crystals surrounded by mononuclear cells, giant cells, and dense fibrous tissue containing small blood vessels (27).

NSAIDs are generally efficacious, and resolution of symptoms is often followed by disappearance of the radiologic calcification and healing of adjacent bone erosions (26,27).

II. INTRA-ARTICULAR BCP CRYSTAL DEPOSITION

A. Acute Calcific (Hydroxyapatite) Arthritis

Intra-articular deposition of HA crystals is a rare cause of acute arthritis (28–31). Rupture of a periarticular HA deposit into an adjacent joint cavity can cause acute HA arthritis, e.g., through a defect in the rotator cuff in patients with ACP of the shoulder (29). Other sites include hips, knee, MTP, wrist, and finger joints. Intra-articular HA crystal deposition is a rare cause of acute and chronic arthritis in patients with polymyositis (30) or mixed connective tissue disease (31).

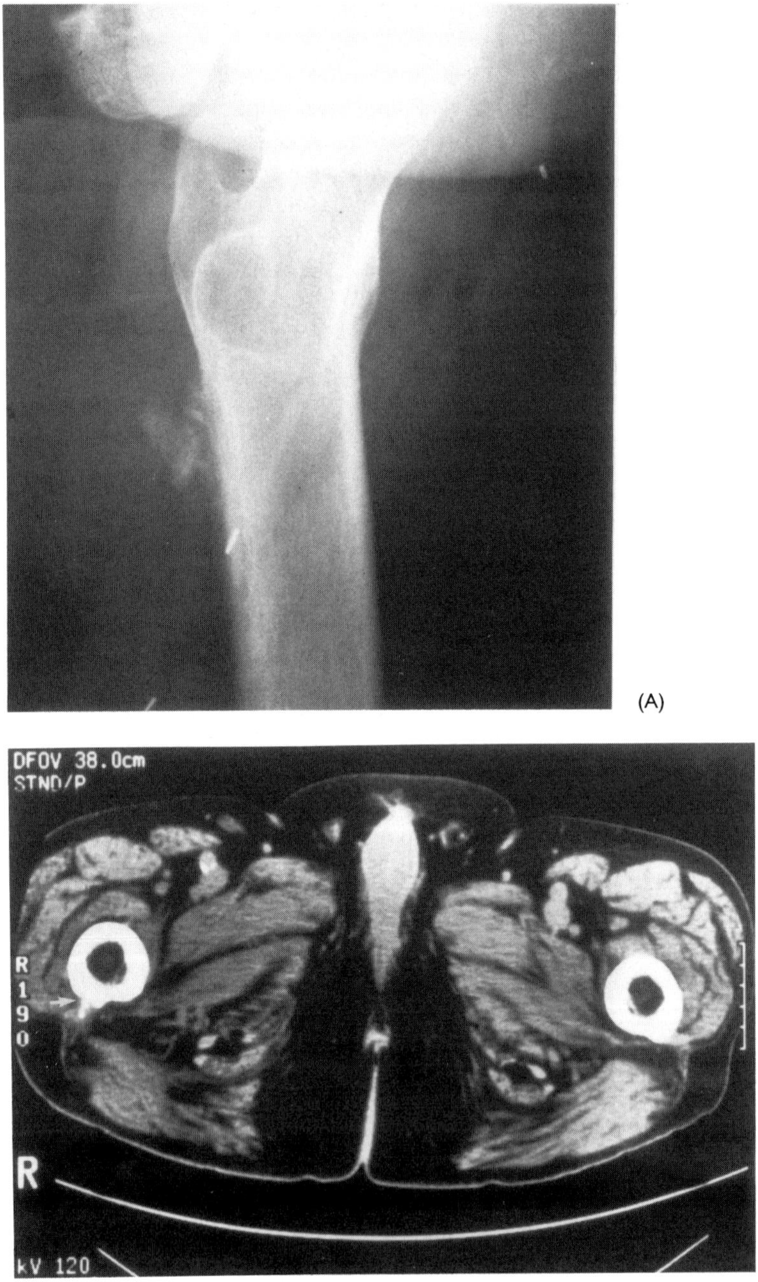

(A)

(B)

FIGURE 3 Calcific tendinitis associated with cortical erosions. (A) Calcific density and underlying cortical erosions at the gluteus maximus tendon insertion into right femur. (B) Axial computed tomographic image showing a crater-like cortical erosion and adjacent dense calcification at the insertion of the gluteus maximus tendon. (Courtesy of Dr. J. Rubenstein, Toronto, Canada.)

Radiographic periarticular and IA calcifications are frequent. Both "inflammatory" and "noninflammatory" synovial effusions containing HA crystals (Figure 4A) have been observed. Massive IA BCP crystal deposition is sometimes associated with "chalky," milky white joint or bursal effusions (Figure 4B) (23,30,32).

Acute apatite arthritis of the 1st MTP joint, associated with milky white synovial effusion, containing extracellular and phagocytosed negatively birefringent HA spherulites about 6 μm in diameter, has recently been reported (Figure 5) (33).

Treatment of acute synovitis due to HA crystals is similar to that of ACP: rest, ice application, and high-dose NSAID therapy.

B. Chronic Apatite Arthropathy, Milwaukee Shoulder-Knee Syndrome, and Apatite-Associated Destructive Arthropathy

Intra-articular deposition of BCP crystals has been linked to a rare, rapidly destructive arthritis affecting the shoulder, knee, and hip, and less commonly the elbow, ankle, and finger joints, in older patients (34–36). The disorder was originally described in the French literature under the terms: "l'epaule senile hemorrhagique," and "l'arthropathie destructrice rapide de l'epaule" (36). In 1981, McCarty and colleagues drew further attention to the entity, when they reported a group of patients with "Milwaukee shoulder syndrome," and emphasized the presence of BCP crystals, particulate collagens, and proteolytic enzymes in joint effusions (34). A variety of other terms have been used to describe the disorder: "apatite-associated destructive arthropathy" (AADA) (35) and "idiopathic destructive arthropathies" (36).

Clinical features of AADA (34–36) include (34–36):

1. Elderly patients, mostly women (90%) in their seventies.
2. Predilection for large joints, including shoulders, knees, and hips. Bilateral and multiple site involvement is not uncommon. The elbow, ankle and finger joints are less frequently affected.
3. Swelling, reduced range of movement, instability, and loss of function of the affected joint but relatively mild pain and little evidence of inflammation.
4. Voluminous "cool" synovial effusions, which are often blood-tinged and "noninflammatory," with low, predominantly mononuclear, leukocyte counts (50–1,000/mm^3), containing particulate collagens, and BCP crystals including carbonate-substituted HA, OCP, and occasionally TCP. Calcium pyrophosphate dihydrate (CPPD) crystals are present in a large proportion of these effusions.
5. A rapidly progressive course with radiographic evidence of accelerated osteoarthritis (OA), extensive juxta-articular bone destruction, and IA osseous bodies. Periarticular calcifications occur in about 50% of patients.

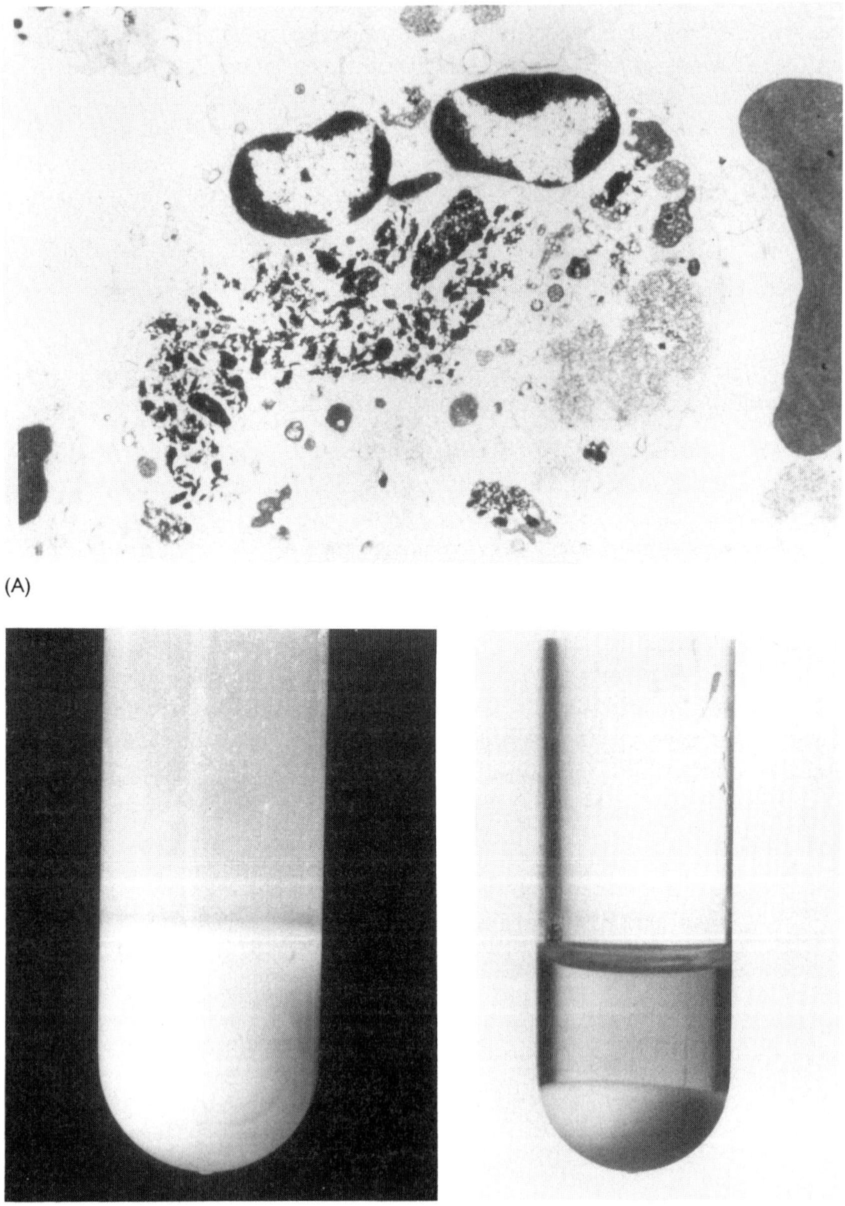

(A)

(B)

(C)

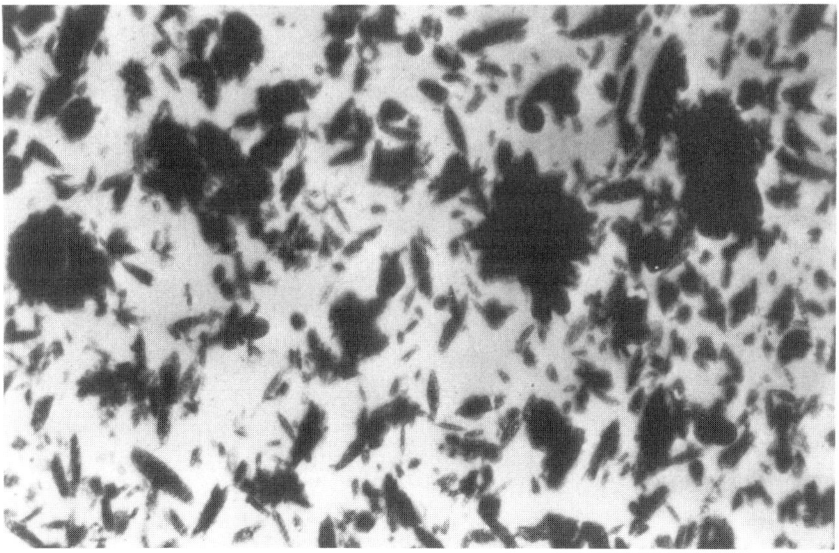

(D)

FIGURE 4 Intraarticular hydroxyapatite (HA) crystal deposition. (A) Acute HA arthritis: transmission electron micrograph of synovial fluid leukocyte showing phagocytosed hydroxyapatite crystals (original magnification × 36,000). (Courtesy of Dr. R.H. Schumacher, Philadelphia, PA.) (B) Massive intraarticular HA crystal deposition: i, milky white "chalky" HA-laden bursal synovial effusion; ii, fluid after standing overnight; iii, transmission electron micrograph of the fluid showing numerous HA crystal aggregates and individual boat-shaped crystals 50–250 nm in length and 1–25nm in width (original magnification × 44,000). (Courtesy of Dr. KPH Pritzker, Toronto, Canada.)

6. Frequent presence of a mild chronic synovitis with synovial lining cell hyperplasia, villous hypertrophy, embedded cartilage and bone fragments, and subsynovial alizarin red-stained calcific deposits of apatite and other BCP crystals, but little or no inflammatory cell infiltrate.
7. Absence of a systemic rheumatic disease, metabolic disorder, osteonecrosis, or other cause of destructive arthritis.

The pathogenesis of AADA is not fully understood (34–36). Although BCP crystals have been linked to this articular disorder, it is unclear whether IA BCP crystal deposition is a primary event or the end stage of cartilage and subchondral bony destruction. Although synthetic BCP crystals are phlogistic when injected into experimental animals, synovial fluid leukocyte counts are no higher in human effusions that contain BCP crystals (as in AADA) than in those that do not (34–36). However, BCP crystals have been shown to stimulate the secretion of collagenase, stromelysin, and neutral proteases from cultured synovial cells.

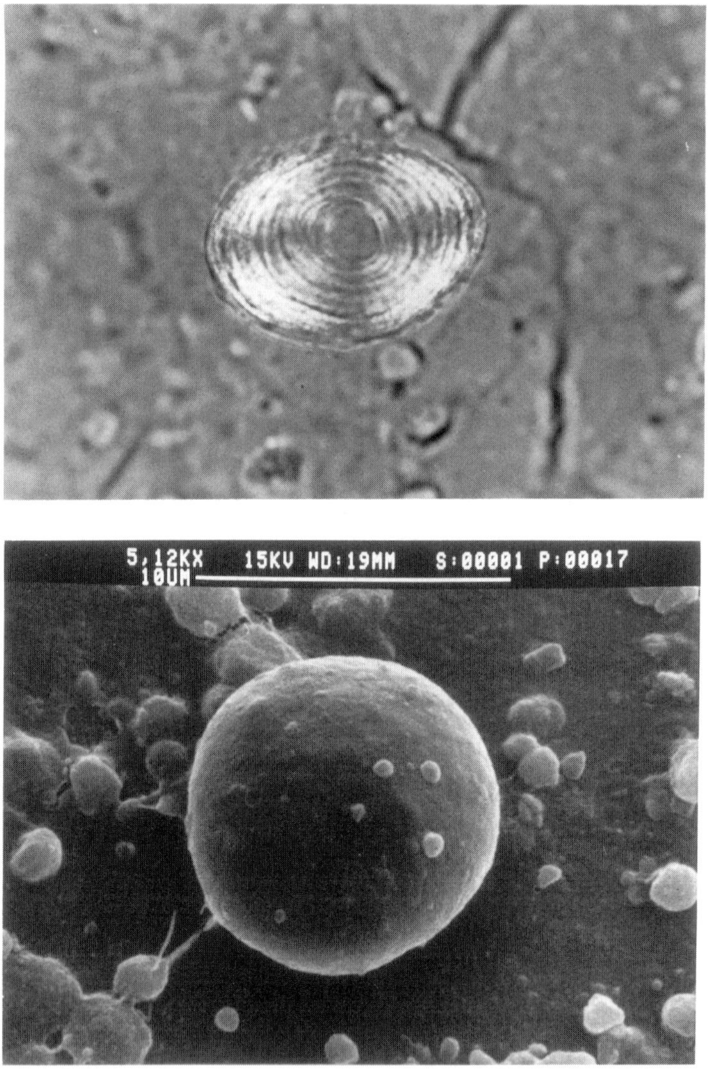

(A)

(B)

FIGURE 5 Acute apatite arthritis of the first MTP joint. (A) Hydroxyapatite spherulite: Maltese cross and concentric rings (× 1600). (B) Scanning electron micrograph of synovial fluid showing a hydroxyapatite spherulite, 13nm in diameter (original × 4080). (Courtesy of Drs. F. Beaudet and R. de Medicis, Sherbrooke, Canada.)

The crystals also enhance synovial proliferation by virtue of their mitogenic properties (34,37). The release of proteases into the joint space can lead to enzymatic "strip-mining" of additional crystals from cartilage, and cause further joint damage with breakdown of IA collagenous structures (cartilage, ligaments, tendons, and adjacent bones) and release of particulate collagens (34,37). However, collagenase and neutral protease activities have been demonstrated in synovial effusions from shoulder joints of some, but not all, patients with AADA (34,40).

Treatment of AADA is similar to that of OA in general (34–36); analgesics, NSAIDs, and physical therapy, including heat and exercises to maintain joint range of movements. Joint aspiration and IA corticosteroid injections may provide temporary relief of pain. Closed-needle tidal irrigation, followed by an IA corticosteroid injection, may be beneficial (39). Proposed mechanisms of action include reduction of BCP crystal population; removal of degradative enzymes, cytokines, and other inflammatory mediators from the joint; and disposal of cartilage and bone "wear particles" (39). Surgical arthroplasty is indicated for those with severe AADA arthritis refractory to conservative management (34–36).

C. Intra-Articular BCP Crystal Deposition in Other Arthritides

BCP crystals are detected in synovial effusions of 26–52.5% of OA joints (40–42). Periarticular and IA radiographic calcifications, and deposits of BCP crystals in the synovium and/or articular cartilage, are frequent. A correlation between the intrasynovial presence of HA crystals and the severity of OA has been recognized (40–42). However, it is unclear whether the crystals are responsible for more severe joint destruction, or merely accompany it (40–42). Although BCP crystal deposition is associated with large joint effusions (42), there is no correlation with clinical signs of inflammation, synovial fluid (SF) leukocytosis, or histologic synovitis (40).

The exact origin of BCP crystals, whether from articular cartilage, subchondral bone, or synovium, and the mechanisms governing their release into the joint fluid, remain poorly understood. The presence of HA crystals in OA synovial effusions does not correlate with synovial fluid concentration of either keratin sulphate (a cartilage proteoglycan constituent) or interleukin-1β (IL-1β), a macrophage-derived cytokine capable of promoting cartilage and bone resorption (42). This suggests that the release of HA crystals is not related to IL-1β–driven cartilage proteoglycan breakdown (42). Searching for BCP crystals in OA effusions is probably of little practical value since their presence does not influence treatment decisions.

Studies of OA joint effusions also indicate that BCP and CPPD crystals are more likely to occur together ("mixed-crystal deposition disease") than either occur alone, and that CPPD crystals tend to correlate with age, whereas BCP crystals appear to correlate with severity of OA (40–43).

Whether BCP crystals contribute to joint damage in these arthritides or merely represent an epiphenomena remains uncertain. Current evidence seems to support the latter hypothesis. Dystrophic calcification may involve both matrix vesicles and mitochondria (44). Calcium (Ca) ion concentration is higher in the extracellular fluid than in the cytosol. This gradient is maintained by impermeability of the cell membrane to ionic Ca, and by the presence of an energy-dependent calcium pump (44). Local tissue injury increases cell membrane permeability, allowing cytosolic influx of sufficient Ca to exceed the capacity of mitochondria to sequester Ca and phosphate (P), and leading to precipitation of cytosolic Ca phosphate (44). This mechanism may explain the occurrence of BCP crystals in damaged joints, whether due to OA, CPPD crystal deposition disease, or other arthritis.

III. SUBCUTANEOUS AND SOFT-TISSUE BCP CRYSTAL DEPOSITION

Ectopic calcification, including calcinosis cutis, is generally classified into four types: metastatic, dystrophic, and idiopathic calcifications and calciphylaxis (45,46). Metastatic calcification occurs in normal tissues as a result of either chronic hypercalcemia (e.g., hyperparathyroidism, vitamin-D overdose, neoplasms) or hyperphosphatemia (e.g., chronic renal failure, hypoparathyroidism), in association with an increased Ca $\times$ P solubility product. Dystrophic calcification, which is associated with normal serum levels of Ca and P, occurs following tissue injury in metabolic diseases (ochronosis, diabetes mellitus, gout) and in connective tissue diseases, including scleroderma, dermatomyositis, mixed connective tissue disease, and occasionally systemic lupus erythematosus (SLE). Idiopathic tumoral calcinosis occurs in normal tissues with normal serum levels of Ca and P. Cutaneous calciphylaxis is a serious but rare condition that occurs in renal dialysis patients with a high Ca $\times$ P product. It is associated with calcification of the medial layer of small vessels and painful, nodular areas of livedo reticularis, which often progress to skin necrosis and ulcerations (45,46).

Subcutaneous calcinosis is more frequent in limited scleroderma (CREST syndrome) than in diffuse cutaneous disease (47) (Figure 6A). The calcifications, which are composed of HA, CHA, and sometimes OCP crystals, are believed to result from microvascular insufficiency and ischemic tissue injury (47). They are commonly asymptomatic, but can cause ulcerations, secondary infection, or recurrent local inflammatory episodes (47).

Dermatomyositis/polymyositis, particularly childhood dermatomyositis, is associated with calcinosis of the deeper structures, including muscles and tendons.

Treatment modalities for calcinosis in scleroderma and polymyositis are

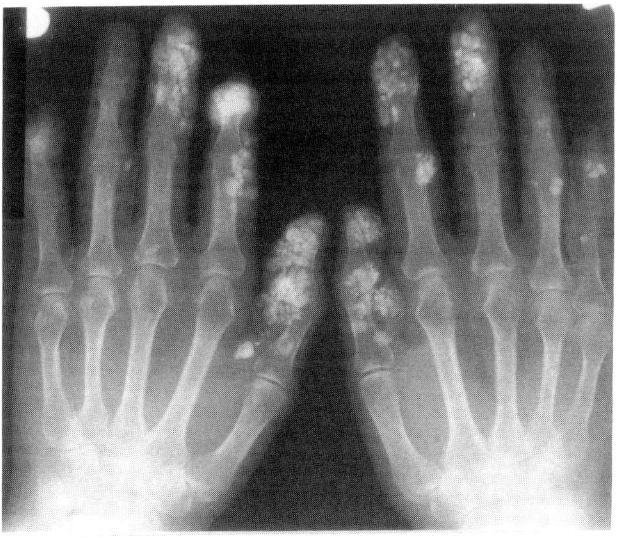

(A)

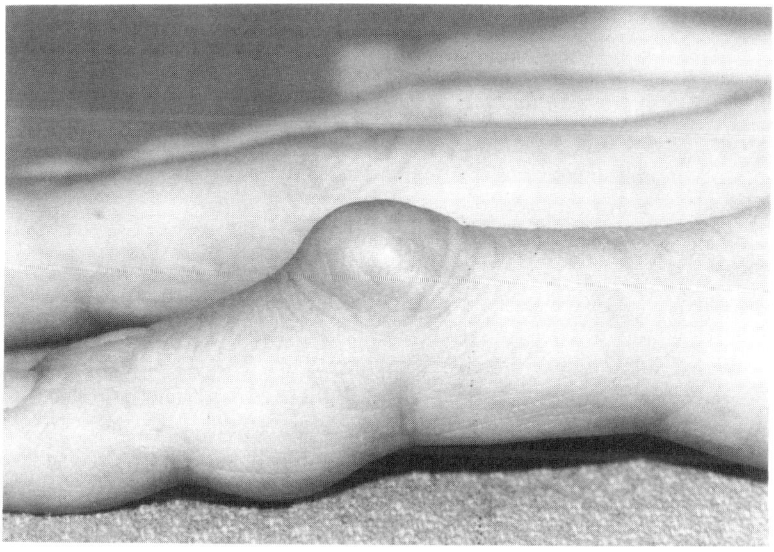

(B)

FIGURE 6 Subcutaneous calcinosis. (A) In a patient with limited cutaneous scleroderma. (B) In a patient with lupus nephritis and renal failure: i, large periarticular and subcutaneous calcific deposits of right index finger; ii, corresponding radiograph.

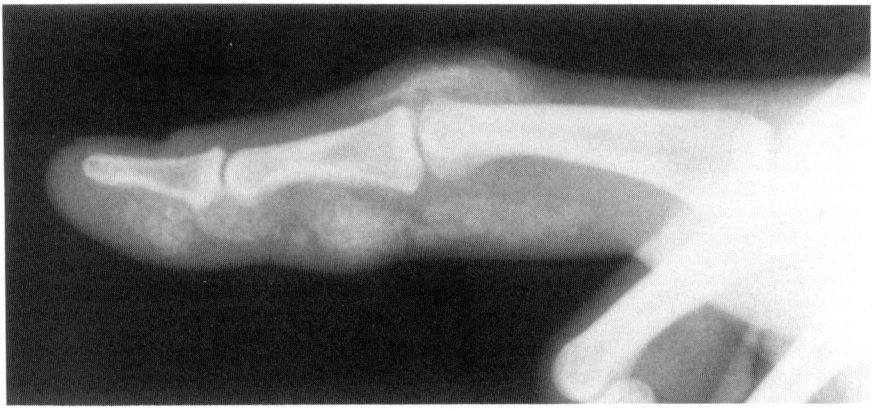

(C)

FIGURE 6 Continued

generally ineffective. A number of drugs have been tried, but proof of their efficacy is lacking. Included among these are low-dose coumadin, bisphosphonates, probenecid, colchicine, aluminum hydroxide, and intralesional corticosteroid injections (47–49). Recently diltiazem, a calcium-channel-blocking drug, by virtue of its vasodilatory effects preventing ischemic tissue injury (47) and its potential role in preserving mitochondrial Ca homeostasis (48), has been shown to be beneficial in the treatment of idiopathic, scleroderma- or dermatomyositis-associated calcinosis (47–49).

Large periarticular "tumoral" tophus-like mass lesions, containing masses of apatite and other BCP crystals, are rare. These may occur as an idiopathic condition (idiopathic tumoral calcinosis) (45,50) or in association with chronic renal insufficiency, SLE (22,45) (Figure 6B) or scleroderma. The idiopathic form frequently affects black children, and is often familial (45,50). Common sites include hips, shoulders, and elbows. It is usually painless, but can cause pressure effects (including carpal tunnel syndrome), recurrent ulcerations, or secondary infection. Surgical excision is indicated in symptomatic patients.

IV. DIAGNOSIS OF BCP CRYSTAL DEPOSITION DISEASE

A. Imaging

Although the radiographic demonstration of periarticular calcifications in ACP is highly diagnostic, radiography is generally both insensitive and nonspecific, revealing only about one-third of periarticular BCP crystal deposits (5,51).

Intra-articular BCP crystal deposition is rarely associated with cartilage calcification (apatite chondrocalcinosis). Synovial or capsular calcification, appearing as amorphus or cloud-like radiodense areas within the joint, is more common (5,51).

Computed tomography (52) or magnetic resonance imaging (MRI) (6,27) may be helpful in revealing small calcific deposits. An added advantage of MRI is its ability to demonstrate edema and inflammation in tissues surrounding the calcification (6,27).

Changes in the periarticular calcific deposits in calcific periarthritis are often associated with abnormalities on technetium-labeled bisphosphonate bone scanning (3).

B. Identification of Apatite and Other BCP Crystals

Unlike CPPD and urate crystals, compensated polarized light microscopy (CPLM) is of limited value in the detection of BCP crystals. HA crystals are too small, ranging in width between 1 and 25 nm and in length between 50 and 250 nm. Their size is below the limits of resolution of light microscopy (1–3). The crystals are nonbirefringent, and have a tendency to aggravate into clumps or microspheroids 1–10 μm in diameter. The crystals exhibit considerable morphologic variation with rod-, plate-, needle-, boat-, and hexagonal-shaped forms (Figure 4). A spherulite form of HA has recently been described in a patient with acute apatite monoarthritis and a milky white synovial effusion (33). Under CPLM, HA spherulites appear as negatively -birefringent Maltese crosses, 4–30μm in diameter (Figure 5) (33).

Although clumps of BCP crystals may be visible by CPLM as nonbirefringent, "shiny laminated coins" (1–3), it is often difficult to distinguish these from SF debris.

Calcium stains, such as alizarin red S, have been used to screen for HA and other calcium-containing crystals in synovial effusions and joint tissues (53,54). A wet-mount technique provides a simple, rapid means of identifying HA clumps, which stain dark red with alizarin. Although the method is sensitive, it is nonspecific for calcium phosphate, and may give false-positive results with CPPD, calcium oxalate, and other Ca-containing crystals (53,54). Identification of intracellular (IC) BCP crystals can be improved by using prefiltered alizarin red S, and fresh, air-dried, alcohol-fixed, permanent cytospin preparations of SF (55). However, the presence of contaminants makes the technique less reliable for identification of extracellular (EC) BCP crystals (55).

Von Kossa phosphate stain, which stains HA crystals dark brown, is both less specific and less sensitive than alizarin red.

Definitive identification of HA and other related BCP crystals often requires the use of one or more specialized techniques, which are largely available in University-affiliated research laboratories (56–62) (Table 3). Transmission electron microscopy (TEM) can be utilized to visualize HA crystals and define their morphology and location whether IC or EC (Figure 5) (1–3,28,56–60). Although TEM lacks specificity, it allows positive identification of the crystals by energy-dispersive, X-ray microprobe elemental analysis (EDXA) for determination of the molar ratio of Ca to P, and comparing it with a known standard (1–3,56–60). The Ca/P ratio is 1.67 for HA, 1.33 for OCP, and 1.5 for TCP.

Scanning electron microscopy (SEM) is less diagnostic than TEM. By SEM, microspheroids of BCP crystals often look like "snowballs" 1.6–18 μm in diameter.

If sufficient calcific material is available (for example from surgically excised calcific deposits, or from "chalky," HA-laden, synovial effusions), X-ray powder diffraction analysis (XRD) can be employed for definitive identification ("finger printing") of HA crystals (1–3,58–62). However, XRD is relatively insensitive for detection of small amounts of BCP crystals in synovial effusions. The diagnostic utility of both EDXA and XRD is limited in calcium deposits containing a mixture of BCP crystals.

Fourier transform infrared (FTIR) spectroscopy is ideally suited for the sequential analysis of a calcific deposit containing a mixture of BCP crystalline phases, but large amounts of the mineral are required (1,59).

^{14}C-ethane-1-hydroxy 1, 1-diphosphonate (^{14}C EHDP) binding assay is a useful, rapid, screening test, for detecting BCP crystals in synovial effusions (1,59,60). TEM examination of synovial fluid pellets that bind ^{14}C EHDP often

TABLE 3 Diagnosis of Basic Calcium Phosphate (BCP) Crystal Deposition Diseases

Imaging
Radiography
Scintigraphy
Computed tomography
Magnetic resonance imaging
Identification of hydroxyapatite and BCP crystals in synovial fluids and tissues
Polarized light microscopy
Alizarin red S calcium stain
Transmission electron microscopy (TEM)
Energy-dispersive X-ray microbe elemental analysis (EDXA)
Scanning electron microscopy (SEM)
Fourier transform infrared (FTIR) spectroscopy
^{14}C-ethane hydroxyl diphosphonate (EHDP) binding assay
Raman microscopy
Atomic force microscopy (AFM)

shows BCP crystal aggregates. These can be further characterized by elemental analysis for molar Ca/P ratio.

Raman microscopy, the analysis of scattered photons after excitation is a promising new method for the identification of crystals in pathologic specimens (61).

Atomic force microscopy (AFM) measures center-to-center intermolecular spacing of different atoms within a crystal, producing a distinct molecular resolution image (62). The technique has recently been used to detect BCP and other microcrystals (less than 1 μm) in synovial effusions (62).

Screening for BCP crystals by alizarin red S and C^{14} EHDP assay and, if indicated, examination by TEM and EDXA of HA-positive SF pellets, are probably sufficient in most clinical settings. XRD and FTIR analysis are valuable research tools, but are impractical for routine use.

V. ANIMAL MODELS OF BCP CRYSTAL DEPOSITION

A. Naturally Occurring Animal Models

Multifocal periarticular calcific deposits, sometimes associated with lameness, have been described in dogs, rats, and horses (63).

A crippling, autosomal recessive, hereditary arthropathy has been described in progressive ankylosis (ank/ank) mice (64). In this murine mutation, IA deposition of HA crystals is associated with apatite-laden synovial effusions, joint inflammation, bridging osteophytes, and multiple joint ankylosis (64).

B. Experimentally Induced Animal Models

The phlogistic potential of HA crystals has been demonstrated in a number of experimental studies (57,65,66). Subcutaneous and IA injection of the crystals induces a self-limited, acute crystal-induced inflammation that peaks in 4–6 hr, and resolves within 24–48 hr. In vitro experiments have demonstrated phagocytosis of HA crystals by neutrophils, with associated degranulation and release of a number of cytokines, inflammatory mediators, and enzymes (17,18,65,66). At equivalent crystal concentrations, urate crystals produce greater degranulation and enzyme release from neutrophils compared to HA crystals (65).

The inflammatory potential of the different BCP crystals, using the synovium-like subcutaneous rat air-pouch model, varies according to their type, specific surface area, and Ca/P ratio (which correlates inversely with crystal solubility) (66). The phlogistic response to the crystals is also influenced by proteins adsorbed to their surfaces (1,17,65,66). For example, the inflammatory reaction is suppressed when a α_2-HS glycoprotein binds to HA crystals (1,17,65). These observations provide a possible explanation for the occurrence of acute crystal-induced inflammation in some, but not all, individuals with periarticular or IA BCP crystal deposits.

Periarticular and subcutaneous calcific deposits can be experimentally induced in the rat by calciphylaxis (67).

Intra-articular calciphylaxis, with cartilaginous and synovial HA crystal deposits but little inflammation, can be produced in the rabbit's knee by the administration of dehydrotachysterol followed by an IA injection of ferric chloride (68).

ACKNOWLEDGMENT

The author wishes to thank Ms. Kathy Carey for secretarial assistance.

REFERENCES

1. P.B. Halverson and D. J. McCarty. Basic calcium phosphate (apatite, octacalcium phosphate, tricalcium phosphate) crystal deposition diseases; calcinosis, In: Arthritis and Allied Conditions (W. Koopman ed.), 13th Edition, Lee and Febiger, Philadelphia, PA, 1997, pp. 2127–2146.
2. G. Faure and G. Daculsi. Calcified tendinitis: a review. *Ann Rheum Dis 42(suppl)*:49–53 (1983).
3. A. G. Fam, K. P. H. Pritzker, J. L. Stein, J. B. Houpt, and A. H. Little. Apatite associated arthropathy: A clinical study of 14 cases and of 2 patients with calcific bursitis. *J Rheumatol 6*:461–471 (1979).
4. C. Sandstrom. Peritendinitis calcarea: common disease of middle life: its diagnosis, pathology and treatment. *Am J Roentgen 40*:1–21, (1938).
5. Resnick. Calcium hydroxyapatite crystal deposition disease. In: Diagnosis of Bone and Joint Disorders (D. Resnick, ed.), 3rd edition, W. B. Saunders, Philadelphia, PA, 1995, pp. 1615–1648.
6. H. Y. Chow, M. P. Recht, J. Schils, and L. H. Calabrese. Acute calcific tendinitis of the hip: Case report with magnetic resonance imaging findings. *Arth Rheum 40*:974–977 (1997).
7. J. Sarkozi and A. G. Fam. Acute calcific retropharyngeal tendinitis: An unusual cause of neck pain. *Arth Rheum 27*:708–710 (1984).
8. D. J. McCarty and R. A. Gatter. Recurrent acute inflammation associated with focal apatite crystal deposition. *Arth Rheum 9*:804–819 (1966).
9. G. Zaphiropoulus. Recurrent calcific periarthritis involving multiple sites. *Proc Roy Soc Med 66*:351–352 (1973).
10. A. G. Fam and J. Rubenstein. Hydroxyapatite pseudopodagra: A syndrome of young women. *Arth Rheum 32*:741–747 (1989).
11. D. Mines and S. B. Abbuhl. Hydroxyapatite pseudopodagra in a young man: Acute calcific periarthritis of the first metatarsophalangeal joint. *Am J Emerg Med 14*:180–182 (1996).

12. G. M. McCarthy, G. F. Carrera, and L. M. Ryan. Acute calcific periarthritis of the finger joints: A syndrome of women. *J Rheumatol 20*:1077–1080 (1993).
13. P. B. Halverson and D. J. McCarty. Clinical aspects of basic calcium phosphate crystal deposition. *Rheum Dis Clin N Am 14*:427–439 (1988).
14. R. B. Cannon and F. R. Schmid. Calcific periarthritis involving multiple sites in identical twins. *Arth Rheum 16*:393–396 (1973).
15. J. C. Marcos, M. A. De Benyacar, O. Garcia-Morteo, A. S. Anturi, et al. Idiopathic familial chondrocalcinosis due to apatite crystal deposition. *Am J Med 71*:557–564 (1981).
16. K. Sarkar, and H. K. Uhthoff. Ultrastructural localization of calcium in calcifying tendinitis. *Arch Pathol Lab Med 102*:266–269 (1978).
17. R. A. Terkeltaub, and M. H. Ginsberg. The inflammatory reaction to crystals. *Rheum Dis Clin N Am 14*:353–364 (1988).
18. J. G. R. Elferink, and M. Deiekauf. A biochemical study of hydroxyapatite crystal induced enzyme release from neutrophils. *Ann Rheum Dis 46*:590–597 (1987).
19. R. W. Evans, H. S. Cheung, and D. J. McCarty. Cultured canine synovial cells solubilize ^{45}Ca-labelled hydroxyapatite crystals. *Arth Rheum 27*:829–832 (1984).
20. R. W. Moskowitz, V. Vertes, A. Schwartz, G. Marshall, and B. Friedman. Crystal induced inflammation associated with chronic renal failure treated with periodic hemodialysis. *Am J Med 47*:450–460 (1969).
21. M. Kessler, B. Grignon, E. Renoult, P. Netter, and A. Gaucher. Complete resolution of large periarticular calcifications after renal transplantation. *J Rheumatol 16*:854–855 (1989).
22. F. M. Grinlinton, J. C. Vuletic, and P. J. Grow. Rapidly progressive calcific periarthritis occurring in a patient with lupus nephritis receiving chronic ambulatory peritoneal dialysis. *J Rheumatol 17*:1100–1103 (1990).
23. A. G. Fam, and K. P. H. Pritzker. Acute calcific periarthritis in scleroderma. *J Rheumatol 19*:1580–1585 (1992).
24. M. K. Dalinka, V. Stewart, J. S. Bomalaski, M. Halpern, and M. E. Kricun. Periarticular calcifications in association with intra-articular corticosteroid injections. *Radiology 153*:615–618 (1984).
25. J.-C. Gerster, and G. H. Fallet. Periarticular hand hydroxyapatite deposition after corticosteroid injection. *J Rheumatol 14*:1156–1159 (1987).
26. C. W. Hayes, D. I. Rosenthal, M. J. Plata, and T. M. Hudson. Calcific tendinitis in unusual sites associated with cortical bone erosions. *Am J Roentgenol* (AJR) *149*:967–970 (1987).
27. P. Fritz, T. Bardin, J.-D. Laredo, J.-M. Ziza, et al. Paradiaphyseal calcific tendinitis with cortical bone erosion. *Arth Rheum 37*:718–723 (1994).
28. H. R. Schumacher, P. V. Cherian, A. J. Reginato, T. Bardin, and S. Rothfuss. Intra-articular apatite crystal deposition. *Ann Rheum Dis 42(suppl. 1)*:54–59 (1983).
29. J. C. Gerster, and D. Fournier. Acute apatite arthritis of the shoulder in a young woman. *Clin Rheumatol 14*:95–99 (1995).
30. I. S. Kazmers, C. D. Scoville, and H. R. Schumacher. Polymyositis associated apatite arthritis. *J Rheumatol 15*:1019–1021 (1988).
31. C. W. Hutton, P. J. Maddison, A. J. Collins, and J. A. Berriman. Intra-articular ap-

atite deposition in mixed connective tissue disease: Crystallographic and technetium scanning characteristics. *Ann Rheum Dis 47*:1027–1030 (1988).

32. K. D. Brandt, and P. R. Krey. Chalky joint effusion: The result of massive synovial deposition of calcium apatite in progressive systemic sclerosis. *Arth Rheum 20*:792–796 (1977).
33. F. Beaudet, R. de Medicis, P. Magny, and A. Lussier. Acute apatite podagra with negative birefringent spherulites in the synovial fluid. *J Rheumatol 20*:1975–1980 (1993).
34. D. J. McCarty, P. B. Halverson, G. F. Carrera, B. J. Brewer, and F. Kozin. "Milwaukee shoulder"-association of microspheroids containing hydroxyapatite crystals, active collagenase, and neutral protease with rotator cuff defects. I. Clinical aspects. *Arth Rheum 24*:464–473 (1981).
35. P. A. Dieppe, M. Doherty, D. G. Macfarlane, C. W. Hutton, et al. Apatite associated destructive arthritis. *Br J Rheumatol 23*:84–91 (1984).
36. L. Zakaoui, H. R. Schumacher, S. Rothfuss, M. Sieck, G. Clayburne. Idiopathic destructive arthropathies: clinical, light and electron microscopic studies. *J Clin Rheumatol 2*:9–17 (1996).
37. G. M. McCarthy, P. G. Mitchell, and H. S. Cheung. The mitogenic response to stimulation with basic calcium phosphate crystals is accompanied by induction and secretion of collagenase in human fibroblasts. *Arth Rheum 34*:1021–1030 (1991).
38. P. A. Dieppe, T. Cawston, E. Mercer, C. V. Campion, et al. Synovial fluid collagenase in patients with destructive arthritis of the shoulder joint. *Arth Rheum 31*:882–890 (1988).
39. R. Caporali, S. Rossi, and C. Montecucco. Tidal irrigation in Milwaukee shoulder syndrome (Letter). *J Rheumatol 21*:1781–1782 (1994).
40. P. A. Gibilisco, H. R. Schumacher, J. L. Hollander, and K. A. Soper. Synovial fluid crystals in osteoarthritis. *Arth Rheum 28*:511–515 (1985).
41. P. B. Halverson, and D. J. McCarty. Patterns of radiographic abnormalities associated with basic calcium phosphate and calcium pyrophosphate dihydrate crystal deposition in the knee. *Ann Rheum Dis 45*:603–605 (1986).
42. G. J. Carroll, R. A. Stuart, J. A. Armstrong, P. D. Breidahl, and B. A. Laing. Hydroxyapatite crystals are a frequent finding in osteoarthritic synovial fluid, but are not related to increased concentrations of keratan sulphate or interleukin Iβ. *J Rheumatol 18*:861–866 (1991).
43. P. Dieppe, G. Campion, and M. Doherty. Mixed crystal deposition. *Rheum Dis Clin N Am 14*:415–426 (1988).
44. H. C. Anderson. Mechanisms of pathologic calcification. *Rheum Dis Clin N Am 14*:303–319 (1988).
45. M. A. M. Cousins, D. B. Jones, M. P. Whyte, and W. W. Monafo. Surgical management of calcinosis cutis universalis in systemic lupus erythematosus. *Arth Rheum 40*:570–572 (1997).
46. R. A. Khafif, C. Delima, A. Silverberg, and R. Frankel. Calciphylaxis and systemic calcinosis. Collective review. *Arch Intern Med 150*:956–959 (1990).
47. S. Vasudevan, B. Simmermann III, and E. V. Lally. Treatment-resistant diffuse calcinosis in scleroderma. *J Clin Rheumatol 2*:227–229 (1996).

48. G. M. A. Palmieri, J. I. Sebes, J. A. Aelion, and M. Moinuddin. Treatment of calcinosis with diltiazem. *Arth Rheum 38*:1646–1654 (1995).
49. M. B. Oliveri, R. Palmero, C. Mautalen, and O. Hubscher. Regression of calcinosis during diltiazem treatment in juvenile dermatomyositis. *J Rheumatol 23*:2152–2155 (1996).
50. R. E. Slavin, J. Wen, D. Kumar, and E. B. Evans. Familial tumoral calcinosis—a clinical, histopathologic, ultrastructural study with an analysis of its calcifying process and pathogenesis. *Am J Surg Pathol 17*:788–802 (1993).
51. I. Watt. Radiology of the crystal-associated arthritides. *Ann Rheum Dis 42(suppl)*:73–80 (1983).
52. H. W. Randle, H. M. Sander, and K. Howard. Early diagnosis of calcinosis cutis in childhood dermatomyositis using computed tomography. *JAMA 256*:1137–1138 (1986).
53. H. Paul, A. J. Reginato, and H. R. Schumacher. Alizarin red S staining as a screening test to detect calcium compounds in synovial fluid. *Arth Rheum 26*:191–200 (1983).
54. C. Gordon, A. Swan, and P. Dieppe. Detection of crystals in synovial fluids by light microscopy; sensitivity and reliability. *Ann Rheum Dis 48*:737–742 (1989).
55. O. Lazcano, C. -Y. Li, R. V. Pierre, J. D. O'Duffy, et al. Clinical utility of alizarin red S stain on permanent preparations to detect calcium-containing compounds in synovial fluid. *Am J Clin Pathol 94*:90–96 (1993).
56. P. R. Crocker, P. A. Dieppe, G. Tyler, S. K. Chapman, and D. A. Willoughby. The identification of particulate matter in biological tissues and fluids. *J Pathol 121*:37–40 (1977).
57. H. R. Schumacher, A. P. Smolyo, R. L. Tse, K. Maurer. Arthritis associated with apatite crystals. *Ann Intern Med 87*:411–416 (1977).
58. P. V. Cherian, and H. R. Schumacher. Diagnostic potential of rapid electron microscopic analysis of joint effusions. *Arth Rheum 25*:98–100 (1982).
59. P. B. Halverson, H. S. Cheung, and D. J. McCarty. "Milwaukee shoulder": Association of microspheroids containing hydroxyapatite crystals, active collagenase and neutral protease with rotator cuff defects: II. Synovial fluid studies. *Arth Rheum 24*:474–483 (1981).
60. D. J. McCarty, J. R. Lehr, and P. B. Halverson. Crystal populations in human synovial fluid: Identification of apatite, octacalcium phosphate, tricalcium phosphate. *Arth Rheum 26*:1220–1224 (1983).
61. N. McGill, P. A. Dieppe, M. Bowden, D. J. Gardiner, and M. Hall. Identification of pathological mineral deposits by Raman microscopy. *Lancet 337*:77–78 (1991).
62. J. M. Blair, L. B. Sorensen, M. F. Arnsdorf, and R. Lal. The application of atomic force microscopy for the detection of microcrystals in synovial fluid from patients with recurrent synovitis. *Sem Arth Rheum 24*:359–369 (1995).
63. G. Ellison, and R. W. Norrdin. Multicentric periarticular calcinosis in a pup. *J Am Vet Med Assoc 177*:542–546 (1980).
64. F. T. Hakim, R. Cranley, K. S. Brown, E. D. Eanes, et al. Hereditary joint disorder in progressive ankylosis (ank/ank) mice. I. association of calcium hydroxyapatite deposition with inflammatory arthropathy. *Arth Rheum 27*:1411–1420 (1984).

65. A. Swan, B. Dularay, and P. Dieppe. A comparison of the effects of urate, hydroxyapatite and diamond crystals on polymorphonuclear cells: A relationship of mediator release to the surface area and adsorptive capacity of different particles. *J Rheumatol 17*:1346–1352 (1990).
66. F. Prudhommeaux, C. Schiltz, F. Liote, A. Hina, et al. Variation in the inflammatory properties of basic calcium phosphate crystals according to crystal type. *Arth Rheum 39*:1319–1326 (1996).
67. H. Selye, G. Gentile, and R. Veilleux. An experimental model of calcareous subdeltoid bursitis induced by calciphylaxis. *Arth Rheum 5*:219–225 (1962).
68. A. J. Reginato, H. R. Schumacher, and C. T. Brighton. Experimental hydroxyapatite synovial and articular cartilage calcification: light and electron microscopic studies. *Arth Rheum 25*:1239–1249 (1982).

23
Inorganic Pyrophosphate Metabolism

IKUKO MASUDA, LAWRENCE M. RYAN, and DANIEL J. MCCARTY
Medical College of Wisconsin
Milwaukee, Wisconsin

Calcium pyrophosphate dihydrate (CPPD) crystal deposition in human articular cartilage is a common age-related event with a 50% prevalence by age 90 (1). CPPD crystals may cause attacks of inflammatory arthritis termed *pseudogout*. Of much greater public health concern are the crystal-associated degenerative changes, especially in large weight-bearing joints and the spine. Degenerative joint disease occurs in most patients with clinically expressed CPPD deposition disease. These associated complications will become more prevalent as the mean age in industrialized countries increases (reviewed in 1). CPPD crystals initiate or amplify cartilage destruction by stimulating synovial lining cell proliferation, as well as synthesis and secretion of neutral proteases and proinflammatory molecules by a variety of cells in articular tissues (reviewed in 2). Prevention or reversal of CPPD crystal deposition should abrogate the progression of joint tissue degeneration. Current knowledge of inorganic pyrophosphate (PPi) metabolism, the key molecule controlling the nucleation and growth of CPPD crystals, is reviewed here.

As calcium is predominantly an extracellular cation, CPPD crystals would be expected to nucleate and grow in an extracellular milieu. But many crystals were found within chondrocytes in a single well-studied case of tumoral CPPD crystal deposition in a temporomandibular joint (3). Crystals were seen in both cytoplasm and mitochondria in healthy-appearing cells. The possibility of an intracellular origin of CPPD crystal nucleation in calcium-rich organelles such as mitochondria remains open as a result of this provocative report. Urinary and plasma PPi levels are normal in patients with CPPD crystal deposition but intracellular PPi [(PPi)i] is increased in cultured skin fibroblasts from both hereditary

(3 different kindred) and sporadic cases (4) and in EB virus-transformed lymphocytes (French kindred) (5). Ectonucleotide pyrophosphohydrolase (NTPPHase) activity in cultured skin fibroblasts was significantly greater than in cells from sporadic, but not hereditary, CPPD crystal deposition disease patients (4).

These data suggest the presence of a generalized metabolic abnormality with phenotypic expression only in cartilage. Synovial fluid PPi levels are higher than plasma levels, even in normal individuals (reviewed in 1). The highest levels are found in degenerative joint diseases. The levels of PPi found correlated not with PPi crystal deposition per se, but with the severity of radiographically evident degeneration (6). The finding of extracellular PPi elaboration by both diseased and normal fibrocartilage and hyaline cartilage in organ culture provided a plausible explanation for the elevated synovial fluid PPi levels and for the site of CPPD crystal deposition (7,8).

Certain molecules have been identified that augment or inhibit PPi elaboration into ambient culture media by cartilage or chondrocytes. Cartilage cultured in serum produced 100% more PPi than tissue cultured in media alone—an effect of transforming growth factor β (TGFβ) in the serum (9). Extracellular PPi elaboration was stimulated by this cytokine in precisely those tissues where CPPD crystals are found—namely hyaline and fibrocartilage, tendon and ligament (10). The outer third of fibrocartilaginous menisci did not elaborate PPi and does not develop CPPD crystal deposits (1). Aged porcine cartilage elaborated more PPi than did cartilage from young pigs (11). Addition of ascorbate stimulated both collagen synthesis and PPi elaboration (12). In contrast, insulin-like growth factor-1 (IGF-1) (13) or interleukin-1 (IL-1) (14) decreased PPi elaboration. Retinoic acid stimulated PPi generation into the culture media (15), whereas inhibitors of protein synthesis (12) or the anion transport inhibitor probenecid (16) reduced it.

These in vitro observations suggest that modulation of cellular PPi by cytokines may underlie CPPD crystal formation production. (PPi)i is produced by many reactions within cells, particularly those involved in the biosynthesis of macromolecules (summarized in 17). Whether this (PPi)i is *secreted* through one or more ion channels, suggested by the probenecid effect, or *coexported* with macromolecules such as collagen, suggested by the ascorbate and protein inhibitor effects, remains unclear (Figure 1).

The identification of chondrocyte NTPPHase as an ectoenzyme (18,19) raised a third intriguing possibility—i.e., that PPi was being produced extracellularly in the tissues (cartilage, tendon, ligament) where CPPD crystal deposition actually occurs. The expression of this enzyme appears to be restricted to articular tissues (20). It is released as an insoluble 127 kD molecule associated with ~100 nm vesicles (21). Even normal cartilage in culture releases these structures (22). Smaller soluble fragments retain NTPPHase activity and appear in both joint fluid (chiefly 61 kD) (23) and plasma (chiefly 100 kD) (24). Western blot study of plas-

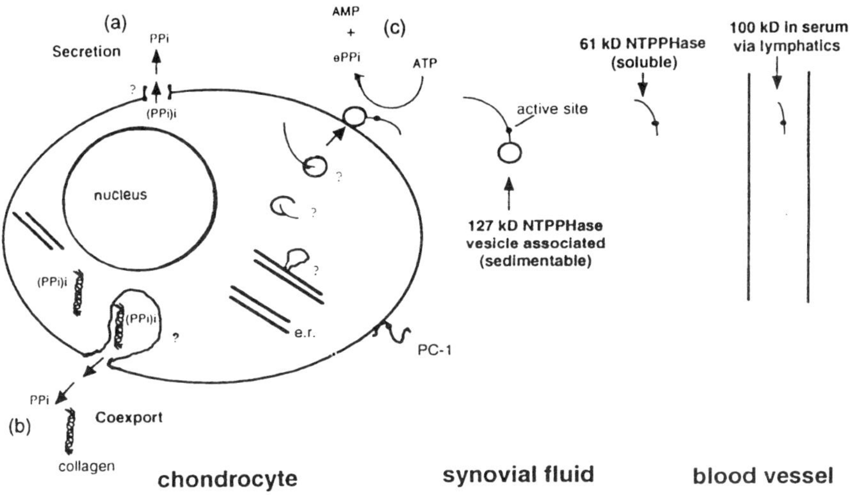

FIGURE 1 Putative pathways in generation of PPi by chondrocytes: (a) PPi leak or secretion from chondrocyte cytoplasm; (b) PPi exported with matrix molecules such as collagen; (c) PPi generated from extracellular ATP by ectoNTPPHases. Tissue specific NTPPHase is shown on chondrocyte membrane, and in vesicles derived from chondrocytes. 127-kD NTPPHase is vesicle associated and sedimentable. Its soluble, enzymatically active 61-kD and 100-kD fragments appear to be derived by limited proteolysis. Other ectoNTPPHases may also be important, such as PC-1, shown here attached to the cell membrane.

mas from 2 normal and 15 patients showed that all NTPPHase activity was due to articular tissue specific NTPPHase (24). The 61 kD fragment has been cloned and sequenced (Figure 2) (25). It has <30% homology with any known protein.

Another ectoNTPPHase has been identified, cloned, and sequenced (26). This enzyme, first found in a plasmacytoma, has been termed PC-1. PC-1 has enzymatic activities other that NTPPHase and it is found in cells from many tissues such as skin fibroblasts, osteocytes, and hepatocytes as well as in chondrocytes (27). PC-1 has been identified in synovial fluids from severely degenerative joints (23,27).

Articular cartilage vesicles (ACV) derived from chondrocytes nucleated and grew monoclinic CPPD crystals in vitro in the presence of extracellular ATP [$(ATP)_e$] (22). These vesicles are analogous to the matrix vesicles at the sites of apatite mineralization in growth plate cartilage. $(ATP)_e$ added to cartilage explants induced formation of perichondral CPPD-like crystals, many of which lay within membranous structures (28). Phosphocitrate, an inhibitor of hydroxyap-

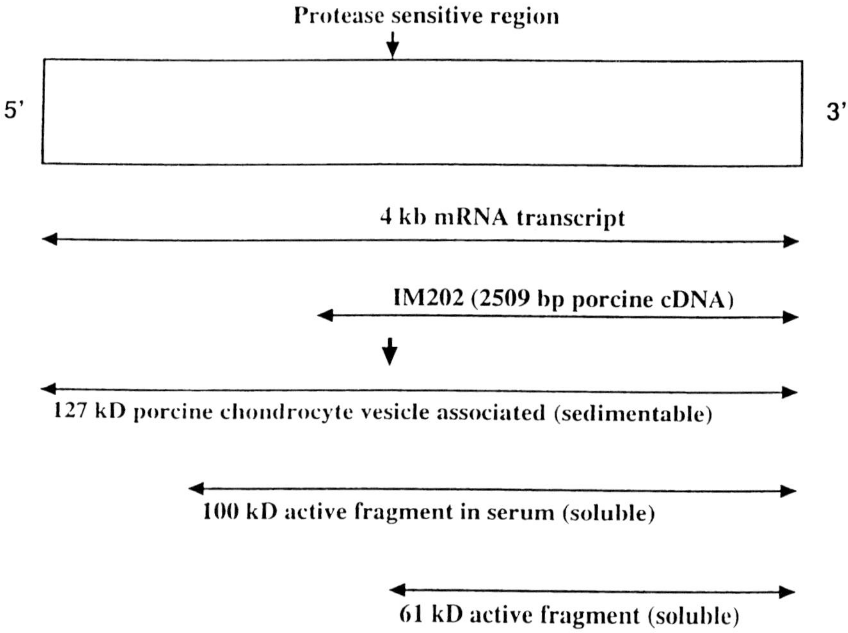

FIGURE 2 Putative molecular model for the synthesis and translocation of tissue specific ectoNTTPHase. The full-length enzyme is transcribed as a 4-kb mRNA. The cDNA IM202 represents its 3-in. portion. The full-length 127-kD NTPPHase is translated, and the secreted membrane-vesicle associated 127-kD NTPPHase is proteolytically processed into soluble, enzymatically active fragments, chiefly 61 kD and 100 kD. The protease sensitive site (RRKRR) for the generation of the 61-kD fragment is immediately upstream of its N-terminal sequence. (From Ref. 25.)

atite and calcium oxalate monohydrate crystal formation in vitro, blocked both ATP- and non-ATP-dependent mineralization in cultured articular cartilage slices, but had no effect on ACV NTPPHase activity (29).

The discovery of ectoNTPPHase prompted a systematic study of plasma and synovial fluid $(ATP)_e$ levels. All plasmas (30) and fluids (31) studied had detectable levels. Synovial fluid $(ATP)_e$ levels were always lower than those in plasma. Mean $(ATP)_e$ levels in fluids from osteoarthritic joints were about half those from degenerative joints that had developed CPPD crystal deposits (~100 vs. ~200 nM), despite higher mean NTPPHase activity in the latter (32). The measured levels in both plasma and synovial fluid are undoubtedly underestimates of the true values because of enzymatic activity occurring during the time of sample collection before transfer into iced tubes containing appropriate inhibitors.

Studies of intra-articular PPi pool and turnover rate in 31 human knee joints showed a production rate of about 0.1 μmol per hour (32). Production of PPi increased with the severity of radiographically evident degeneration, reaching about 0.6 μmol per hour in severely damaged joints with large effusions. In all instances, clearance of radiolabelled PPi injected into a joint was log linear for at least 3 hr, indicating a single pool. Presumably the 3–4 mm thick articular cartilages became part of the pool during the initial 15 min period of mixing by barbotage. That the synovial fluid and cartilage were part of the same pool should have suggested that the former was in fact producing PPi as efficiently as the latter.

The finding of both ectoNTPPHase and its substrate $(ATP)_e$ in synovial fluid provided a possible explanation for this seeming paradox. Samples of cell-free synovial fluid were therefore pH adjusted and incubated under physiologic conditions in vitro (34). The rate of disappearance of $(ATP)_e$ added to stirred samples to approximate the mean ex-vivo ATP levels previously measured was used to calculate the rate constant. ATP was then added using an infusion pump to maintain a steady state level of 100 nM (osteoarthritis) or 200 nM (CPPD crystal deposition). In all fluids in these two conditions, ATP was stoichiometrically converted to PPi. Fluids from CPPD crystal patients produced six times more PPi than did those from osteoarthritis. Rates of hydrolysis of PPi were relatively insignificant, averaging only 4%.

The rate of PPi production by synovial fluid in vitro multiplied by the pool volume previously estimated by dilution of radiolabelled PPi injected into knee joints (33) yielded rough estimates of PPi production of 0.3–1.8 μmoles per hour, about three times the rates determined by the in vivo pool and turnover studies.

The total hyaline and fibrocartilage mass in a normal human knee was estimated at 37 g by measurements on a skeleton. PPi elaborated into culture medium by four normal human articular cartilages was about 100 ρ mol per mg wet weight per hour. At this rate, basal PPi production by cartilage in a normal knee would be 0.37 μmoles per hour. Thus three different methods used to estimate PPi production are of the same order of magnitude (34). Taken together, these data suggest that virtually all PPi production is from $(ATP)_e$ via ectoNTPPHase.

These quantitative data (Table 1) must be reconciled with the evidence already cited for: (1) generalized elevated (PPi)i levels, (2) the effects of stimulants and inhibitors on extracellular elaboration of PPi by cultured cartilage or chondrocytes, and (3) the increased ectoNTPPHase activity in cultured skin fibroblasts from patients with sporadic CPPD crystal deposition.

We postulate that the driving force underlying CPPD crystal deposition is the availability of $(ATP)_e$ of intracellular origin. A generalized metabolic abnormality that increases intracellular ATP generation could explain the observed elevation of (PPi)i via the NTPPHase present in the endoplasmic reticulum prior to its translocation (35). Perhaps the increased ATP production occurs in mitochondria

TABLE I Quantitative Estimates of PPi Synthesis in Human Knee Joints

1. In vivo pool and turnover of radiolabelled PPi showed single intrasynovial PPi pool that included the synovial fluid; 0.1 μ to 0.6 μmol PPi hr^{-1} was produced by human knee joints, proportional to the severity of radiographically evident degeneration.
2. Plasma $(ATP)_e$ showed diurnal variation with mean levels about 600 μM, well above synovial fluid values (approximately 100 μM in OA and 200 μM in CPPD). At these steady-state levels, $(ATP)_e$ was stoichiometrically converted to PPi by cell-free synovial fluids. Sixfold more PPi was produced by CPPD fluids. At these rates, 0.3–1.8 μmoles of PPi would be produced in vivo by the entire pool per hour.
3. Normal human cartilage PPi elaboration in vitro was about 10 ρmol per mg wet weight per hour; 0.37 μmoles of PPi per hour would be produced by a normal human knee with an estimated total cartilage mass of 37 g.

as suggested by the observations of Dijkgraaf et al. (3). The original description of increased pyrophosphohydrolase activity in degenerated cartilage from CPPD deposition vis-a-vis osteoarthritic cartilage also found increased 5' nucleotidase activity, which might imply excessive accumulation of extracellular adenosine monophosphate (36). $(ATP)_e$ is present even in normal subjects although the physiologic mechanism(s) of its release from cells is unknown. Perhaps, in tissues such as cartilage that normally elaborate PPi, the cellular outflux of ATP is augmented if the intracellular level is abnormally elevated. Skin fibroblasts do not normally elaborate detectable PPi, and therefore may not generate $(ATP)_e$, even under abnormal conditions. Could an increased intracellular ATP level induce increased synthesis of ectoPC-1, the activity of which we presumably measured in fibroblasts from patients with sporadic CPPD crystal deposition? If so, why did this not occur in fibroblasts from patients with hereditary forms of this condition?

We further speculate that PPi, known to be a potent inhibitor of apatitic crystal nucleation and growth (37), is elaborated by tissues that are attached to bone to prevent their mineralization. CPPD crystal deposition in this view is a result of a normal physiologic defense mechanism gone awry. As the vital processes leading to $(ATP)_e$ and extracellular PPi generation become clarified, it may be possible to prevent CPPD crystal formation by modulating PPi production pharmacologically.

REFERENCES

1. L. M. Ryan, and D. J. McCarty. Calcium pyrophosphate crystal deposition disease; Pseudogout; Articular chondrocalcinosis, *Arthritis and Allied Conditions* (W. Koopman, ed.), 13th ed., Williams and Wilkins, Baltimore, MD, pp. 2103–2125 (1996).

2. H. S. Cheung, and L. M. Ryan. Role of crystal deposition in matrix degradation, *Joint Cartilage Degradation: Basic Research and Clinical Implication* (F. Woessner and D. S. Howell, eds.), Marcel Dekker, Inc., New York, NY, pp. 209 (1993).
3. H. C. Dijkgraaf, R. S. B. Liem, L. G. M. deBont, and G. Boering. Calcium pyrophosphate dihydrate deposition disease: A review of the literature and a light and electron microscopic study of the temporo mandibular joint with numerous intracellular crystals in the chondrocytes. *Osteoarthritis and Cartilage 3*:35–45 (1995).
4. L. M. Ryan, R. L. Wortmann, B. Karas, M. P. Lynch, and D. J. McCarty. Pyrophosphohydrolase activity and inorganic pyrophosphate content of cultured human skin fibroblasts: Elevated levels in some patients with calcium pyrophosphate dihydrate deposition disease, *J Clin Invest 77*:1689 (1986).
5. G. Lust, G. Faure, P. Netter, A. Gaucher, and J. E. Seegmiller. Evidence of a generalized metabolic defect in patients with hereditary chondrocalcinosis. *Arthritis Rheum 24*:1517 (1981).
6. D. C. Silcox and D. J. McCarty. Elevated inorganic pyrophosphate concentrations in synovial fluid in osteoarthritis and pseudogout. *J Lab Clin Med 83*:518 (1974).
7. D. S. Howell, O. Muniz, J. C. Pita, and J. E. Enis. Extrusion of pyrophosphate into extracellular media by osteoarthritic cartilage incubates. *J Clin Invest 56*:1473 (1975).
8. L. M. Ryan, H. S. Cheung, and D. J. McCarty. Release of pyrophosphate by normal mammalian articular hyaline and fibrocartilage in organ culture. *Arthritis Rheum 24*:1522 (1981).
9. A. K. Rosenthal, H. S. Cheung, and L. M. Ryan. Transforming growth factor β1 stimulates inorganic pyrophosphate elaboration by porcine cartilage. *Arthritis Rheum 34*:904 (1991).
10. A. K. Rosenthal, B. A. McCarty, H. S. Cheung, and L. M. Ryan. A comparison of the effect of transforming growth factor β1 on pyrophosphate elaboration from various articular tissues. *Arthritis Rheum 36*:539 (1993).
11. A. K. Rosenthal and L. M. Ryan. Ageing influences TGFβ-induced pyrophosphate elaboration by cartilage. *Mech Aging Development 75*:35 (1994).
12. L. M. Ryan, I. Kurup, and H. S. Cheung. Stimulation of cartilage inorganic pyrophosphate elaboration by ascorbate. *Matrix: Collagen and Related Res. 11*:276 (1991).
13. U. Olmez, L. M. Ryan, I. V. Kurup, and A. K. Rosenthal. Insulin-like growth factor-1 suppresses pyrophosphate elaboration by transforming growth factor β1-stimulated chondrocytes and cartilage. *Osteoarthritis and Cartilage 2*:149 (1994).
14. M. Lotz, F. Rosen, G. McCabe, F. Blanco, J. Dudler, J. E. Seegmiller, and R. Terkeltaub. Interleukin 1 beta suppresses transforming growth factor-induced inorganic pyrophosphate (PPi) production and expression of the PPi-generating enzyme PC-1 in human chondrocytes. *Proc Natl Acad Sci USA 92*:10364 (1995).
15. A. K. Rosenthal and L. A. Henry. Retinoic acid stimulates pyrophosphate elaboration by cartilage and chondrocytes. *Calcif Tissue Int 59*:128 (1996).
16. A. K. Rosenthal and L. M. Ryan. Probenecid inhibits transforming growth factor-β1 induced pyrophosphate elaboration by chondrocytes. *J Rheumatol 21*:896 (1994).
17. A. Kornberg. On the metabolic significance of phosphorylytic and pyrophosphorylytic reactions. *Horizons in Biochemistry* (M. Kasha and D. Pullman, eds.), Academic Press, New York, NY (1962).

18. L. M. Ryan, R. L. Wortmann, B. Karas, and D. J. McCarty. Cartilage nucleoside triphosphate (NTP) pyrophosphohydrolase: I. Identification as an ectoenzyme. *Arthritis Rheum* 27:913 (1984).
19. A. Caswell, and R. G. G. Russell. Identification of ectonucleoside triphosphate pyrophosphatase in human articular chondrocytes in monolayer culture. *Biochem Biophys Acta 847*:40 (1985).
20. A. Cardenal, I. Masuda, A. L. Haas, and D. J. McCarty. Specificity of a porcine 127 kD nucleotide pyrophosphohydrolase for articular tissues. *Arthritis Rheum 39*:245 (1996).
21. I. Masuda, J. Hamada, A. L. Haas, L. M. Ryan, and D. J. McCarty. A unique ectonucleotide pyrophosphohydrolase associated with porcine chondrocyte-derived vesicles. *J Clin Invest 95*:699 (1995).
22. B. A. Derfus, J. W. Rachow, N. S. Mandel, A. L. Boskey, M. Buday, V. M. Kushnaryov, and L. M. Ryan. Articular cartilage vesicles generate calcium pyrophosphate dihydrate-like crystals in vitro. *Arthritis Rheum 35*:1520 (1992).
23. I. Masuda, A. Cardenal, W. Ono, J. Hamada, A. L. Haas, and D. J. McCarty. Nucleotide pyrophosphohydrolase in human synovial fluids. *J Rheumatol 24*:1588 (1997).
24. A. Cardenal, I. Masuda, A. L. Haas, W. Ono, and D. J. McCarty. Identification of a nucleotide pyrophosphohydrolase from articular tissues in human serum. *Arthritis Rheum 39*:252 (1996).
25. I. Masuda, B. D. Halligan, J. T. Barbieri, A. L. Haas, L. M. Ryan, and D. J. McCarty. Molecular cloning and expression of a porcine chondrocyte nucleotide pyrophosphohydrolase. *Gene 197*:277 (1997).
26. I. Funakoshi, H. Kato, K. Horie, T. Yano, Y. Hori, H. Kobayashi, T. Inoue, H. Suzuki, S. Fukui, M. Tsukahara, T. Kajii, and I. Yamashina. Molecular cloning of cDNAs for human fibroblast nucleotide pyrophosphatase. *Arch Biochem Biophys 295*:180 (1992).
27. R. Huang, M. Rosenbach, R. Vaughn, D. Provvedini, N. Rebbe, S. Hickman, J. Goding, and R. Terkeltaub. Expression of the murine plasma cell nucleotide pyrophosphohydrolase PC-1 is shared by human liver, bone and cartilage cells. *J Clin Invest 94*:560 (1994).
28. L. M. Ryan, I. V. Kurup, B. A. Derfus, and V. M. Kushnaryov. ATP-induced chondrocalcinosis. *Arthritis Rheum 35*:1520 (1992).
29. H. S. Cheung, I. V. Kurup, J. D. Sallis, and L. M. Ryan. Inhibition of calcium pyrophosphate dihydrate crystal formation in articular cartilage vesicles and cartilage by phosphocitrate. *J Biol Chem 271*:28082 (1996).
30. L. M. Ryan, J. W. Rachow, B. A. McCarty, and D. J. McCarty. Adenosine triphosphate levels in human plasma. *J Rheumatol 23*:214 (1996).
31. L. M. Ryan, J. W. Rachow, and D. J. McCarty. Synovial fluid ATP: A possible substrate for generation of inorganic pyrophosphate in calcium pyrophosphate dihydrate (CPPD) crystal deposition disease. *J Rheumatol 18*:716 (1991).
32. J. W. Rachow, L. M. Ryan, D. J. McCarty, and P. B. Halverson. Synovial fluid inorganic pyrophosphate concentration and nucleotide pyrophosphohydrolase activity in basic calcium phosphate deposition arthropathy and Milwaukee shoulder syndrome. *Arthritis Rheum 31*:408 (1988).

33. M. Camerlain, D. J. McCarty, D. C. Silcox, and A. Jung. Inorganic pyrophosphate pool size and turnover rate in arthritis joints. *J Clin Invest 55*:1373 (1975).
34. W. Park, I. Masuda, A. Cardenal-Escarcena, D. L. Palmer, and D. J. McCarty. Inorganic pyrophosphate generation from adenosine triphosphate by cell-free human synovial fluid. *J Rheumatol 23*:665 (1996).
35. R. Terkeltaub, M. Rosenbach, F. Fong, and J. Goding. Causal link between nucleotide pyrophosphohydrolase overactivity and increased intracellular inorganic pyrophosphate generation demonstrated by transfection of cultured fibroblasts and osteoblasts with plasma cell membrane glycoprotein-1: Relevance to calcium pyrophosphate dihydrate deposition disease. *Arthritis Rheum 37*:934 (1994).
36. J. O. Tenenbaum, O. Muniz, H. R. Schmacher, A. E. Good, and D. S. Howell. Comparison of phosphohydrolase activities from articular cartilage in calcium pyrophosphate deposition disease and primary osteoarthritis. *Arthritis Rheum 24*:294 (1981).
37. H. Fleisch and R. G. G. Russell. Pyrophosphate and polyphosphates. *Pharmacology of the Endocrine System and Related Drugs* (H. Rasmussen, ed.), Pergamon Press, New York, NY, pp. 61–100 (1970).

24

Calcium Oxalate and Other Miscellaneous Crystal Related Arthropathies

ANTONIO J. REGINATO and GERALD F. FALASCA
Cooper Hospital/University Medical Center, Robert Wood Johnson Medical School at Camden, University of Medicine and Dentistry of New Jersey, Camden, New Jersey

In addition to monosodium urate and calcium pyrophosphate crystals, a large number of crystalline materials have been identified in synovial or bursal fluids, synovium, bone, and muscle of patients with arthritis and other musculoskeletal complaints (1) (Table 1). These crystals are found less often than monosodium urate, calcium pyrophosphate, and hydroxyapatite, but may sometimes be confused with them by inexperienced observers (2). The identification of these crystals in synovial fluid also may provide the clue of a systemic disease such as in the case of cryoglobulinemia, Fabry's disease, and hypereosinophilic syndrome (3). Some of these crystals may be associated with pseudovasculitic syndromes as is seen with cholesterol embolization (4), cryoglobulinemia (5), primary and secondary oxalosis (6,7), amyloidosis (8), Fabry's disease (9), and hypereosinophilic syndrome (10). Diseases such as primary hyperoxaluria type 1 provide important biochemical and molecular genetic lessons to be applied to the study of other human enzymatic diseases associated with crystalline deposits (11).

In this chapter we will provide an update about those musculoskeletal syndromes associated with calcium oxalate, cholesterol, cryoglobulins, Charcot-Leyden crystals, and synthetic corticosteroids crystals (1,2). The remaining crystals of Table 1 have only been described in synovial fluid, synovium, muscle, or bone in isolated case reports, which have been summarized in detail in previous reviews (1–3).

TABLE I Crystals Uncommonly Found in Joints, Muscles, or Bones

Calcium Oxalate
Cholesterol
Lipid liquid crystals
Other crystalline lipids
Cryoglobulins
Lysophospholipase (Charcot-Leyden)
Synthetic corticosteroid
Miscellaneous Crystals
Cystine
Xanthine
Hypoxanthine
Aluminum
Hemoglobin
Hematoidin
Amyloid

I. OXALATE GOUT/CALCIUM OXALATE DEPOSITION DISEASE

Oxalate gout* is a rare metabolic disorder that may be a result of familial enzymatic defects leading to increased oxalate production or end-stage renal disease necessitating long-term dialysis (1–3). The musculoskeletal manifestations of oxalate gout have been confused in the past with those of monosodium urate (MSU), calcium pyrophosphate dihydrate (CPPD), and apatite gouts (Figure 1). Patients with oxalate gout may present a variety of articular and nonarticular manifestations due to calcium oxalate deposits. These deposits may also induce life-threatening organ involvement such as reversible arterial spasm (6), chronic peripheral vascular insufficiency and gangrene (7), cardiomyopathy (12), complete heart block (13), peripheral neuropathy (14), cerebral edema with focal areas of necrosis, aseptic meningitis (15), and aplastic anemia (16).

*In this review, the term *gout* is used to refer to any disease attributable to the deposition of crystals in tissues.

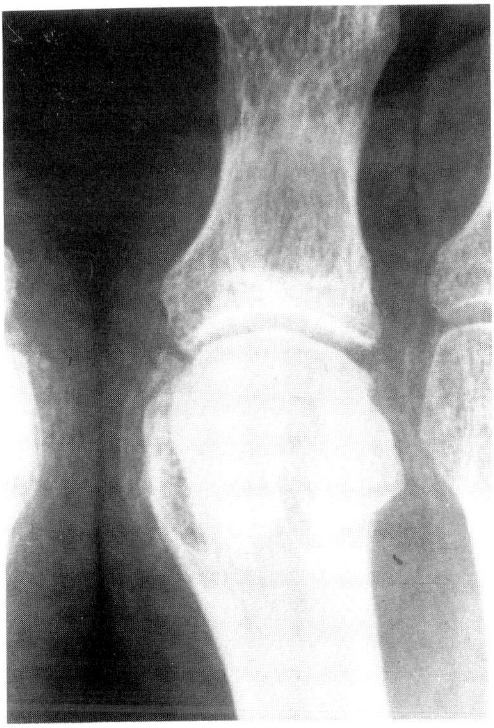

FIGURE 1 Synovial and articular calcifications observed in one patient with podagra due to secondary oxalosis. (From Ref. 1.)

II. PRIMARY OXALOSIS

Primary hyperoxaluria type 1 (PH1) is a rare and potentially lethal autosomal recessive inborn error of glyoxylate metabolism caused by a deficiency of the liver-specific peroxisomal enzyme alanine glyoxylate aminotransferase (AGT) (17–19) (Figure 2). The disease is characterized by increased synthesis and excretion of oxalate and glyoxylate due to a blockage of glyoxylate alternative pathways. These patients present with urolithiasis or nephrocalcinosis at an early age and, in severe cases, renal failure followed by rapidly progressive systemic oxalosis. The disease has a striking clinical and biochemical heterogeneity (20–21). From the clinical point of view, the disease shows a wide variation of age of disease onset (1–57 years), severity of clinical manifestations, degree of hyperoxaluria and hyperglycolic aciduria, rates of progression to systemic oxalosis, pyridoxine response, and age of death (1–65 years). These patients also show

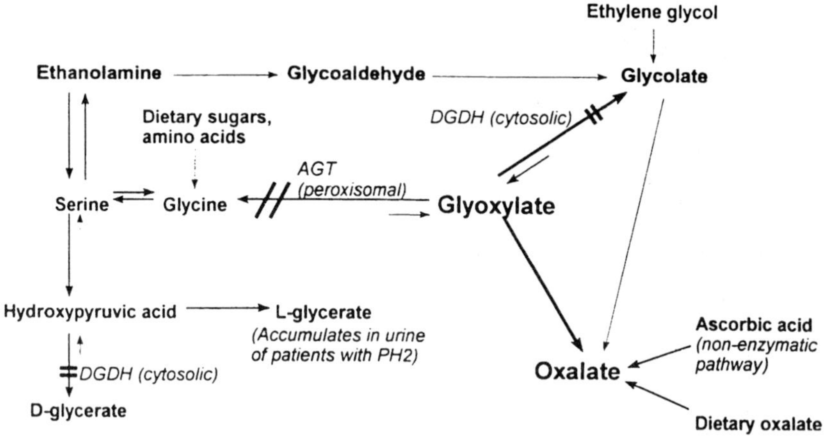

FIGURE 2 Simplified metabolic pathways leading to oxalate production. The major defect in PH1 is a defect in activity of peroxisomal alanine:glyoxylate aminotransferase (AGT) leading to accumulation of glyoxylate. In PH2, the major defect appears to be loss of D-glycerate dehydrogenase/glyoxylate reductase (DGDH) activity leading to accumulation of L-glycerate in the urine as well as oxalate. (Modified from Ref. 113.)

a wide variation in enzymatic activity, subcellular distribution, and genetic coding sequence for AGT (21–25). Several point mutations, all occurring at conserved position in the coding region of the AGT gene, have been identified in these patients (17,22–24) (Figure 3). The most common mutation found so far leads to a Gly170→Arg amino acid substitution (17,22–24). The enzymatic defect can be diagnosed by determining the activity of AGT in liver tissue obtained through a needle biopsy, but cloning and sequencing of the human AGT gene now provides the possibility of prenatal screening, using genomic linkage analysis and mutation analysis from DNA isolated from chorionic villi during the first trimester (26). Most of the prenatal diagnoses of PH1 by liver biopsy have been performed during the second trimester (25).

Primary hyperoxaluria type 2 (PH2) is also autosomal recessive but is much less common than PH1. It seems to result from a defect in hydroxypyruvate metabolism due to a liver enzymatic deficiency of glyoxylate reductase (GR), which also has D-glycerate dehydrogenase activity (19,27–30) (Figure 2). Both of these enzymatic activities appear to be attributed to a single enzyme. Deficiency of D-glycerate acid dehydrogenase activity presumably causes accumulation of its substrate, hydroxypyruvate, which is then converted to L-glycerate by the action of L-lactic acid dehydrogenase. L-glycerate is not found in normal urine but is characteristically found in PH2. Deficiency of glyoxylate reductase activity presumably causes impaired conversion of glyoxylate to glycolate. Conversion of

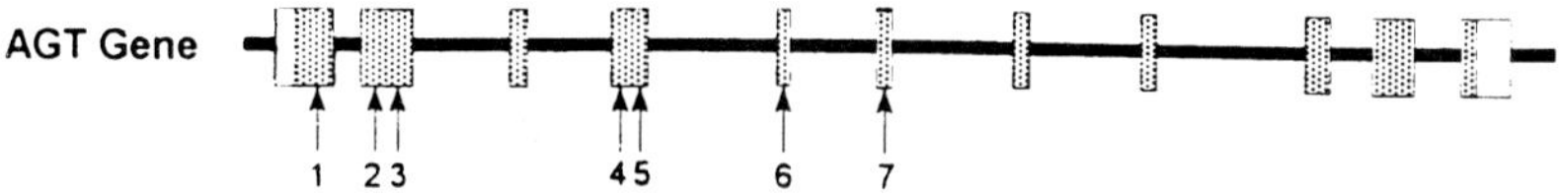

Mutation Number	Base Substitution	Amino Acid Substitution
1	G243 → A	Gly-41 → Arg
2	C320 → G	Tyr-66 → Ter (predicted)
3	G367 → A	Gly-82 → Glu
4	T576 → A	Phe-152 → Ile
5	G630 → A	Gly-170 → Arg
6	C682 → T	Ser-187 → Phe
7	T735 → C	Ser-205 → Pro

FIGURE 3 Diagrammatic representation of the human AGT gene (not drawn to scale). Shaded areas represent the eleven exons. Unshaded boxes represent the 5' and 3' untranslated regions. Arrows show the positions of the of known PH1 mutations. (Modified from Ref. 22.)

glyoxylate to oxalate by L-lactic acid dehydrogenase would explain the observed hyperoxaluria (Figure 2). Decreased activity of D-glycerate acid dehydrogenase has been found in leukocytes of patients with this type of hyperoxaluria (19).

Sixteen of the 21 patients previously reported with type 2 hyperoxaluria initially had renal calculi between 6 months and 24 years of age (27–30). Five affected relatives seemed to have had no symptoms and were identified only because their siblings also had the disorder. This suggests that this subset of asymptomatic patients may be more common than originally suspected (25–30). Thus PH2 may be a much more benign disease with a better long-term prognosis in terms of renal function than PH1. A third type, PH3, is due to primary increased absorption of oxalate from the small bowel (17).

In PH1 and PH2 the renal insufficiency is associated with rapid, progressive calcium oxalate crystal deposits in kidney, myocardium, skin, bone, and blood vessels (17,19). Oxalate crystals have been described in the synovium, tendon sheaths, articular cartilage, and bone (1,2,17). Table 2 summarizes the reported clinical, radiological, and pathological musculoskeletal manifestations of PH1 (3).

III. ACQUIRED OXALOSIS

Oxalic acid is the metabolic end product of glycine, serine, other amino acids, and ascorbic acid (19) (Figure 2). Large amounts of oxalate are also found in certain foods such as spinach and rhubarb (15). Oxalate is readily absorbed after ingestion. It is removed from the body almost entirely by glomerular filtration

TABLE 2 Skeletal Manifestation Observed in 29 Patients with Primary Hyperoxaluria Type 1 and End-Stage Renal Disease[a]

Skeletal manifestations		Number of patients
Bone Pain		22
I.	Dense bones	18
II.	Osteitis fibrosa cystica	14
III.	Osteomalacia	3
IV.	Fracture/separation of epiphysis[b]	3
V.	Vertebral fractures	3
VI.	Multiple fractures	1
VII.	Spinal stenosis	1
Joint Pain		18
I.	Polyarticular pain	10
II.	Acute Arthritis	8
III.	Chronic arthritis	7
IV.	Finger destructive arthropathy[c]	8
V.	Chondrocalcinosis	4
VI.	Chronic shoulder destructive arthropathy	1
Tendon/Bursa Pain		9
I.	Calcific flexor finger tendon sheaths	9
II.	Calcified olecranon bursitis	2
III.	Arterial spasm	1
IV.	Hypercalcemia	6
V.	Livedo reticularis	1

[a]Patients ranged in age from 6 to 60 yr and had been managed on dialysis for 1.7 to 7 yr (mean 6.7 yrs). From references 44–47.
[b]Children only.
[c]Cutaneous calcinosis in three.
Sources: Refs. 44–47.

and secretion into the proximal tubule. Hyperoxalemia, hyperoxaluria, oxalate kidney stones, and crystalline tissue deposits may be the result of contributing factors affecting oxalate metabolism (1,3,19) (Table 3). Excessive oxalate in the diet (15,19) or increased absorption in patients with chronic inflammatory bowel disease, small bowel resection, intestinal bypass (31), and external biliary drainage (32) can lead to hyperoxalemia and oxalate kidney deposits, but so far no calcium oxalate crystals have been isolated in the joint fluid of patients with enteric oxalosis (3). Methoxyflurane, ethylene glycol, ascorbic acid, and xylitol are all metabolized to oxalate (19). Fatal oxalate poisoning after eating 20–100 g of stems and leaves of raw rhubarb has been reported in 2- to 6-year-old children (15).

Thiamine and pyridoxine deficiencies may inhibit glyoxylate metabolism, increasing oxalate production (19). *Aspergillus niger* can synthesize oxalic

TABLE 3 Types of Oxalosis

Familial	I.	Primary hyperoxaluria Type 1: AGT deficiency Type 2: GR deficiency Type 3: Increased oxalate absorption
Acquired	I.	Diet rich in oxalate
	II.	Ingestion or administration of oxalate precursors: ascorbic acid, ethylene glycol, xylitol
	III.	Increased absorption: small bowel resection or bypass, inflammatory bowel disease, external biliary drainage.
	IV.	Increased production: deficiency of thiamine or pyridoxine, *Aspergillus niger* infection.
	V.	Dystrophic: retinal damage, lymph node granulomas.

TABLE 4 Clinical Manifestations in 14 Reported Patients with Secondary Oxalosis Due to End Stage Renal Disease and Dialysis

Manifestation	Number of patients
Bone Pain	12
Joint Pain	12
Arthritis	11
Acute	3
Chronic	11
Skin oxalate deposits	8
Myocardiopathy	3
Obliterative vascular disease	3
Periodontitis	1

Sources: Refs. 1, 38, 39.

acid, which may crystallize in infected tissues and in aspergillomas (2,33). Chronic renal failure can lead to serum oxalate levels 4–8 times greater than normal (19,34,35). Oxalate serum levels parallel those of creatinine, becoming saturated when levels of the latter reach 8–9 mg/dl (35). Secondary oxalosis complicating renal failure has been reported infrequently, and estimating the frequency of this occurrence on the basis of published series is difficult (36–39) (Table 4). In some series, the administration of large doses of ascorbic acid was considered a significant aggravating factor (37,39).

The formation of calcium oxalate crystals in biologic fluids and tissues results when the limits of solubility are exceeded. In the urine, the degree of saturation of calcium oxalate expressed in terms of the ionic concentration of calcium and oxalic acid is the single most important factor in the formation of oxalate stones (19,35). Similar mechanisms may operate in serum and other tissues. In some organs, such as kidney, myocardium, thyroid, retina, and lymph nodes (in the setting of granulomatous inflammation), and in *Aspergillus niger* infections, oxalic acid is produced locally, so that local acid concentration may exceed those of serum (33,40–43). This may account for the calcium oxalate crystal formation in idiopathic calcium urolithiasis (40), aspergillosis (33), dystrophic retinal damage (41), and lymph nodes affected by a variety of granulomatous diseases such as sarcoidosis, Crohn's disease, and other mycobacterial infections that are associated with normal serum oxalate (42).

IV. CLINICAL MANIFESTATIONS

Diffuse bone pain, vertebral compression fractures, symmetric acute or chronic arthritis involving the proximal interphalangeal and metacarpophalangeal joints

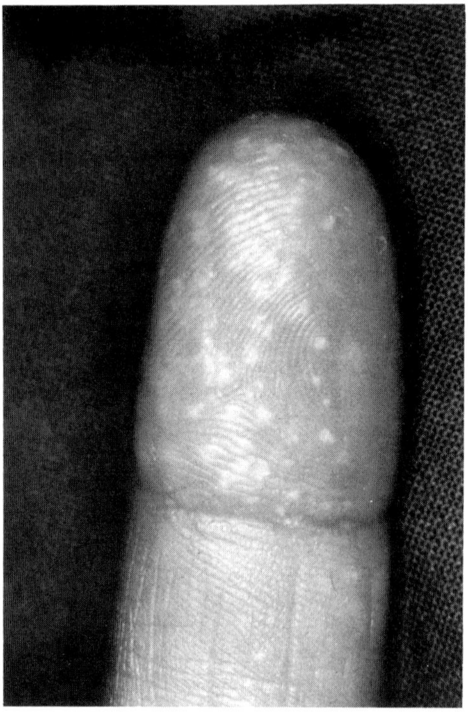

FIGURE 4 Miliary calcinosis due to oxalate deposition in a patient receiving hemodialysis. (From Ref. 39.)

with or without flexor tenosynovitis, associated miliary calcified skin deposits of digits, and vascular calcification are the most characteristic clinical presentations (Figure 4). Acute or chronic effusion of large joints involving knees, elbows, or ankles, podagra, Achilles tenosynovitis, and a bursitis also have been described (3,37,39). A patient with primary oxalosis and hyperostosis presented with central spinal stenosis due to oxalate crystal deposits in the ligamentum flavum, similar to that reported in patients with apatite and calcium pyrophosphate crystal deposition diseases (43).

In most patients, the acute synovitis usually follows a chronic course, responding poorly to colchicine, nonsteroidal anti-inflammatory agents, intra-articular corticosteroids, and even increasing the frequency of dialysis (37–39). Synovial fluid obtained from acute and chronic effusions has been clear or bloody with normal viscosity (2,37,39). Abundant clumps of extracellular polymorphic oxalate crystals are often seen but intracellular crystals are less commonly observed (2).

Oxalate crystals in synovial fluid may present as polymorphic crystals composed of calcium oxalate monohydrate (whewellite) or they may adopt a characteristic dipyramidal shape (like a letter envelope) formed by calcium oxalate dihydrate

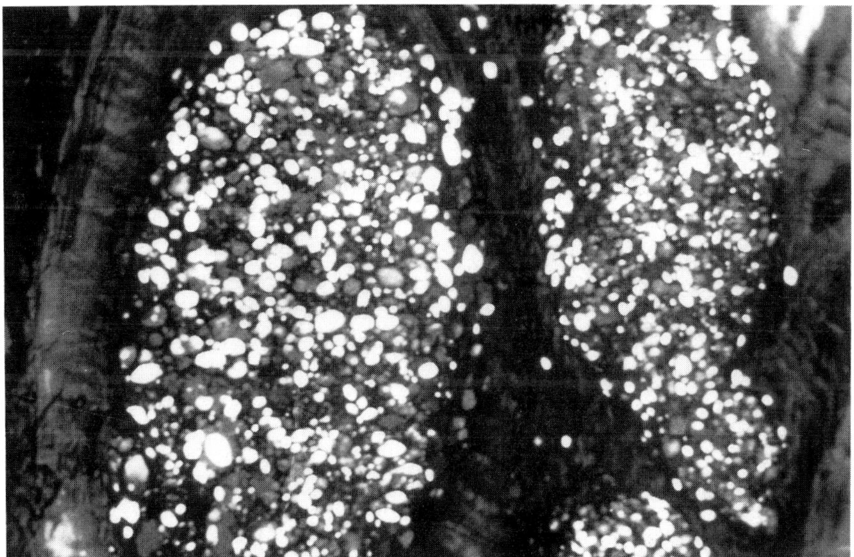

FIGURE 5 Calcium oxalate deposit in the articular cartilage obtained from the first metatarsophalangeal joint shown in Figure 1. Compensated, polarized light × 180. (From Ref. 39.)

(weddellite) (2). Polymorphic crystals may appear as broken squares, chunks, short rods, stretched ovals, dumbbells, and even microspherules mimicking small calcium pyrophosphate crystals or hydroxyapatite clumps. Sizes range from 5–30 μm and they may show an intense birefringence with positive elongation.

V. RADIOGRAPHIC MANIFESTATIONS

The radiographic manifestations of primary and secondary oxalosis are similar and characteristically involve the hands and feet, with miliary skin calcification as well as digital arteries, periarticular, and intra-articular calcifications (3,37–39,43–47) (Figure 1). Rosette-like areas of bony sclerosis in hands and feet, metaphyseal sclerotic bands, diffuse osteosclerosis, hyperostosis, pathologic fractures, multiple bilateral fractures, separation of epiphysis, and pseudoarthrosis may be seen alone or in combination with the bony changes of renal osteodystrophy (39,43). Large shallow areas of subperiosteal resorption and bone erosions can be seen without evidence of secondary hyperparathyroidism (48–52). Chondrocalcinosis of both small and large joints and periarticular calcified masses have also been described (37,39,50) (Figure 1).

VI. OXALATE DEPOSITS IN SYNOVIUM, CARTILAGE, AND BONE

Most synovium has been obtained from patients with chronic synovitis and has shown mild synovial cell hyperplasia with hyperemia and pleomorphic calcium oxalate crystals lying in a mildly fibrotic interstitium with scarce mononuclear cells and a few giant cells. In articular cartilage and menisci, oxalate crystals appear packed in the cartilage matrix or surrounded by cystic areas (37,39). Bone histology in most patients with oxalosis shows oxalate crystalline deposits surrounded by giant cell granulomas and bone marrow fibrosis (3,51). These deposits correlate with radiologic areas of subperiosteal resorption endosteal erosions, pseudo fractures, or localized osteosclerosis resulting from deposits of radiopaque calcium oxalate crystals in the bone marrow (3,43–49). Calcium oxalate crystal deposits in bone may provoke the formation of giant cells granulomas, stimulate osteoclastic bone reabsorption, and may induce hypercalcemia (48,49).

In patients with oxalosis due to end-stage renal disease managed with long-term dialysis, serum oxalate levels range from around 168±36 mg/l, about eight times higher than normal. Most patients with secondary oxalosis and renal failure have low serum calcium and high phosphorous, although a few may present hypercalcemia in the absence of secondary hyperparathyroidism (48,49).

VII. MANAGEMENT

The efficacy of the management of PH1 depends upon early diagnosis (3,53). Before renal failure occurs, there are several medical interventions that may be effective in preventing and minimizing renal and extrarenal oxalate crystal deposition (53,54). These measures include maintenance of a high urine output with a daily water intake of about 3–4 l/m^2/day. Water intake is adjusted in accordance with oxalate excretion in order to decrease the oxalate urinary level below 250 μmol/l and should be distributed evenly during day and night (53). Patients should avoid high oxalate foods such as tea, chocolate, spinach, and rhubarb. The diet should provide only the minimum requirement of Vitamins C and D (3). Nonspecific inhibitors of crystallization and/or crystal aggregation such as neutral orthophosphate (54), pyrophosphate, magnesium oxide, and potassium citrate (54,55) can be used to increase the solubility of calcium oxalate. Pharmacological doses of pyridoxine are indicated in some patients with PH1 (54), because pyridoxine is a coenzyme for AGT that stimulates the conversion of glyoxylate to glycine (Figure 2).

Early renal transplantation preceded by aggressive preoperative hemodialysis and the use of a living, related graft donor have been tried to make renal transplantation more successful. However, the kidney transplantation experience has been disappointing due to graft oxalosis (56). Combined liver-kidney transplantation is the treatment of choice for children with PH1 and advanced renal failure (53,57–59). The liver provides enough enzyme to lower oxalate production into the normal range and induce resolution of life threatening myocardiopathy (59), and oxalate osteopathy (53). According to one study, patients with primary oxaluria and end-stage renal failure managed with dialysis present relentless oxalate bone deposits and should be considered for combined liver and kidney transplantation as soon as they develop renal failure (59,60). The use of gene therapy in this inborn error of metabolism awaits further technical advances in the field (11).

Acute and chronic arthropathy due to oxalate crystals has been managed with nonsteroidal anti-inflammatory drugs (NSAIDs), intra-articular corticosteroid injections, and colchicine with poor to mediocre improvement (3,37,39). In those patients with hypercalcemia, corticosteroids and mithramycin were both effective in normalizing the serum calcium (48). Acute vasospastic phenomena have been controlled with continuous infusion of sodium nitroprusside with a maximum dose of 2.6 μg/kg/min followed by the administration of nifedipine (6).

VIII. SYNDROMES ASSOCIATED WITH CHOLESTEROL CRYSTALS AND OTHER CRYSTALLINE LIPIDS

A. Cholesterol Crystals

Cholesterol crystals are occasionally identified in rheumatoid arthritis joints, pleural and pericardial fluid (3,61,62), rheumatoid nodules (3,63), bursal effusions (3,62,63), subcutaneous tissues as cholesterol tophaceous deposit (64) or in the skin of patients with scleroderma (65), or tumoral calcinosis in patients with dermatomyositis (66). They are rarely observed in the synovial fluid from patients with osteoarthritis (67), chronic tophaceous gout (3), systemic lupus erythematosus (SLE) (3,61), and in a variety of other chronic effusions (3,62,66,68,69). Cholesterol crystal clefts are also found in rheumatoid nodules (63), xanthomas (70,71), and necrobiotic xanthogranulomas with paraproteinemia (72). Table 5 summarizes these and other conditions associated with cholesterol crystal deposition.

The few studies performed on synovial fluid of patients with arthritis associated with hyperlipoproteinemia have failed to show cholesterol or other crystalline lipids (3,72). Xanthomas often develop in the Achilles tendon and extensor tendon sheaths of the hands of patients with familial hypercholesterolemia (71,72). Incompletely characterized rod-like crystals have been identified in a patient with hyperlipoproteinemia with acute Achilles tendinitis (70), while cholesterol type crystals have been observed in other patients with olecranon bursitis (A.

TABLE 5 Conditions Associated with Cholesterol Crystals

Skin
Xanthomas
Necrotic xanthogranulomas with paraproteinemia
Cholesterol tophus
MSU tophus
Calcific exudate (scleroderma, dermatomyositis
Rheumatoid nodules, rheumatoid nodulosis
Joints, Bursae, and Tendons
Rheumatoid arthritis
SLE
Ankylosing spondylitis
Severe degenerative joint disease
Chronic tophaceous gout
Hyperbetalipoproteinemia
Bone
Unicameral bone cyst
Bone granulomatosis (Erdheim-Chester disease)
Pleural/Pericardial Effusions
Rheumatoid arthritis
Malignancy
Tuberculosis
Arteries
Atheromas
Cholesterol emboli

J. Reginato; unpublished observation). The syndrome of multiple cholesterol emboli is often an underdiagnosed clinical entity that may present with a constellation of systemic manifestations mimicking necrotizing vasculitis (74).

Synovial fluid containing cholesterol crystals often has a golden-honey or yellow-brown color (3), but cholesterol crystals have also been observed in chalky calcific exudate obtained from the skin of patients with scleroderma or dermatomyositis (3,64,65). Cholesterol crystals in synovial fluid are extracellular but are often associated with intra- and extracellular birefringent lipid droplet with features of "Maltese crosses". Cholesterol crystals show two morphologic forms (2,3): (1) highly birefringent, large, flat, rectangular plates with one or more notched corners, ranging from 8 to 100 μm (2) (Figure 6); and (2) rod- or needle-shaped, strongly birefringent crystals with either positive or negative elongation, ranging in size from 2 to 20 μm. Needle-shaped crystals may be confused with MSU, while short plates can be confused with CPPD crystals (3).

Many factors are probably involved in the formation of cholesterol crystals in inflamed tissues including increased cholesterol synthesis, in situ bleeding, lipid release from damaged cell membranes and organelles, and abnormal intra-

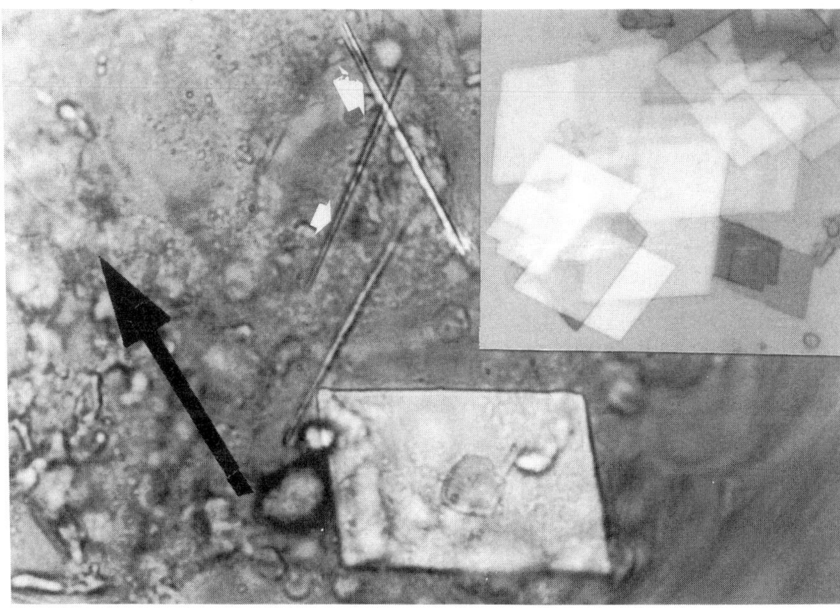

FIGURE 6 Cholesterol crystals showing the characteristic needle (arrows) and notched plate (inset) shapes. Large arrow shows axis of slow vibration of compensator. Compensated, polarized light × 300.

cellular transport of lipids resulting from chronic inflammation and/or infection (3,61,62). The capability of synthetic cholesterol crystals to induce moderate acute and chronic inflammation in skin, subcutaneous tissue, and knee joints of rabbits has been demonstrated in several studies (75). Cholesterol crystals however, have not been observed inside human phagocytes, as occurs with MSU, CPPD, or basic calcium phosphate (BCP) crystals. Although cholesterol crystals may activate serum complement (75), which might potentiate inflammation and aggravate joint destruction in rheumatoid arthritis (RA) and even osteoarthritis (OA), there is as yet no clinical evidence to support this concept (3).

B. Lipid Liquid Crystals

Lipid liquid crystals represent states of matter having characteristics of both liquid and solids (3,76). These inclusions are formed by phospholipids or by other polar molecules which can also be arranged as liquid crystals and display intense birefringence (2,3).

As already noted, birefringent Maltese crosses occasionally have been found in synovial or bursal fluids of patients with RA in association with cholesterol crystals (3). They have been found in synovial fluid of acute unexplained monarthritis (76–78) or polyarthritis (79), acute olecranon bursitis (3), hemarthrosis (3,76), and pigmented villonodular synovitis (80), and during an acute rheumatoid arthritis flare (81).

Under compensated polarized light, these microspherules have an intense double-positive birefringence. Sizes range from 2 to 8 μm. In atherosclerotic plaque, bile, and synovial fluid, these liquid lipid microspherules precede the formation of cholesterol crystals (2). They are commonly seen inside cells, stain with Sudan black B, and are dissolved completely in 1:1 alcohol-ether (3). Smaller microspherules may appear to be anisotropic (nonbirefringent). These birefringent Maltese crosses of positive elongation formed by phospholipid and cholesterol must be differentiated from the birefringent MSU microspherules of negative elongation formed by MSU crystals, seen rarely in patients with gout, and also from talcum powder crystals that may contaminate synovial fluids when gloves are used during arthrocentesis (3). The latter consist of magnesium silicate or starch granules and show a strong birefringence with positive elongation, but their outlines are more irregular than the MSU and lipid crystal microspherules (3). Birefringent microspherules with positive elongation formed by glycosphingolipids can be seen in the urine of patients with Fabry's disease, but so far these birefringent microspherules have not been seen in the synovial fluid of the few patients described with Fabry's disease arthropathy (3,82,83).

All patients described have experienced the acute onset of monarticular synovitis similar to that seen in other crystal-associated arthritis (3,76–79). The knee was most commonly involved, although wrist involvement was noted in one instance (73). Synovial fluid was inflammatory, with white cell counts ranging from 10,000 to 45,000/μL with 75–90% neutrophils. About 10–20% of these contain doubly birefringent microspherules (2). Arthritis in all patients subsided completely within a week after NSAIDs were given. Synovium was obtained in only two patients with acute synovitis (2,79), mild inflammatory changes with rare lymphocytic, mononuclear, or PMN cell infiltrates were seen in both cases, and in one specimen, intracellular birefringent microspherules were seen inside mononuclear cells (79).

Synthetic lipid liquid crystals injected into rabbit knees induced either acute or subacute synovitis (84). The origin of these microspherules in articular tissues is unknown. Injection of autologous blood into rabbit knee joints was associated with formation of Maltese crosses (85). Similar spherules seen in human joints may be formed by lipids derived from breakdown of membranes of platelets, erythrocytes, leukocytes, and even from serum lipids (3).

C. Other Crystalline Lipids

Other crystalline lipids, thought to be fatty acids, have been described in skin fat necrosis of newborns (2,3). Identical structures have been observed in synovial fluid of patients with OA associated with large bone cysts, in hemarthrosis, and in synovial fluid examined several days after arthrocentesis (2,3,86,87). Such crystals may have either a strongly positive or a strongly negative birefringence and may present with needle, plate, or rod shapes. Some may form clumps or rosettes (2,3). The rod-shaped and needle-shaped crystals can be confused with CPPD or MSU crystals.

D. Cryoglobulin Crystals

Paraprotein and cryoglobulins can crystallize within plasma cells of patients with multiple myeloma (3,88). Similar crystals can be seen independent of plasma cells in the renal glomeruli, tubules, lungs, skin, liver, spleen, lymph nodes, adrenals, testes, and cornea of patients with multiple myeloma and cryoglobulinemia (3,5,88–96). These deposits can be associated with variable degrees of organ failure (3,5,88). They may also occur in coronary, renal, and other arteries and induce thrombosis and infarction mimicking vasculitis (5,88,92–94). Similar crystalline deposits have been observed in peripheral vessels of patients with essential cryoglobulinemia and purpura, and in the necrotic skin lesions (3,5) as well as in the synovial membrane in association with chronic oligoarthritis or symmetric erosive peripheral and axial polyarthritis mimicking rheumatoid arthritis (2,90–93). Two of these patients also had, at the same time, an occlusive crystal induced vasculopathy (92,93).

Paraprotein crystals are characterized by their large size, ranging from 3 to

60 μm or more, and their polymorphic shapes, which may vary with the cooling process used (2). They usually appear as hexagonal, diamond-shaped, or polygonal crystals, but they may resemble squares, rectangles, rhomboids, or needles (2,3,88,95). They may show either a strongly positive or a strongly negative birefringence. They stain with Giemsa or with hematoxylin and eosin. Transmission and electron microscopic studies of amorphous, gelatinous and crystalline cryoglobulins have shown the ability of this crystal to form macromolecular nets and trap cells (95). This morphological property of cryoglobulin crystals may explain their ability to induce vascular occlusion and also to induce granulomatous inflammation (96).

Episodic joint pain followed by an erosive, chronic, symmetric polyarthritis involving joints of the hands, feet, and one ankle has been observed in one patient with cryoprecipitable immunoglobulin G (IgG) in his serum and cryoglobulin crystals in joint fluid and synovium (90). Another patient with erosive polyarthritis and crystallized monoclonal cryoglobulin also has been reported (2), and in two recent reports, two patients presented with polyarthritis and vasculitis mimicking rheumatoid disease (92,93). Two patients with multiple myeloma and corneal paraprotein crystalline deposits presented with foot arthritis, including podagra (3). Arthritis and arthralgias associated with cryoglobulinemia but without paraprotein crystals in synovial fluid have also been reported (2,97).

E. Charcot-Leyden Crystals

Charcot-Leyden crystals are formed in the cytoplasm of disrupted eosinophils and are found in the sputum of asthmatic patients; the tissue of patients with hypereosinophilia and other eosinophilic disease processes such as eosinophilic bone granuloma and hypereosinophilic syndrome; the stools of patients with parasitic infections and granulocytic leukemia; and the synovial fluid of patients with eosinophilic synovitis (3,10,98–101). Circulating Charcot-Leyden crystals have been observed in patients with hypereosinophilic syndrome, and crystalline deposits were found in thrombosed vessels and in the renal glomeruli (10,102).

Eosinophilic synovitis associated with Charcot-Leyden crystals on wet synovial fluid preparation has been documented in seven patients with history of allergic reactions and dermatographism (98,100,101). These patients developed painless monarthritis after minor trauma without concurrent allergic symptoms. Joint swelling was seen in the knee of seven patients and in the first metatarsophalangeal joint of another patient. Each episode subsided within 1 to 2 weeks without therapy; three patients had recurrent episodes. Synovial fluid was mildly inflammatory, with leukocyte counts of 10,850 ± 3,665/μL and up to 46% eosinophils. Charcot-Leyden crystals were seen inside cells on wet preparations.

Charcot-Leyden crystals are bipyramidal, hexagonal-shaped crystals formed by a lysophospholipase or phospholipase B (99, 102). Crystal sizes range from 17 to 25 μm. With hematoxylin and eosin stain, they appear fairly eosinophilic; with Giemsa stain, they appear light purple or pink; and under fluorescent microscopy, these crystals appear as bright yellow-green fluorescent needles (103). The fluorescent technique seems to be more sensitive than light microscopy for the detection of Charcot-Leyden crystals (103).

F. Synthetic Corticosteroids Crystals

Intra-articular corticosteroid injection have been used in the management of arthritis during the last 46 years. They might remain inside joints for weeks and months and can be confused with calcium pyrophosphate or MSU crystals (104, 105). If after an injection of corticosteroid crystal the same hypodermic needle is used to put the fluid in a tube, abundant intracellular and extracellular crystals may be seen in the fresh preparation (2). Corticosteroid crystals are characterized by having intense birefringence with crystals present in the same preparation having either positive or negative elongation (2, 105). Other clues for recognizing corticosteroid crystals include their presence in large amounts and irregular shapes and sizes. Because they vary in shape and birefringence, it is recommended to become familiar with the shape and birefringence of the particular type of corticosteroid crystals used in practice (2) (Table 6).

Corticosteroid injections can be associated with a variety of iatrogenic

Table 6 Some Synthetic Corticosteroid Crystals

Crystal	Shape	Size (μM)	Birefringence	Predominant elongation	Look-alike crystals[a]
Prednisolone tebutate (Hydeltra T.B.A.®)	Small, pleomorphic, branched	<8	Intense	Positive	CPPD, oxalate
Methylprednisolone acetate (DepoMedrol®)	Small, pleomorphic	<5	Intense	Positive	Dot-like MSU
Triamcinolone acetonide (Kenalog®)	Small, pleomorphic	<5	Intense	—	Dot-like MSU
Triamcinolone hexacetonide (Aristopan®)	Rod, square	15–60	Intense	Negative	MSU
Betamethasone (Celestone Soluspan®)	Rod	10–20	Intense	Negative	MSU

[a]Data are from Ref. 1.

CPPD = calcium pyrophosphate dihydrate; MSU = monosodium urate.

complications, which include septic arthritis due to inadvertent joint contamination, acute crystal induced synovitis, skin atrophy, giant periarticular calcification mainly observed in children, tendon rupture, urticaria, throat constriction, angioedema, petechial rash, and shock (106–109). Progressive destructive finger arthropathy and aseptic bone necrosis also have been observed in those patients receiving frequent injections (107). Inappropriate repeated injections may lead to "steroid arthropathy," characterized by an accelerated rate of joint destruction and radiographic evidence of Charcot joint-like arthropathy. Debate continues regarding the time interval to be regarded as "safe" between repeated injections (110–111).

In two patients with coexistent rheumatoid arthritis and sickle cell, corticosteroid injections precipitated a sickle cell crisis (112). Anaphylactoid reaction to synthetic corticosteroid or their vehicle has been reported in several patients (110). We have seen a patient who developed leukocytoclastic vasculitis that recurred upon rechallenge with intra-articular corticosteroid injection and that was confused with rheumatoid vasculitis.

G. Miscellaneous Crystals

Cystine crystals have been described in the bone of one patient with cystinosis, while in other patient with arthritis no crystals were found in the synovial fluid. Cystine crystalline deposits have been found in muscles of patients with cystinosis presenting with muscle weakness and wasting (1–3).

Arthritis has been described in two patients with xanthinuria, mimicking acute gout, but no synovial fluid analysis was performed. Hypoxanthine and xanthine crystal have been identified in tender muscles of patient with xanthinuria. Xanthine, hypoxanthine, and oxipurinol crystals have also been identified in the muscle of patients with Lesch-Nyhan syndrome and lymphoma managed with allopurinol (1–3).

Aluminum crystals have been identified in the calcification front of bone of patients with hemodialysis and aluminum-induced osteomalacia, but no such crystals have been identified in the synovial fluid (1–3). The role of aluminum in inducing arthritis in patients in chronic dialysis remains speculative.

Hemoglobin and hematoidin crystals have been seen rarely in hemorrhagic synovial fluids and in an occasional patient with sickle cell arthropathy (1–3).

REFERENCES

1. A. J. Reginato, and B. Kurnik. Calcium oxalate and other crystals associated with kidney diseases and arthritis. *Semin Arth Rheum 18*:198–224 (1989).
2. H. R. Shumacher and A. J. Reginato. Atlas of synovial fluid and crystal identification. Lea and Febiger, Philadelphia, PA, 1991.

3. A. J. Reginato. Calcium oxalate and other crystals or particles associated with arthritis, *Arthritis and Allied Conditions*, (W. J. Koopman, ed.), Williams and Wilkins, Baltimore, MD, 13th ed., pp. 2147–2168 (1997).
4. M. C. Smith, M. K. Ghose, and A. R. Henry. The clinical spectrum of renal cholesterol embolization, *Am J Med 71*:174–180 (1981).
5. G. C. Stone, B. A. Wall, I. R. Oppliger, M. H. Wener, S. L. Jolly, A. Aguirre, R. Dwyer, and P. A. Simkin. A vasculopathy and deposition of lambda light chain crystals, *Ann Intern Med 110*:275–278 (1989).
6. R. Van Damme-Lombaerts, W. Proesmans, G. Alexandre, M. VanDyck, M. Serrus, and G. Wilms. Reversible arterial spasm in an adolescent with primary oxalosis, *Clin Neph 30*:235–238 (1988).
7. G. S. Arbus and S. Sniderman. Oxalosis with peripheral gangrene, *Arch Pathol 97*:107–110 (1974).
8. J. C. Jennette, D. S. Sheps, and D. D. McNeill. Exclusively vascular systemic amyloidosis with visceral ischemia, *Arch Pathol Lab Med 106*:323–327 (1982).
9. D. L. Jardine, M. A. Fitzpatrick, W. D. Troughton, and A. B. Tie. Small bowel ischaemia in Fabry's disease, *J Gastroenterol Hepatol 9*:201–204 (1994).
10. P. Honsoon, T. J. Burton, and J. M. Van der Bel-Kahn. Circulating Charcot-Leyden crystals in hypereosinophilic syndrome, *Am J Clin Pathol 75*:236–243 (1981).
11. C. J. Danpure. Molecular and cell biology of primary hyperoxaluria type 1, *Clin Investig 72*:725–727 (1994).
12. R. D. Lewis, H. A. Lowenstam, and G. R. Rossman. Oxalate nephrosis and crystalline myocarditis: case report with postmortem and crystallographic studies, *Arch Pathol Lab Med 98*:149–155 (1974).
13. R. R. West, W. R. Salyer, and G. M. Hutchins. Adult onset primary oxalosis with complete heart block, *Johns Hopkins Med 133*:195–200 (1973).
14. P. J. Moorhead, D. J. Cooper, and W. R. Timperley. Progressive peripheral neuropathy in a patient with primary hyperoxaluria, *Br Med J 2*:312–313 (1975).
15. P. Sanz and R. Reig. Clinical and pathological findings in fatal plant oxalosis: a review, *Am J Forensic Med Pathol 13(4)*:342–345 (1992).
16. D. E. Hricik and R. Hussain. Pancytopenia and hepatosplenomegaly in oxalosis, *Arch Intern Med 144*:167–168 (1984).
17. R. W. E. Watts. Primary hyperoxaluria type I, *Q J Med 87*:593–600 (1994).
18. C. J. Danpure, P. R. Jennings, and R. W. E. Watts. Enzymological diagnosis of primary hyperoxaluria type 1 by measurement of hepatic alanine: glyoxylate aminotransferase activity, *Lancet 1*:289–293 (1987).
19. R. E. Hillman. Primary hyperoxaluria, *The Metabolic and Molecular Bases of Inherited Diseases* (C. R. Scriver, ed.), 6th ed., McGraw-Hill, New York, NY, 1989, pp. 933–944.
20. P. J. Wise, C. J. Danpure, and P. R. Jennings. Immunological heterogeneity of hepatic alanine: glyoxylate aminotransferase in primary hyperoxaluria type I, *FEBS Lett 222*:17–20 (1987).
21. C. J. Danpure. Molecular and clinical heterogeneity in primary hyperoxaluria type I, *Am J Kidney Dis 17*:366–369 (1991).
22. C. J. Danpure. Molecular and cell biology of primary hyperoxaluria type I, *Clin Investig 72*:725–727 (1994).

23. C. J. Danpure, P. R. Jennings, P. Fryer, P. E. Purdue, and J. Allsop. Primary hyperoxaluria type 1: genotypic and phenotypic heterogeneity, *J Inherited Metab Dis 17*:487–499 (1994).
24. C. J. Danpure, G. M. Birdsey, G. Rumsby, M. J. Lumb, P. E. Purdue, and J. Allsop. Molecular characterization and clinical use of polymorphic tandem repeat in an intron of the human alanine: glyoxylate aminotransferase gene, *Human Genetics 94*:55–64 (1994).
25. B. Hoppe, C. J. Danpure, G. Rumsby, P. Fryer, P. R. Jennings, N. Blau, G. Schubiger, T. Neuhaus, and E. Leumann. A vertical (pseudodominant) pattern of inheritance in the autosomal recessive disease primary hyperoxaluria type I: lack of relationship between genotype, enzymatic phenotype, and disease severity, *Am J Kidney Dis 29(1)*:36–44 (1997).
26. C. J. Danpure and G. Rumsby. Strategies for the prenatal diagnosis of primary hyperoxaluria type I, *Prenat Diagn 16(7)*:587–98 (1996).
27. H. E. Williams and L. H. Smith Jr. L-glyceric aciduria: A new genetic variant of primary hyperoxaluria, *N Engl J Med 278*:233–238 (1968).
28. R. A. Chalmers, B. M. Tracey, J. Mistry, K. D. Griffiths, A. Green and M. H. Winterborn. L-Glyceric aciduria (primary hyperoxaluria type 2) in siblings in two unrelated families, *J Inherit Metab Dis 7(suppl2)*:133–134 (1984).
29. L. E. Seargeant, G. W. deGroot, L. A. Dilling, C. J. Mallory, and J. C. Haworth. Primary oxaluria type 2 (l-glyceric aciduria): a rare cause of nephrolithiasis in children, *J Pediat 118*:912–914 (1991).
30. P. T. Chlebeck, D. S. Milliner, and L. H. Smith. Long-term prognosis in primary hyperoxaluria type 2(l-glyceric aciduria), *Am J Kidney Dis 23(2)*:255–259 (1994).
31. V. S. Chadwick, K. Modha, and R. H. Dowling. Mechanism for hyperoxaluria in patients with ileal dysfunction, *N Engl J Med 289*:172–176 (1973).
32. M. C. Kaye, S. B. Streem, and P. M. Hall. Enteric hyperoxaluria associated with external biliary drainage, *J Urol 151*:396–397 (1994).
33. W. Louthrenoo, Y. S. Park, L. Philippe, and H. R. Shumacher Jr. Localized peripheral calcium oxalate crystal deposition caused by Aspergillus niger infection, *J Rheumatol 17*:407–412 (1990).
34. E. M. Worcester, Y. Nakawaga, D. A. Bushinsky, and F. L. Coe. Evidence that serum calcium oxalate supersaturation is a consequence of oxalate retention in patients with chronic renal failure, *J Clin Invest 77*:1888–1896 (1986).
35. D. V. Weber. Urinary saturation measurements in calcium nephrolithiasis, *Ann Intern Med 90*:180–184 (1979).
36. B. Celasun, M. Safali, and M. Yenicesu. Secondary oxalosis of bone in a dialysis patient, *Scand J Urol Nephrol 29*:211–214 (1995).
37. G. S. Hoffman, H. R. Schumacher, H. Paul, V. Cherian, R. Reed, A. G. Ramsey, and W. A. Franck. Calcium oxalate microcrystalline-associated arthritis in end stage renal disease, *Ann Intern Med 97*:36–42 (1982).
38. G. Abuelo, S. T. Schwartz, and A. J. Reginato. Cutaneous oxalosis after long term hemodialysis, *Arch Int Med 152*:1517–1520 (1992).
39. A. J. Reginato, J. L. Ferreiro Seoane, C. Barbazan Alvarez, J. Mitja Piferrer, L. Vi-

dal Meijon, R. Pascual Turon, F. Vasconez, E. R. Rivera, G. Clayburne, and S. Rothfuss. Arthropathy and cutaneous calcinosis in hemodialysis oxalosis, *Arth Rheum 29*:1387–1396 (1986).

40. R. A. Hautman. Intrarenal distributiuon of oxalic acid, calcium, sodium, and potassium in man, *Eur J Clin Invest 10*:173–176 (1980).
41. I. Pecorella, A. C. McCartney, S. Lucas, L. Michaels, A. Ciardi, U. DiTondo, and A. Garner. Histological study of oxalosis in the eye and adnexa of AIDS patients, *Histopathology 27(5)*:431–438 (1995).
42. P. J. Symmans, K. Brady, and C. E. Keen. Calcium oxalate crystal deposition in epithelioid histiocytes of granulomatous lymphandenitis: analysis by light and electronmicrospy, *Histopathology 27(5)*:423–429 (1995).
43. R. Q. Knight, R. F. Taddonio, F. B. Smith, S. Weseley, and H. M. Pecker. Oxalosis: cause of degenerative spinal stenosis. A case report and review of the literature, *Orthopedics 11(6)*:955–958 (1988).
44. C. L. Benhamou, T. Bardin, D. Tourliere, L. Voisin, M. Audran, C. Edouard, M. H. Lafage, J. L. Sebert, M. C. de Vernejoul, D. Wendling, et al. Attiente osseuse de l-oxalose primitive. Etude de 20 cas. (Bone involvement in primary oxalosis. Study of 20 cases). *Rev Rheum Mal Osteoartic 58*:763–769 (1991).
45. C. M. Schnitzler, J. A. Kok, D. W. Jacobs, P. D. Thomson, F. J. Milne, J. M. Mesquite, P. C. King, and V. A. Fabian. Skeletal manifestations of primary oxalosis, *Pediatr Nephrol 5*:193–199 (1991).
46. E. Ring, H. Wendler, M. Ratschek, and G. Zobel. Bone disease of primary hyperoxaluria in infancy, *Pediatr Radiol 20*:131–133 (1989).
47. P. Desmond and O. Hennessy. Skeletal abnormalities in primary oxalosis, *Australasian Radiol 37*:83–85 (1993).
48. C. Canavese, M. Salomone, C. Massara, M. Portigliatti-Barbos, A. Cadario, I. Pavan, M. Marangella, et al. Primary oxalosis mimicking hyperarathyroidism diagnosed after long-term hemodialysis, *Am J Nephrol 10*:344–349 (1990).
49. C. Toussaint, L. DePauw, C. Tielemans, and D. Abramowicz. Hypercalcemia complicating systemic oxalosis in primary hyperoxaluria type 1, *Nephrol Dial Transplant 10(suppl 8)*:17–21 (1995).
50. H. R. Shumacher, A. J. Reginato, and S. Pullman. Synovial fluid oxalate deposition complicating rheumatoid arthritis with amyloidosis and renal failure: demonstration of intracellular oxalate crystals, *J Rheumatol 14*:361–366 (1987).
51. G. Gherardi, A. Poggi, S. Sisca, V. Calderaro, and E. Bonucci. Bone oxalosis and renal osteodystrophy, *Arch Pathol Lab Med 104*:105–111 (1980).
52. D. L. Day, J. I. Scheinman, and J. Mahan. Radiological aspects of primary hyperoxaluria, *Am J Roentgenol 146(2)*:395–401 (1986).
53. M. Broyer, P. Jouvet, P. Niaudet, M. Daudon, and Y. Revillon. Management of oxalosis, *Kidney Int 49(suppl 53)* :S93–S98 (1996).
54. D. S. Milliner, J. T. Eickholt, E. J. Bergstralh, D. M. Wilson, and L. H. Smith. Results of long-term treatment with orthophosphate and pyridoxine in patients with primary hyperoxaluria, *N Engl J Med 331*:1553 (1994).
55. E. Leumann, B. Hoppe, and T. Neuhaus. Management of hyperoxaluria: efficacy of oral citrate administration, *Pediatr Nephrol 7*:207–211 (1993).

56. M. Broyer, F. P. Brunner, H. Bryngner, S. R. Dykes, J. H. Ehrich, W. Fassbinder, et al. Kidney transplantation in primary oxalosis: data from the EDTA registry, *Nephrol Dialysis Transplant* 5:332–336 (1990).
57. J. Uribarri, C. H. Miller, and L. Burrows. Combined liver-kidney transplantation for the genetic disorder primary hyperoxaluria type 1, *Mt Sinai J Med 61*:32–36 (1994).
58. T. E. Bunchman, H. Majors, G. Majors, J. J. Gardner, J. DeVee, E. M. Dennerll, J. L. Hesford, C. L. Mitchell, and J. D. Punch. The infant with primary hyperoxaluria and oxalosis: from diagnosis to multiorgan transplantation, *Adv Ren Replace Ther 3(4)*:315–325 (1996).
59. B. S. Fyfe, D. H. Israel, A. Quish, A. Squire, L. Burrows, C. Miller, S. K. Sharma, S. Muthy, and J. Machac. Reversal of primary hyperoxaluria cardiomyopathy after combined liver and renal transplantation, *Am J Cardiol 75(2)*: 210–212 (1995).
60. M. Marangella, C. Vitale, M. Petrarulo, A. Tricerri, E. Cerelli, A. Cardario, M. P. Barbos, and F. Linari. Bony content of oxalate in patients with primary hyperoxaluria or oxalosis-unrelated renal failure, *Kidney Int 48(1)*:182–187 (1995).
61. M. B. Lazarevic, J. L. Skosey, J. Vitic, V. Mladenovic, B. L. Myones, J. Popovic, and W. I. Swedler. Cholesterol crystals in synovial and bursal fluid. *Sem Arth Rheum 23*:99–103 (1993).
62. C. M. Wise, R. E. White, and C. A. Agudelo. Synovial fluid lipid abnormalities in various disease states: review and classification, *Semin Arth Rheum 16*:222–230 (1987).
63. G. Rodriguez, A. J. Reginato, O. J. Rillo, and J. A. Barcat. Cholesterol crystals in rheumatoid nodulosis, *Rev Esp Rheumatol 20*:403(abstract) (1993).
64. A. G. Fam. Subcutaneous cholesterol crystal deposition and tophus formation, *Arth Rheum 32*:1190–1191 (1989).
65. P. A. Saxe and R. D. Altman. Subcutaneous cholesterol mimicking calcinosis cutis in systemic sclerosis, *J Rheumatol 18*:743–745 (1991).
66. J. Corts, L. Castellanos, A. J. Reginato, and H. R. Schumacher. Tumoral calcinosis containing hydroxyapatite and cholesterol crystals associated with dermatomyositis, *Arth Rheum 35*:S76(abstract) (1992).
67. A. G. Fam, K. P. H. Pritzker, P. T. Cheng, and A. H. Little. Cholesterol crystals in osteoarthritic joint effusions, *J Rheumatol 8*:273–280 (1981).
68. J. W. Riordan and P. A. Dieppe. Cholesterol crystals in shoulder synovial fluid, *Br J Rheumatol 26*:430–432 (1987).
69. J. F. Van Offel, L. S. DeClerck, and I. E. Kersschot. Cholesterol crystals and IgE-containing immune complexes in rheumatoid pericarditis, *Clin Rheumatol 10*:78–80 (1991).
70. H. R. Schumacher and R. Michaels. Recurrent tendinitis and achilles tendon nodule with positively birefringent crystals in a patient with hyperlipoproteinemia, *J Rheumatol 16*:1387–1389 (1989).
71. H. S. Kruth. Lipid deposition in human tendon xanthoma, *Am J Pathol 121*:311–315 (1985).
72. M. C. Finan and R. K. Winkelmann. Necrobiotic xanthogranuloma with paraproteinemia. A review of 22 cases, *Medicine 65*:376–388 (1986).

73. K. L. Schmidt, H. W. Leber, and G. Schutterle. Arthropathies bei primarer Oxalose-Krystallsynovitis oder Osteopathie, *Dtsch Med Wochenschr 19*:106 (1981).
74. M. C. Smith, M. K. Ghose, and A. R. Henry. The clinical spectrum of renal cholesterol embolization, *Am J Med 71*:174–180 (1981).
75. K. P. H. Pritzker, A. G. Fam, S. A. Omar, and S. K. Gertzbein. Experimental cholesterol crystal arthropathy, *J Rheumatol 8*:281–290 (1981).
76. A. J. Reginato, H. R. Schumacher, D. A. Allan, and J. L. Rabinowitz. Acute monoarthritis associated with lipid liquid crystals, *Ann Rheum Dis 44*:537–643 (1985).
77. D. C. Trostle, H. R. Schumacher Jr., T. A. Medsger, and W. N. Kapoor. Lipid microspherule-associated acute monoarticular arthritis, *Arth Rheum 29*:1166–1168 (1986).
78. G. C. Gardner and R. A. Terkeltaub. Acute monoarthritis associated with intracellulr positively birefringent Maltese cross appearing spherules, *J Rheumatol 16*:394–396 (1989).
79. P. A. Schlesinger, M. T. Stillman, and L. Peterson. Polyarthritis with birefringent lipid within synovial fluid macrophages: case report and ultrastructural study, *Arth Rheum 25*:1365–1368 (1982).
80. K. Ugai, M. Kurosaka, and K. Hirohata. Lipid microspherules in synovial fluid of patients with pigmented villonodular synovitis, *Arth Rheum 31*:1442–1446 (1988).
81. C. H. Rivest, M. Hazeltine, G. Gariepy, and R. DeMedicis. Acute polyarthritis associated with birefringent lipid microspherules occuring in a patient with long standing rheumatoid arthritis, *J Rheumatol 19*:617–620 (1992).
82. K. J. Sheth and G. C. Bernhard. The arthopathy of Fabry's disease, *Arth Rheum 22*:781–783 (1979).
83. S. O. Paira, S. Roverano, J. L. Iribas, and H. A. Barcelo. Joint manifestations of Fabry's disease, *Clin Rheumatol 11*:562–565 (1992).
84. S. J. Choi, H. R. Schumacher Jr., G. Clayburne, M. S. Rothfuss, and M. Sieck. Liposome-induced synovitis in rabbits: light and electon microscopic studies, *Arth Rheum 29*:889–896 (1986).
85. S. J. Choi, H. R. Schumacher, and G. Clayburne. Experimental hemarthrosis produces mild inflammation associated with intracellular Maltese crosses, *Ann Rheum Dis 45*:1025–1028 (1986).
86. A. J. Freemont and J. Denton. Synovial fluid findings early in traumatic arthritis, *J Rheumatol 15*:881–882 (1988).
87. A. J. Freemont. What is the significance of synovial fluid lipid crystals in an isolated monarthritis? *Br J Rheumatol 31*:183–184 (1992).
88. T. L. Dornan, J. W. Blundell, A. G. Morgan, R. P. Burden, W. G. Reeves and R. E. Cotton. Widespread crystallization of paraprotein in myelomatosis, *Q J Med 222*:659–667 (1985).
89. S. Nishi, M. Ueno, S. Suzuki, R. Kawasawa, H. Hayashi, H. In, T. Saitou, et al. Glomerulonephritis with various crystalline deposits, *Am J Nephrol 13*:271–274 (1993).
90. D. R. Langlands, R. L. Dawkins, L. R. Matz, T. J. Cobain, P. Goatcher, J. M. Papadimitriou, and M. L. Cohen. Arthritis associated with crystalizing cryoprecipitable IgG paraprotein, *Am J Med 68*:461–465 (1980).

91. H. S. An, T. C. Namey, and K. Kim. Essential cryoglobulemia associated with intense and persitent synovitis of the knees, *Clin Orthop Rel Res 215*:173–178 (1987).
92. L. Albert, R. Inman, D. A. Gordon, B. Chiu, E. Amdemichael, and A. Katz. Cryocrystalglobulinemia mimicking rheumatoid arthritis and vasculitis, *J Rheumatol 23(7)*:1272–1277 (1996).
93. T. Papo, L. Musset, T. Bardin, B. Bucki, C. Jorgensen, E. Dion, A. Quillard, C. deGennes, J. Sany, P. Godeau, and J. C. Piette. Cyrocrystalglobulemia as a cause of systemic vasculopathy and widespread erosive arthropathy, *Arth Rheum 39(2)*:335–340 (1996).
94. H. Hasegawa, T. Ozawa, N. Tada, Y. Taguchi, K. Ohno, T. Chou, and T. Watanabe. Multiple myeloma-associated vasculopathy due to crystalglobulin or polyarteritis nodosa, *Arth Rheum 39*:330–334 (1996).
95. D. N. Podell, C. H. Packman, J. Maniloff, and G. N. Abraham. Characterization of monoclonal IgG cryoglobulins: fine structural and morphological analysis, *Blood 69*:677–681 (1987).
96. C. W. Denko. Cryoglobulin induced inflammation, *Agents Actions 17*:92–96 (1985).
97. A. Rubens-Duval and G. Kaplan. Articular manifiestaitons of cryogobulinemias (French), *Revue du Rhumatisme et des Maladies Osteo-Articulares 41(10)*:605–613 (1974).
98. J. P. Brown, M. Rola-Pleszczynski, and H. A. Menard. Eosinophillic synovitis: Clinical observations on a newly recognized subset of patients with dermatographism, *Arth Rheum 29*:1147–1151 (1986).
99. P. F. Weller, D. Bach, and K. F. Austen. Human eosinophil lysophospholipase, the sole protein component of Charcot-Leyden crystals, *J Immunol 128*:1346–1350 (1982).
100. M. Dougados, L. Benhamou, and B. Amor. Charcot-Leyden crystals in synovial fluid, *Arth Rheum 26*:1416 (1983).
101. H. A. Menard, R. DeMedicis, A Lessier, and J. Brown. Charcot-Leyden crystals in synovial fluid, *Arth Rheum 24*:1591–1593 (1981).
102. A. M. Dvorak, P. F. Weller, R. A. Monahan-Early, L. Letouneau, and S. J. Ackerman. Ultrastructural localization of Charcot-Leyden crystal protein (lysophospholipase) and peroxidase in macrophages, eosinophils, and extracellular matrix of the skin in the hypereonsinophillic syndrome, *Lab Investig 62*:590–607 (1990).
103. H. J. Carson, R. J. Buschmann, P. Weisz-Carrington, and Y. S. Choi. Identification of Charcot-Leyden crystals by electron microscopy, *Ultrastruct Pathol 16*:403–411 (1992).
104. J. Holander, et al. Hydrocortisone and cortisone injected into arthritis joints, *JAMA 147*:1629 (1951).
105. C. B. Kahn, J. L. Hollander, and H. R. Shumacher. Corticosteroid crystals in synovial fluid, *JAMA 211*:807–809 (1970).
106. D. J. McCarty Jr. and J. M. Hogan. Inflammatory reaction after intra-synovial injection of microcrystalline adreno-corticosteroid esters, *Arth Rheum 7*:359 (1969).
107. G. N. Chandler and V. Wright. Deleterious effect of intra-articular hydrocortisone, *Lancet 2*:661–663 (1958).

108. J. S. Peller and E. J. Bardana Jr. Anaphylactoid reaction to corticosteroid: case report and review of the literature, *Ann Allergy 54(4)*:302–305 (1985).
109. E. Toussirot, P. Kremer, A. Benmansour, and D. Wendling. Giant calcification in soft tissue after shoulder corticosteroid injection, *J Rheumatol 23(1)*:181–182 (1996).
110. R. B. Greer III. Into the knee with needles and steroids, *Orthop Rev 22*:1302 (1993).
111. W. J. McCune. Injection of corticosteroids into joints (letter), *Orthop Rev 23*:299 (1994).
112. D. D. Gladman and C. Bombardier. Sickle cell crisis following intraarticular steroid therapy for rheumatoid arthritis, *Arth Rheum 30(9)*:1065–1068 (1987).
113. D. L. Earnest. Enteric hyperoxaluria. *Adv Intern Med 24*:407–427 (1979).

Index